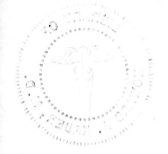

EVOLVING CONCEPTS IN GASTROINTESTINAL MOTILITY

Evolving Concepts in

Gastrointestinal Motility

« »

Malcolm C. Champion

MB FRCPC FRCP(UK)
University of Ottawa, Division of Gastroenterology,
Ottawa Civic Hospital, Ottawa, Ontario, Canada

William C. Orr

PhD, FACG
Thomas N. Lynn Institute for Healthcare Research,
Integris/Baptist Medical Center of Oklahoma,
University of Oklahoma Health Sciences Center,
Oklahoma City, Oklahoma, USA

Blackwell Science

© 1996 by
Blackwell Science Ltd
Editorial Offices:
Osney Mead, Oxford OX2 0EL
25 John Street, London WC1N 2BL
23 Ainslie Place, Edinburgh EH3 6AJ
238 Main Street, Cambridge
  Massachusetts 02142, USA
54 University Street, Carlton
  Victoria 3053, Australia

Other Editorial Offices:
Arnette Blackwell SA
  224, Boulevard Saint Germain
  75007 Paris, France

Blackwell Wissenschafts-Verlag GmbH
  Kurfürstendamm 57
  10707 Berlin, Germany

  Zehetnergasse 6
  A-1140 Wien
  Austria

First published 1996

Set by DP Photosetting, Aylesbury, Bucks
Printed in Great Britain at
the Alden Press, Oxford and Northampton
and bound by Hartnolls Ltd, Bodmin,
Cornwall

The Blackwell Science logo is a
trade mark of Blackwell Science Ltd,
registered at the United Kingdom
Trade Marks Registry

DISTRIBUTORS

  Marston Book Services Ltd
  PO Box 269
  Abingdon
  Oxon OX14 4YN
  (*Orders:* Tel: 01235 465500
           Fax: 01235 465555)

USA
  Blackwell Science, Inc.
  238 Main Street
  Cambridge, MA 02142
  (*Orders:* Tel: 800 215-1000
           617 876-7000
       Fax: 617 492-5263)

Canada
  Copp Clark, Ltd
  2775 Matheson Blvd East
  Mississauga, Ontario
  Canada, L4W 4P7
  (*Orders:* Tel: 800 263-4374
           905 238-6074)

Australia
  Blackwell Science Pty Ltd
  54 University Street
  Carlton, Victoria 3053
  (*Orders:* Tel: 03 9347 0300
           Fax: 03 9349 3016)

Catalogue records for this title
are available from the British Library
and the Library of Congress

ISBN 0-86542-944-8

Contents

Contributors

James M. Becker MD, James Utley Professor, Chairman, Department of Surgery, Boston University School of Medicine. Surgeon-in-Chief, Boston University Medical Center Hospital and Boston City Hospital, Boston, Massachusetts, USA

Malcolm C. Champion MB, FRCPC, FRCP (UK), Associate Professor, University of Ottawa, Division of Gastroenterology, Ottawa Civic Hospital, Ottawa, Ontario, Canada

Michael D. Crowell PhD, Director, Center for Physiologic Studies, Thomas N. Lynn Institute for Healthcare Research, Integris/Baptist Medical Center of Oklahoma. Associate Professor of Biological Psychology, University of Oklahoma Health Sciences Center, Oklahoma City, Oklahoma, USA

Robert S. Fisher MD, Professor of Medicine, Chief, Gastroenterology Section, Director, Functional Gastrointestinal Disease Center, Temple University School of Medicine, Philadelphia, Pennsylvania, USA

Robert C. Heading BSc MD FRCP, Reader in Medicine, The University of Edinburgh. Consultant Physician, Centre for Liver and Digestive Disorders, Royal Infirmary of Edinburgh, Edinburgh, Scotland

Peter J. Kahrilas MD, Professor of Medicine, Division of Gastroenterology and Hepatology, Northwestern University Medical School, Chicago, Illinois, USA

Richard W. McCallum MD, FRACP (AUST), FACG, Paul Janssen Professor of Medicine, Program Director, Division of Gastroenterology, Hepatology, and Nutrition, University of Virginia School of Medicine, Charlottesville, Virginia, USA

John G. Moore MD, Chief, Gastroenterology Section, Department of Veterans Affairs Medical Center. Professor of Medicine, University of Utah School of Medicine, Salt Lake City, Utah, USA

William C. Orr PhD FACG, President and Chief Operating Officer, Thomas N. Lynn Institute for Healthcare Research, Integris/Baptist Medical Center of Oklahoma. Adjunct Professor of Psychiatry and Behavioral Sciences, University of Oklahoma Health Sciences Center, Oklahoma City, Oklahoma, USA

Eamonn M.M. Quigley MD, FRCP, Associate Professor and Chief, Section of Gastroenterology and Hepatology, University of Nebraska Medical Center, Omaha, Nebraska, USA

Lawrence R. Schiller MD, Director, Gastrointestinal Physiology Laboratory, Baylor University Medical Center, Dallas, Texas, USA

André J.P.M. Smout MD, Professor of GI Motility, Department of Gastroenterology, Utrecht University Hospital, Utrecht, The Netherlands

W. Grant Thompson MD, FRCP(C), Chief, Division of Gastroenterology, Ottawa Civic Hospital. Professor of Medicine, University of Ottawa, Ottawa, Ontario, Canada. Visiting Professor, University of Bristol (1994–95)

Preface

Evolving Concepts in Gastrointestinal Motility was inspired by the need for an up-to-date text to reflect the many recent advances in gastrointestinal (GI) motility. The importance of GI motility in explaining GI symptoms and diseases has become increasingly recognized over the past two decades. Coincident with this increased awareness of motility disorders was the recognition that controlling acid secretion was not necessarily the solution to many upper GI problems. This textbook reviews significant developments in technological assessment, physiology, diagnosis, and pharmacologic treatment of GI motility disorders. Less common as well as common clinical syndromes are covered, along with the potential roles of visceral sensation and perception and sleep in the pathogenesis of motility disorders.

Advances in available instrumentation to monitor motility disorders have highlighted the role of dysmotility in many GI diseases. This is particularly so with 24-hour ambulatory monitoring of the upper GI tract in patients with gastroesophageal reflux disease; but the understanding of other conditions, including gastroparesis, intestinal pseudo-obstruction, and irritable bowel syndrome, has also been advanced. There has also been heightened awareness of the symptoms and symptom complexes associated with different motility disorders. This has resulted in criteria for the diagnosis of several common intestinal diseases. It is generally recognized that symptom complexes associated with motility disorders should be more clearly defined, and the value of such criteria needs to stand the test of time. In this book, we attempt to identify common motility disorders, highlight the relationships between these disorders and clinical symptoms, and point out areas where further research is needed to advance the understanding and treatment of these conditions.

The importance of the enteric nervous system as a major controlling factor of GI motility has resulted in a better understanding of the neurophysiology of intestinal motility. Ongoing research into enteric neurotransmitters has and will continue to discover newer modalities that can pharmacologically inhibit or stimulate intestinal motility. The application of basic research to whole-gut motility and motility abnormalities is emphasized throughout the text.

It is axiomatic that advances in therapy are preceded by advances in our understanding of the pathophysiology. Our current interest in visceral sensation and perception has emerged from a better understanding of the enteric nervous system and its multiplicity of excitatory and inhibitory networks. Visceral perception remains an area of intense investigation, and the rapid expansion of research in recent years has enhanced our understanding of GI symptoms. In addition, research has created new horizons in the development of effective therapeutic modalities. These include more potent prokinetic agents, drugs to manipulate visceral perception both centrally and peripherally, and better definition of the role of biofeedback. The role of surgery also has become better defined.

The title of this text reflects the rapid growth in knowledge of GI motility. We anticipate that our understanding will continue to evolve at an ever-increasing pace. This will hopefully result in the necessity for future editions of *Evolving Concepts in Gastrointestinal Motility*.

The editors and the authors wish to acknowledge the very capable and diligent efforts of Sifor Ng in the editing and completion of this textbook, and Julie Jones of Blackwell Science for turning our manuscript into a published textbook in such a short period of time.

M.C. Champion
W.C. Orr

Evolving Concepts in Gastrointestinal Motility: A Review of Past Progress

Richard W. McCallum

We need to reflect back only to the start of this century to highlight the remarkable progress that has been made in the study of gastrointestinal (GI) motility. Advances have relied on a confluence of research in smooth-muscle physiology, electrophysiology, neurohormonal regulation of the GI tract, anatomic/mechanical factors, flow dynamics, as well as basic molecular and cellular biology. Increasingly sophisticated instrumentation, biomedical engineering, and pharmaceutical research have also added to this rich harvest over the past 50 years. Hence, progress in GI motility has proceeded from the contributions of a wide range of disciplines. This may help explain the unpredictable and seemingly erratic growth in knowledge of different areas of the gut. A central theme to the progress that will be recounted in this chapter is the recognition, evolution, and greater understanding of the enteric nervous system, where more than 10^6 neurons intercommunicate and integrate messages from the gut and brain to organize and coordinate the minute-to-minute control which we call gut motility.

The quantitation of gut motility has been a constant goal during this era, particularly the study of peristaltic contractions by means of pressures in the gut lumen. The measurement of intraluminal pressures started with the use of balloons inflated in the stomach and intestine. In the 1950s, open-tipped catheters began to be used to study the esophagus. Subsequent improvements include the continuous-perfusion catheters with the low-compliance Arndorfer pump, and development of the Dent sleeve which have facilitated the study of sphincters. At the turn of the century, gastric flow could be imaged by means of contrast radiography [1]. By the 1980s, scintigraphy enabled flow studies throughout the GI tract to be performed routinely in clinical practice. Scintigraphy also has enabled quantitation of esophageal and gastric emptying as well as small-bowel and colonic transit.

Scientific investigation of gut wall movement began with the use of miniature force transducers sewn to the luminal wall. Electromyography has also been used to enhance our understanding of wall movement. Recent studies [2] suggest that prolonged scanning with magnetic resonance imaging (MRI) can be used to correlate gut wall motion with intraluminal pressures and other physiologic parameters.

Concomitant with advances in instrumentation for measuring motility, basic research has focused on the neurohormonal regulation and myogenic components of GI motility. In the 1930s, it was believed that gut motor activity occurred as a result of opposition between excitatory parasympathetic (cholinergic) and inhibitory sympathetic (adrenergic) nerves. Electrical field stimulation of gut muscle preparations led to the discovery of nonadrenergic noncholinergic (NANC) nerves as the predominant intrinsic inhibitory nerves of the GI tract [1]. The identity of the NANC neurotransmitter, perhaps vasoactive intestinal polypeptide (VIP) or nitric oxide, remains to be identified definitively. In the gut, electrical slow waves govern the rhythmicity of contractions, and slow waves of the stomach and small bowel began to be studied extensively by muscle electrophysiologists in the 1950s and 1960s.

W.B. Cannon and F.T. Murphy in 1906–7 reported that gastric emptying and intestinal motility may be depressed by both central nervous system and local mechanisms [3]. In 1943, Wolf and Wolff suggested that certain emotional states can increase gastric motility (as well as secretion and vascularity). There is ongoing research into the influence of GI peptides and hormones on the migrating motor complex (MMC). In a review 10 years after the demonstration of the migrating complex, Wingate [4] noted that neural and hormonal factors are involved in regulation, but 'details remain blurred' — an observation that holds true today.

Motility research from the esophagus to the colon

Esophageal motility

The phenomena of esophageal peristalsis and lower esophageal sphincter (LES) dynamics were first described on fluoroscopy at the start of this century, when contrast radiography was used to study the movement of ingested material from the proximal to the distal esophagus. However, radiation exposure limited the duration of observation. The *in vivo* recording of esophageal contractions was enhanced by balloon kymography. Balloon kymography extended the period of observation, but was associated with artificial stimulation of almost continuous contractile activity, hence limiting any interpretation [5]. Around the middle of the 20th century, Code and Ingelfinger used water-filled, open-tipped catheters and external transducers to identify the nature of the response to deglutition in the esophagus [5]. Intraluminal pressure sensors placed at different levels of the esophagus measured the primary peristaltic wave occurring after swallowing.

It was not until Harris *et al.* [6] developed a technique of constant slow infusion within intraluminal catheters that contractile pressures in the esophagus could be quantitated more accurately. Subsequent work by Castell [7] and Dodds [8] determined that accurate recording of esophageal peristaltic pressures required more rapid perfusion rates into intraluminal catheters, and current techniques make use of a low-compliance, pneumohydraulic pressure system or small intraluminal strain gauge transducers. Dodds [8] showed that a lumen-occluding peristaltic contraction on X-ray was required for the orderly esophageal transit of a barium bolus; otherwise, there would be no identifiable pressure response on manometry.

The presence of a physiologic sphincter at the esophagogastric junction – the LES – that would allow aboral passage of a swallowed bolus, yet maintain closure and minimize retrograde flow of gastric contents was established by W.B. Cannon at the start of this century. Subsequent investigations up to the present time have evaluated anatomic, neurogenic, myogenic, and hormonal determinants of LES tone.

The influence of the diaphragm on LES tone was postulated long before 1988, when Mittal *et al.* [9] established the role of the muscles of the right crus of the diaphragm in producing changes in resting LES pressure during inspiration. LES tone is primary myogenic. However, LES relaxation in response to swallowing appears to be neurally mediated. Experimental animal data have shown relaxation on vagal stimulation and complete inhibition of LES relaxation with administration of tetrodotoxin. The neurotransmitter involved remains to be discovered. At present, investigators [10, 11] have presented convincing arguments in favor of nitric oxide with a potential role for VIP as a cofactor.

Investigation of hormonal influences on the LES was stimulated by the report of an increase in resting LES pressure on administration of pentagastrin [12]. However, subsequent studies [13, 14] by McCallum and colleagues investigating physiologic infusions of gastrin 17 (G-17) and gastrin 34 (G-34), as well as careful assessment of gastrin levels and LES pressure in different clinical settings, found that gastrin was not a regulator of LES pressure. In healthy subjects, both G-17 and G-34 stimulated LES pressure, with a more prolonged LES response to G-34 [14]. Nevertheless, changes in serum G-17 and G-34 in physiologic concentrations did not affect LES pressure significantly. Whether gastrin plays a more subtle or supportive role in the control of LES pressure remains to be determined. If gastrin is not a major determinant, then concepts about the pathogenesis of LES disorders may have to be revised. For the present, the 'gastrin era' is over, in that no minute-to-minute control is assigned to the gastrin level.

Other GI peptides have since been found to exert inhibitory (glucagon and secretin) as well as stimulatory (motilin and substance P) effects on basal LES pressure. It should be noted that these effects were demonstrated with pharmacologic rather than physiologic levels of these peptides.

Gastric motility

Nineteenth-century physicians believed that the digestive tract was at rest during fasting. 'When [the chyme] is all transferred to the duodenum, the motions of the stomach cease,' wrote William Beaumont [15]. The MMC, which is also referred to as the migrating myoelectric complex, was first clearly described by Code and Szurszewski [16] in canine studies in the USA and by Ruckebusch [17] in sheep studies in France. The USA investigators noted that a complex was always present somewhere in the bowel during fasting.

Pioneers in the study of periodic gastric motor activity included Boldyreff, who noted periodic gastric contractions that could be inhibited by feeding. It was Boldyreff who in 1901–3 may have made the first definitive experimental study of the fasting complex [4]. In 1913, A.J. Carlson published a description of three types of gastric motor activity.

The MMC was first described in humans in 1975 by Stanciu and Bennett [18] and in 1977 by Vantrappen *et al.* [19]. In addition, differences in fasting and fed patterns of gut motility were firmly established. The concept of three phases of MMC is best exemplified at night, but is not unique to sleep. It is seen in all states of prolonged fasting, and cycle frequency ranges from 1 to 2.5 hours. The first phase III usually begins about 3 hours after a meal and is responsible for emptying nondigestible solids from the stomach. Thereafter, the major role of the MMC in prolonged fasting states is to maintain upper gut sterility by sweeping bacteria in the upper small bowel downstream and transporting gastric acid from the stomach into the proximal gut.

In the 1970s the study of gastric flow was advanced by the discovery of phenomena such as sieving — the separation of solids and liquids by the antrum [20] — and passive relaxation. Abrahamson [21] and others advanced the study of reflex mechanisms inducing vagally-mediated relaxation. Progress was also made in the correlation of luminal flow with motility. One result has been a call for more precise terminology to describe gastric motor events [22]. Gastric emptying of solids and liquids occurs separately, involving different areas of the stomach. The antrum was thought to undergo orderly peristaltic contractions and act as a pump, while the proximal segment functions more as a reservoir. This view of a two-compartment stomach was reinforced in the 1960s by results of electrophysiologic studies.

Intubation techniques are useful for measuring gastric emptying of liquids. However, limitations on patient tolerance of the procedure as well as difficulties in assessing solid emptying have reduced the popularity of intubation tests in clinical practice. Radioscintigraphy has provided a noninvasive, more physiologic means of quantitating gastric emptying with greater reliability.

Pioneer work by Meyer *et al.* [23] was followed by a double-isotope technique that enabled simultaneous quantitation of solid and liquid emptying. The use of radionuclide test meals raised many methodologic questions, including the decay rate of the isotope being used. In the future, counts may be obtained at intermittent intervals rather than by maintaining patients in a fixed position for a period of time. By enabling an individual to move between scans, interval scanning approaches can facilitate the study of elderly or disabled patients and free up gamma camera time; a downside is potential variation in the area of interest assumed by the computer to be the stomach. The principle of uniformity of method is critical in measuring gastric emptying. Furthermore, numerical results depend on the method of analysis. Before measurement of gastric emptying can be established as a clinical test, a method must be decided on, a normal range established for an individual laboratory, and the technique kept consistent.

Both catheter perfusion techniques and probes containing transducers are available to study gastric motor activity. While perfusion catheters are less expensive and easy to obtain, transducers are thinner probes which pass through the nose more easily and remain tolerable for longer periods; by not disturbing the luminal surface, transducers provide 'physiologic' recordings.

Studies using electrogastrography (EGG), a noninvasive technique that can measure gastric slow wave and spike activity, were first reported in the 1950s. In 1968 Nelsen and Kohatsu [24] reported the absence of a one-to-one relationship between myoelectric findings and gastric contractions; thus, EGG could determine the frequency of gastric contractions, but not when the contractions were occurring. It had been suggested that the EGG amplitude reflected the proximity of the gastric antrum to the abdominal surface on which the electrodes were positioned; in 1980 Smout *et al.* [25] showed that the EGG amplitude increases when contractions occur.

Interpretation of EGG data has progressed from visual to spectral analysis. Quantitative analysis — determining the dominant frequency of the EGG, the percent of time in which normal gastric slow waves are observed, and the percent of tachygastrias, bradygastrias, and other arrhythmias — was introduced only recently [26, 27]. EGG changes have been described in patients with delayed gastric emptying as well as artificially induced nausea [28, 29].

Small bowel motility

The beginnings of research into intestinal motility may be traced to the work of W.B. Cannon, who at the start of this century described basic patterns of intestinal movements in animal studies using barium-contrast radiography. W.P. Chapman and W.L. Palazzo were the first to record migrating complexes in the small bowel, in 1949 [4]. In 1954 W.T. Foulk *et al.* first reported periodicity in the human duodenum of regular phasic contractions alternating with quiescence.

By the 1940s, gut pressure activity was monitored predominantly with intraluminal balloons and intraluminal catheter systems [30]. For a number of reasons, investigations utilizing these systems were relatively short in duration and monitored only a few locations in the intestine. Limitations of the balloon system include poor patient compliance, a slow response rate, and the recording of summed rather than individual pressures. Both the initial nonperfused and subsequent perfused catheter systems were insensitive to less than lumen-occluding pressures. Until 1977, perfused systems required high flow rates, which in itself produced artifacts. Then, Arndorfer *et al.* [31] introduced a low-flow, low-compliance perfusion system that enabled multiple-port prolonged recording. The Arndorfer system stimulated changes in research focus, from the analysis of waveforms for consideration of whole organ function.

Experience with intestinal manometry has been extensive and has resulted in the identification of motility patterns in health and disease. Of great interest has been the suggestion that manometry may be useful for diagnosing the irritable bowel syndrome (IBS). Small bowel motility is difficult to record, however, and it should be cautioned that studies of proximal small bowel motility have demonstrated considerable regional variations and that the location of a probe can itself affect the type of motility pattern recorded. Small bowel motility has been shown to be affected by a number of variables, including stress, changes in hormone levels, and sleep. In the sleeping state, migrating complex cycles are associated with phase III bursts separated by absolute quiescence. Current technology enables 24-hour ambulatory manometric recording, which affords the advantage of better recording of MMC activity and circadian variations. Advantages of stationary recordings include more reliable positioning of catheters in the antrum and thus an accurate measurement of the fed motor response.

Colonic motility

Motility may be less well understood in the colon than in any other area of the GI tract. In 1904 W.B. Cannon reported the observation of anti-peristalsis in the large intestine. Electrophysiologic studies have also demonstrated this phenomenon. Manometry was used by Almy *et al.* [32] to demonstrate the effect of emotions and stressors on left-colon motility in patients with IBS.

Colonic transit has been examined via ingestion of radio-opaque markers that were then serially imaged on radiography. Instillation of radioisotope directly into the cecum has permitted colonic imaging clearly distinguished from overlying small bowel activity [33]. Scintigraphy has proved to be useful in quantifying transit of radiotracers via such techniques as calculation of geometric centers of activity. The management of idiopathic constipation has benefited from use of scintigraphy. Recently, mass peristaltic movements were described which have been termed high-amplitude propagated contractions (HAPC) [34] typically associated with, or in close proximity to, bowel movements. The uses of markers and scintigraphic techniques to assess colon transit has been combined with ano-rectal motility studies to diagnose, stratify and treat constipation.

Sphincter of Oddi motility

The sphincter of Oddi (SO) constitutes an adaptive mechanism for maintaining low pressure within the biliary and pancreatic ductal systems. Basal SO pressure, which exceeds resting duodenal pressure by an average of 15 mmHg, is considered the primary factor in monitoring flow from either system. Superimposed on the basal pressure are phasic SO contractions, of about 4 per minute, which remove debris from the sphincteric zone. The role of SO dysfunction in clinical disorders requires elucidation. In both the biliary and pancreatic systems, patients have been classified for clinical study into three 'working groups' each, with type I patients evincing a higher prevalence of SO dysfunction than type III patients. SO motility remains very much a research technique and should be confined to centers attempting to standardize and advance the area. Therapeutic decision-making remains an area for active research.

Some landmarks in the study of motility disorders

Achalasia and other esophageal motility disorders

Achalasia was known as simple ectasia or cardiospasm before 1957, when Code and coworkers demonstrated abnormal LES relaxation on esophageal manometry [35]. The absence of distal esophageal peristalsis characteristic of this disorder was confirmed by other studies. The discovery of decreased enteric ganglia in the myenteric plexus (denervation of the distal esophagus) and denervation sensitivity has contributed to our understanding of achalasia [36].

The development of perfused catheters and solid-state transducers has enabled the establishment of manometric criteria for achalasia. The nature of the aperistalsis in achalasia has been the subject of speculation following the report of Vantrappen et al. [37] of the return of peristaltic contractions after pneumatic esophageal dilatation.

With improved manometric techniques, a prevalent manometric entity in patients with unexplained chest pain has been the 'nutcracker esophagus,' or high-amplitude peristaltic contractions. Nutcracker esophagus has been described as an example of altered visceral afferent sensitivity and overlaps the broader group of nociception disorders best illustrated by the IBS and 'nonulcer' dyspepsia. Such terms as the *irritable esophagus* emerged from the work of Clouse et al. [38]; treatment approaches evolved to include use of antidepressants as adjuvant therapy in these patients.

Gastroesophageal reflux disease (GERD)

In GERD, gastric contents are displaced retrograde into the esophagus and, in some instances, the tracheobronchial tree. The primary pathogenic factor in GERD was once thought to be a proximally displaced esophagogastric junction, as represented by a hiatus hernia. In 1971 Cohen and Harris [39] suggested that a low basal LES pressure was more important in the development of chronic heartburn. By the 1970s, the primacy of the smooth-muscle LES as the major antireflux barrier was generally accepted, and GERD is now recognized primarily as a motility disorder. The role of hiatus hernia in GERD remains controversial. It is regarded not as the initiator of gastroesophageal junction incompetence, but rather as interfering with and prolonging esophageal acid clearance [40, 41].

LES research initially focused on the phenomenon of low basal pressures. More recently, attention has centered on transient relaxations of the LES (TLESRs). In 1982 Dodds *et al.* [42] reported that the LES relaxed spontaneously both in healthy subjects and, with greater frequency, in patients with reflux disease. Prolonged manometric recordings by these investigators using a 6 cm Dent sleeve showed that TLESRs were frequent and of short duration, with clearance of acid reflux achieved by secondary peristalsis. The most likely inducer of a transient relaxation was identified by Holloway *et al.* [43] and Mittal and McCallum [44] as being distention of the proximal stomach and fundus. This in turn can be incorporated into the observation by McCallum *et al.* [45] regarding slow gastric emptying in GERD patients and their propensity for greater gastric residual volume and hence more distention.

Twenty-four-hour pHmetry

Even though dysmotility has a primary role in GERD, simply measuring motility disorders in these patients is inadequate to describe the complex pathophysiology of GERD. Efforts initiated in the mid-1970s have led to the development of prolonged pH monitoring of stomach contents (i.e. acid, pepsin, and bile) in the esophagus. Pioneer researchers include Johnson and DeMeester [46, 47], who described various parameters of 24-hour esophageal acid contact time in patients with GERD and healthy controls. Intragastric pH monitoring had been attempted using telemetric techniques such as with a Heidelberg capsule, but Johnson and DeMeester were the first to apply this concept to the esophagus in patients with GERD. These prolonged studies, which have evolved to the point that they allow completely ambulatory recordings, have provided remarkable insights into the pathogenesis of GERD.

DeMeester *et al.* [46] first described the differences in pattern of reflux during the day (upright position) and at night (supine position). The daytime reflux pattern is predominantly postprandial and consists of repeated short episodes of reflux; nocturnal reflux, albeit less frequent, tends to be associated with a marked prolongation of acid clearance. In the late 1970s, these investigators demonstrated that the more severe forms of esophagitis were associated with supine reflux, occurring predominantly during sleep.

These observations have spawned a proliferation of research regarding various aspects of esophageal acid mucosal contact and the resulting developing of mucosal damage and symptoms. Numerous studies have assessed the pathogenic role of sleep in GERD — work discussed in Chapter 12. In addition, the ambulatory monitoring technique has provided a unique opportunity to correlate reflux events with production of symptoms. This has led to a variety of techniques to describe and quantify the relationship between reflux events and symptoms [48–50]. Although the appropriate techniques for determining the true relationship between reflux events and reports of symptoms remain somewhat controversial, the discussion itself would never have evolved without the availability of 24-hour pHmetry.

Endoscopy may be a highly specific diagnostic test for GERD, but it is not very sensitive [51]. A significant proportion — perhaps as many as 60% [52, 53] — of GERD patients do not have esophagitis and thus would go undiagnosed with endoscopy. Prolonged esophageal pH monitoring is effective not only in confirming the presence of GERD in 'endoscopy-negative' patients, but also in achieving reproducible findings in patients with atypical as well as classic GERD symptoms [49].

More recently, investigators have evaluated the effectiveness of prolonged esophageal pH monitoring of shorter duration than 24 hours. Comparisons have been made, for example, with a 3-hour postprandial monitoring period. Evaluation of such shorter-duration pH monitoring for the diagnosis of GERD has met with mixed results [54, 55]. Logically, monitoring pH solely during a postprandial period (when the subject is upright) would be less sensitive than 24-hour monitoring, because individuals who reflux solely or predominantly in the supine position would have negative findings. It does not appear likely that there is a correlation between upright (daytime) and supine (nocturnal) reflux. Recognizing these limitations, some researchers are investigating the recording of pH over a combination monitoring schedule; for example, monitoring during a postprandial (upright) period followed by a monitoring period with the subject lying supine.

Twenty-four-hour pHmetry is used extensively in the evaluation of new pharmacologic agents to treat GERD. There is also considerable research work in the development of animal models to assess the relative contribution of gastric contents in producing esophageal mucosal damage [56]. Such studies have documented the role of prolonged esophageal acidification, and the relative contribution of pepsin, bile acids, and pancreatic enzymes in producing esophageal mucosal damage. These data and the persistent observation of patients who seem to be refractory to powerful gastric acid suppression have led to considerable recent interest in bile acids and their role in the production of esophagitis and, particularly, Barrett's esophagus [57, 58].

Barrett's esophagus

About one or two in every ten patients with esophagitis develop a severe complication such as stricture or Barrett's esophagus. There is considerable interest in the latter because the most common epithelial type in Barrett's — specialized intestinal metaplasia — is associated with a strong predisposition for adenocarcinoma [59]. Barrett's is the result of attempts at mucosal repair by the esophagus. Neither symptom frequency nor severity is predictive of mucosal damage, although a long history of symptoms appears to correlate with Barrett's esophagus [60]. Reviving a controversy of the 1950s, there are some recent data to suggest a genetic predisposition for Barrett's [61].

Because severe GERD is frequently associated with large hiatal hernias and significant esophageal inflammation, an endoscopic diagnosis of Barrett's esophagus was fraught with methodologic difficulties. Arbitrary diagnostic criteria were promulgated for the purposes of entering patients into clinical trials, and subsequently such criteria were adopted by clinicians. For a number of reasons, the diagnostic criteria for Barrett's have evolved from 'an esophagus lined extensively by gastric epithelium' to 'one lined by any extent of intestinal epithelium' [62]. Efforts are ongoing to propose a classification scheme to better minimize diagnostic difficulties [62].

Conclusion

The objectives of more precise measurement of motor abnormalities and correlation of dysmotility with other parameters of disease activity are to understand pathophysiology better and improve the clinician's ability to evaluate and treat patients with motility-related disorders. As an example of the former, combined 24-hour ambulatory pH and manometric monitoring in patients with reflux esophagitis suggests that motor abnormalities precede rather than are the consequence of mucosal inflammation [63]. Recent studies in chronic intestinal dysmotility syndrome patients suggest that autonomic status may be a more reliable predictor of patient response to prokinetic therapy than manometric parameters [64]. Already, increasingly sophisticated technology has begun to yield more effective strategies for treatment as well as enhanced understanding of the pathophysiologic mechanisms underlying GI motility disorders. As we approach the end of the twentieth century, GI motility is no longer the 'forgotten factor' but rather the first factor that needs to be considered.

References

1 Christensen J. History of the evolution of ideas in gastrointestinal motility. In: Kirsner JB, ed. *The Growth of Gastroenterologic Knowledge During the Twentieth Century*. Philadelphia: Lea & Febiger, 1994:140–58.

2 Evans DF, Lamont G, Stehling MK *et al*. Prolonged monitoring of the upper gastrointestinal tract using echo planar magnetic resonance imaging. *Gut* 1993;**34**:848–52.

3 Davenport HW, Walter B. Cannon's contribution to gastroenterology. *Gastroenterology* 1972;**63**:878–89.

4 Wingate DL. Backwards and forwards with the migrating complex. *Dig Dis Sci* 1981;**26**:641–66.

5 Castell DO. Esophageal motility and benign disorders. In: Kirsner JB, ed. *The Growth of Gastroenterologic Knowledge During the Twentieth Century*. Philadelphia: Lea & Febiger, 1994:3–10.

6 Harris LD, Winans CS, Pope CE II. Determination of yield pressures: a method for measuring anal sphincter competence. *Gastroenterology* 1966;**50**:754–60.

7 Hollis JB, Castell DO. Amplitude of esophageal peristalsis as determined by rapid infusion. *Gastroenterology* 1972;**63**:417.

8 Kahrilas PJ, Dodds WJ, Hogan WJ. The effect of peristaltic dysfunction on esophageal volume clearance. *Gastroenterology* 1988;**94**:73.

9 Mittal RK, Rochester DF, McCallum RW. Electrical and mechanical activity in the human lower esophageal sphincter during diaphragmatic contraction. *J Clin Invest* 1988;**81**:1182–9.

10 Goyal RK, Rattan S. VIP as a possible neurotransmitter of non-cholinergic non-adrenergic inhibitory neurones. *Nature* 1980;**288**:378–80.

11 Sanders KM, Ward SM. Nitric oxide as a mediator of nonadrenergic noncholinergic neurotransmission. *Am J Physiol* 1992;**262**:G379–92.

12 Castell DO, Harris LD. Hormonal control of gastroesophageal–sphincter strength. *N Engl J Med* 1970;**282**:886–9.

13 McCallum RW, Walsh JH. Relationship between lower esophageal sphincter pressure and serum gastrin concentration in Zollinger–Ellison syndrome and other clinical settings. *Gastroenterology* 1979;**76**:76–81.

14 Jensen DM, McCallum RW, Corazziari E, Elashoff J, Walsh JH. Human lower esophageal sphincter responses to synthetic human gastrins 34 (G-34) and 17 (G-17). *Gastroenterology* 1980;**79**:431–8.

15 Beaumont W. *Experiments and Observations on the Gastric Juice, and the Physiology of Digestion*. Plattsburgh: FP Allen, 1833.

16 Szurszewski JH. A migrating electric complex of the canine small intestine. *Am J Physiol* 1969;**217**:1757–63.

17 Ruckebusch Y, Laplace JP. La motricite intestinale chez le mouton: phenomenes mecaniques et electriques. *CR Soc Biol* 1967;**161**:2517.

18 Stanciu C, Bennett JR. The general pattern of gastroduodenal motility: 24-hour recordings in normal subjects. *Rev Med Chir Soc Med Nat Iasi* 1975;**79**:31–6.

19 Vantrappen G, Janssens J, Hellemans J, Ghoos Y. The interdigestive motor complex of normal subjects and patients with bacterial overgrowth of the small intestine. *J Clin Invest* 1977;**59**:1158–66.

20 Meyer JH, Thomson JB, Cohen MB, Shadchehr A, Mandiola SA. Sieving of solid food by the canine stomach and sieving after surgery. *Gastroenterology* 1979;**76**:804–13.

21 Abrahamson H. Studies on the inhibitory neuronal control of gastric motility. *Acta Physiol Scand* 1973;**390**(Suppl.):1–38.

22 Horowitz M, Dent J. The study of gastric mechanics and flow: a Mad Hatter's tea party starting to make sense? *Gastroenterology* 1994;**107**:302–6.

23 Meyer JH, MacGregor MB, Gueller R. ^{99m}Tc-tagged chicken liver as a marker of solid food in the human stomach. *Am J Dig Dis* 1976;**21**:296.

24 Nelsen TS, Kohatsu S. Clinical electrogastrography and its relationship to gastric surgery. *Am J Surg* 1968;**116**:215–22.

25 Smout AJPM, van der Schee EJ, Grashuis JL. What is measured in electro-gastrography? *Dig Dis Sci* 1980;**25**:179–87.

26 Chen JZ, McCallum RW. Clinical applications of electrogastrography. *Am J Gastroenterol* 1993;**88**:1324–36.

27 Chen JZ, McCallum RW, eds. *Electrogastrography: Principles and Applications.* New York: Raven Press, 1994.

28 Lin ZY, Pan J, McCallum RW, Chen JDZ. Do gastric myoelectrical abnormalities predict delayed gastric emptying? *Gastroenterology* 1995;**108**:A639.

29 Xu LH, Koch KL, Summy-Long J et al. Hypothalamic and gastric myoelectrical responses during vection-induced nausea in healthy Chinese subjects. *Am J Physiol* 1993;**265**:E578–84.

30 Quigley EMM. Intestinal manometry in man: a historical and clinical perspective. *Dig Dis* 1994;**12**:199–209.

31 Arndorfer RC, Stef JJ, Dodds WJ, Linehan JH, Hogan WJ. Improved infusion system for intraluminal esophageal manometry. *Gastroenterology* 1977;**73**:23–7.

32 Almy TP, Abbot FK, Hinkle LE Jr. Alterations in colonic function in man under stress: IV. Hypomotility of the sigmoid colon, and its relationship to the mechanism of functional diarrhea. *Gastroenterology* 1950;**15**:95–103.

33 Krevsky B, Malmud LS, D'Ercole F, Maurer AH, Fisher RS. Colonic transit scintigraphy: a physiologic approach to the quantitative measurement of colonic transit in humans. *Gastroenterology* 1986;**91**:1102–12.

34 Bassotti G, Crowell M, Whitehead W. Contractile activity of the human colon: lessons from 24 hour studies. *Gut* 1993;**34**:129–33.

35 Creamer B, Olsen AM, Code CF. The esophageal sphincters in achalasia of the cardia (cardiospasm). *Gastroenterology* 1957;**33**:293–301.

36 Cassella RR, Brown AL Jr, Sayre GP, Ellis FH Jr. Achalasia of the esophagus: pathologic and etiologic considerations. *Ann Surg* 1964;**160**(3):474–87.

37 Vantrappen G, Janssens J, Hellemans J, Coremans G. Achalasia, diffuse esophageal spasm, and related motility disorders. *Gastroenterology* 1979;**76**:450–7.

38 Clouse RE, McCord GS, Lustman PJ, Edmundowicz SA. Clinical correlates of abnormal sensitivity to intraesophageal balloon distention. *Dig Dis Sci* 1991;**36**:1040.

39 Cohen S, Harris LD. Does hiatus hernia affect competence of the gastroesophageal sphincter? *N Engl J Med* 1971;**284**:1053–6.

40 Mittal RK, Lange RC, McCallum RW. Identification and mechanism of delayed esophageal acid clearance in subjects with hiatus hernia. *Gastroenterology* 1987;**92**:130–5.

41 Sloan S, Kahrilas PJ. Impairment of esophageal emptying with hiatal hernia. *Gastroenterology* 1991;**100**:596–605.

42 Dodds WJ, Dent J, Hogan WJ et al. Mechanisms of gastroesophageal reflux in patients with reflux esophagitis. *N Engl J Med* 1982;**307**:1547–52.

43 Holloway RH, Hongo M, Berger K, McCallum RW. Gastric distention: a mechanism for postprandial gastroesophageal reflux. *Gastroenterology* 1985;**89**:779–84.

44 Mittal RK, McCallum RW. Characteristics and frequency of transient relaxations of the lower esophageal sphincter in patients with reflux esophagitis. *Gastroenterology* 1988;**95**:593–9.

45 McCallum RW, Berkowitz DM, Lerner E. Gastric emptying in patients with gastro-esophageal reflux. *Gastroenterology* 1981;**80**:285–91.

46 DeMeester TR, Johnson LF, Joseph GJ, Toscano MS, Hall AW, Skinner DB. Patterns of gastroesophageal reflux in health and disease. *Ann Surg* 1976;**184**:459–69.

47 Johnson LF. New concepts and methods in the study and treatment of gastro-esophageal reflux disease. *Med Clin North Am* 1981;**65**:1195–222.

48 Weusten BLAM, Roelofs JMM, Akkermans LMA, Van Berge Henegouwen GP, Smout AJPM. The symptom-association probability: an improved method for symptom analysis of 24-hour esophageal pH data. *Gastroenterology* 1994;**107**:1741–5.

49 Wiener GJ, Morgan TM, Copper JB *et al.* Ambulatory 24-hour esophageal pH monitoring: reproducibility and variability of pH parameters. *Dig Dis Sci* 1988;**33**:1127–33.

50 Orr WC. The physiology and philosophy of cause and effect. *Gastroenterology* 1994;**107**:1878–901.

51 Klauser AG, Heinrich C, Schindlbeck NE, Muller-Lissner SA. Is long-term esophageal pH monitoring of clinical value? *Am J Gastroenterol* 1989;**84**:362–6.

52 Schnell T, Sontag S, Wanner J, Chintam R, Chejfec G, O'Connell S, Moroni B. Endoscopic screening for Barrett's esophagus (BE), esophageal adenocarcinoma (AdCa) and other mucosal changes in ambulatory subjects with symptomatic gastroesophageal reflux (GER). *Gastroenterology* 1985;**88**:A1576.

53 Winters C, Spurling TJ, Chobanian SJ *et al.* Barrett's esophagus: a prevalent, occult complication of gastroesophageal reflux disease. *Gastroenterology* 1987;**92**:118–24.

54 Fink SM, McCallum RW. The role of prolonged esophageal pH monitoring in the diagnosis of gastrophageal reflux. *JAMA* 1984;**252**:1160–4.

55 Johnsson F, Joelsson B, Isberg P-E. Ambulatory 24 hour intraesophageal pH monitoring in the diagnosis of gastroesophageal reflux disease. *Gut* 1987;**28**:1145–50.

56 Johnson LF, Harmon JW. Experimental esophagitis in a rabbit model: clinical relevance. *J Clin Gastroenterol* 1986;**8**(Suppl.1):26–44.

57 Kauer WK, Peters JH, DeMeester TR, Ireland AP, Bremner CG, Hagen JA. Mixed reflux of gastric and duodenal juices is more harmful to the esophagus than gastric juice alone: the need for surgical therapy re-emphasized. *Ann Surg* 1995;**222**:525–31.

58 Champion G, Richter JE, Vaezi MF, Singh S, Alexander R. Duodenogastro-esophageal reflux: relationship to pH and importance in Barrett's esophagus. *Gastroenterology* 1994;**107**:747–54.

59 Reid BJ, Weinstein WM, Lewin KJ *et al.* Endoscopic biopsy can detect high-grade dysplasia or early adenocarcinoma in Barrett's esophagus without grossly recognizable neoplastic lesions. *Gastroenterology* 1988;**94**:81–90.

60 Tuohy CD, Allen V, Sampliner RE, Aicken M, Garewal H. Can symptoms alone differentiate patients with Barrett's esophagus from patients with gastroesophageal reflux disease lacking Barrett's? *Gastroenterology* 1990;**98**:A141.

61 Phillips RW, Wong RKH. Barrett's esophagus: natural history, incidence, etiology, and complications. *Gastroenterol Clin North Am* 1991;**20**:791–816.

62 Spechler SJ, Goyal RK. The columnar-lined esophagus, intestinal metaplasia, and Norman Barrett. *Gastroenterology* 1996;**110**:614–21.

63 Timmer R, Breumelhof R, Nadorp JHSM, Smout AFPM. Oesophageal motility and gastro-oesophageal reflux before and after healing of reflux oesophagitis: a study using 24 hour ambulatory pH and pressure monitoring. *Gut* 1994;**35**:1519–22.

64 Camilleri M, Balm RK, Zinsmeister AR. Determinants of response to a prokinetic agent in neuropathic chronic intestinal motility disorder. *Gastroenterology* 1994;**106**:916–23.

<< 2 >>

Esophageal Motility Disorders: Pathogenesis, Diagnosis, Treatment

Peter J. Kahrilas

The esophagus, a muscular tube with a sphincter at each end, is the pathway between the pharynx and the stomach. The neuromuscular function of the esophagus (motility) has the simplest of goals, which can be summarized as maintaining emptiness in the face of numerous intrusions from above or below. Primary esophageal peristalsis sweeps the esophagus clear after distention by pharyngeal contents during swallowing; secondary peristalsis eliminates air or fluid refluxed from the stomach. The upper esophageal sphincter (UES) contracts during inspiration to exclude inspired air from the digestive tract; elements of the gastroesophageal junction contract in response to transient increases in intra-abdominal pressure, preventing gastroesophageal reflux. A pervasive attribute of esophageal motility disorders is that they break this cardinal rule of preserving emptiness. Retention of material within the esophagus and the excessive entry of material into the esophagus are abnormal. These dysfunctions can be categorized as disorders of peristalsis or of sphincter competence. The main dysfunction of sphincter competence occurs with reflux disease, an entity covered in Chapters 3 and 4. This chapter will focus on less common causes of sphincter dysfunction and on disorders of esophageal peristalsis.

Neuromuscular anatomy

The esophageal body is a 20–22 cm tube composed of skeletal (striated) and smooth muscle. In humans, the proximal 5% of the esophageal body, including the UES, is striated; the middle 35–40% is mixed, with an increasing proportion of smooth muscle distally; and the distal 50–60% consists entirely of smooth muscle [1, 2]. The bundles of the outer, longitudinal muscle arise from the cricoid cartilage, receiving slips from the cricopharyngeus, and pass dorsolaterally to fuse posteriorly about 3 cm below the cricoid cartilage. The inner muscle layer is formed of a circular muscle sheath running the length of the esophagus. The circular muscle ring that functions as the lower esophageal sphincter (LES) angles obliquely upward from the lesser to the greater curvature of the stomach and is contiguous with the circular muscle of the esophageal body [3]. The maximal thickness of the LES occurs at the greater curvature of the stomach. Towards the stomach, the LES is split into two segments: one forms short transverse muscle clasps around the esophagus, and the other forms long oblique loops in the stomach (gastric sling fibers). The LES is normally situated within the esophageal hiatus of the diaphragm which, in its most common configuration, is formed entirely by the fibers of the right diaphragmatic crus [4]. Recent studies [5] suggest that extrinsic compression of the LES by the diaphragmatic crus represents a component of intraluminal LES pressure.

Both the striated- and smooth-muscle portions of the esophagus contain a nerve network (the myenteric plexus) between the longitudinal and circular muscle layers (Figure 2.1) [6]. In the smooth-muscle portion, these enteric neurons are the relay neurons between the vagus and the smooth muscle; the function of these neurons in the striated-muscle esophagus is obscure. A second nerve network, the submucosal or Meissner's plexus, is situated between the muscularis mucosa and the circular muscle layer. However, this network is sparse in the human esophagus, with only a few ganglion cells [7].

The extrinsic innervation of the esophagus occurs via the vagus nerve. Fibers innervating the striated muscle are axons of lower motor neurons with cell bodies in the nucleus ambiguus; innervation of the smooth-muscle esophagus is provided by the dorsal motor nucleus of

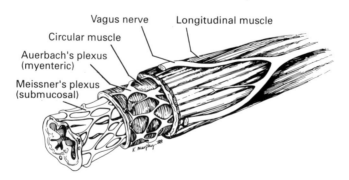

Fig. 2.1 Neuromuscular anatomy of the esophagus. Two nerve networks are interposed between the muscular layers. The myenteric plexus receives input from the vagus nerve and controls contractile activities of the major muscular layers. The submucosal plexus contains only sparse neurons. (From Kahrilas [6]. Courtesy of David W. Gelfand MD and Joel E. Richter MD from the book *Dysphagia*, Igaku-Shoin Medical Publishers, New York, NY; 1989.)

the vagus [8, 9]. The cricopharyngeus muscle receives its motor nerve supply from the pharyngeal branch of the vagus [10, 11]. Efferent nerve fibers reach the cervical esophagus via the pharyngoesophageal nerve [12]. Histologic studies [13, 14] have shown that vagal efferents synapse directly on striated muscle neuromuscular junctions. The vagus nerves provide sensory innervation in the cervical esophagus via the superior laryngeal nerve with cell bodies in the nodose ganglion. In the remainder of the esophagus, sensory fibers travel via the recurrent laryngeal nerve or, in the most distal esophagus, via the esophageal branches of the vagus. Many free nerve endings have been observed in the mucosa, submucosa, and muscular layers [15–17]. A few encapsulated structures resembling spindles have also been described in humans. These vagal afferents are strongly stimulated by esophageal distention.

The upper esophageal sphincter

The UES is variably considered to be an esophageal or a pharyngeal structure (pharyngoesophageal sphincter or segment). The confusion is justified as the sphincter functions as an integral part of both the esophagus and the pharynx. In humans, the zone of maximal pressure is approximately 1 cm long and corresponds precisely to the fluoroscopically determined location of the cricopharyngeus muscle [18]. The UES is distinct from more rostral pharyngeal structures in that it is a tonically contracted segment. Resting pressure within the UES exhibits marked radial asymmetry: anterior and posterior pressures are greater than lateral pressures. The slit-like configuration of the sphincter explains this asymmetry; indeed, the radial asymmetry disappears following laryngectomy [19]. Intraluminal UES pressure is also affected by the measurement technique. The less movement applied to the recording catheter during measurement, the lower the recorded pressures [20]. The lowest pressures are obtained with a stationary recording device; even then, further adaptation and diminution of intraluminal pressure are demonstrable during prolonged recordings. A physiologic correlate of this sensitivity to intraluminal recording devices has been observed in animal experiments, in which intubation of the sphincter prompts vigorous electromyographic (EMG) activity in the cricopharyngeus muscle [21, 22].

A common observation during intraluminal UES recordings or cricopharyngeal EMG recordings is that the UES contracts in synchrony with inspiration, a response that probably prevents inhalation of air into the esophagus. Inspiratory augmentation is most evident during periods of low

UES pressure and is often undetectable during periods of higher sphincter pressures, presumably because it is obscured by more vigorous responses. Balloon distention of the esophagus stimulates UES contraction; the effect is more pronounced with proximal balloon positions [20]. However, when the pattern of distention induced by gas reflux is imitated by using a long cylindrical balloon or by rapid injection of air into the esophagus, relaxation, rather than contraction, of the UES occurs (Figure 2.2) [23]. Thus, the

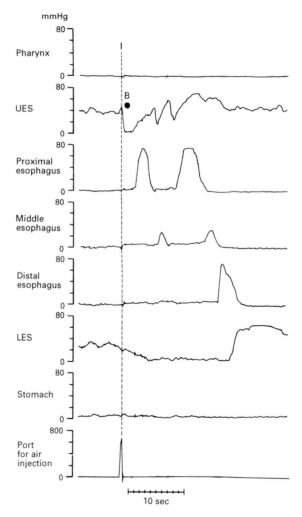

Fig. 2.2 UES relaxation induced by the rapid injection of air into the midportion of the esophagus. UES pressure was continuously recorded by a sleeve sensor. The timing of air insufflation is indicated by the vertical dotted line. Note that an LES relaxation was also induced by the esophageal distention but that it occurred after the UES relaxation. B indicates the timing of the perception of a belch. (From Kahrilas *et al.* [23].)

esophageal response to the sudden distention of a considerable length of the esophageal body is the opposite of the response to balloon distention of a discrete segment. Stress increases UES pressure in humans [24], whereas anesthesia [25] or sleep [26] virtually eliminates it. Although early manometric studies [27, 28] suggested that the UES contracted in response to esophageal acidification, more recent studies [29] have been unable to confirm this, despite 30 minutes of esophageal acid perfusion. Probably the most relevant observation is that spontaneous gastroesophageal acid reflux has no effect on continuously recorded UES pressure in either normal volunteers [26] or individuals with peptic esophagitis [29].

Esophageal peristalsis

Esophageal peristalsis becomes evident shortly after the pharyngeal contraction traverses the UES. The peristaltic contraction moves from the proximal striated muscle to the distal smooth muscle of the esophagus at a speed of 2–4 cm/s. The longitudinal muscle of the esophagus also contracts at the onset of peristalsis. The net effect is a transient shortening of the structure by 2.0–2.5 cm [30, 31]. Primary peristalsis is initiated by a swallow, whereas secondary peristalsis can be elicted in response to luminal distention at any level of the esophagus. The mechanical correlate of peristalsis is a stripping wave that 'milks' the esophagus clean, from its proximal to its distal end (Figure 2.3). The velocity of the stripping wave corresponds exactly to the speed of the manometrically recorded contraction: the point of the inverted 'V' seen fluoroscopically at each esophageal locus occurs with the upstroke of the pressure wave [32]. However, the relationship between the manometrically recorded contractile wave and the movement of the bolus is more complex, as suggested in Figure 2.4 [33]. In the normal setting, the intraluminal sensor detects an increased intraluminal pressure only in association with luminal closure. Immediately before closure, however, an intrabolus pressure is recorded. The magnitude of the intrabolus pressure in any particular setting depends on the outflow resistance: the greater the outflow resistance, the greater will be the recorded intrabolus pressure prior to luminal closure. However, manometric recordings of intrabolus and intraluminal pressure within a sealed lumen can be distinguished accurately only by the use of concurrent fluoroscopic imaging [34].

Recent detailed analyses of the vigor and propagation of esophageal peristalsis have concluded that its progression through the tubular

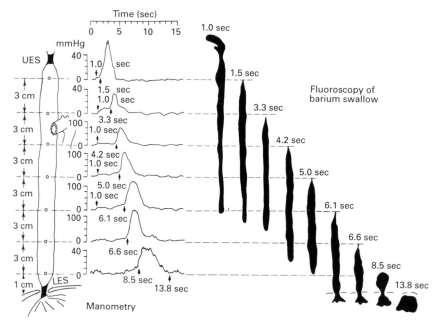

Fig. 2.3 The relationship between manometric and fluoroscopic recordings of esophageal peristalsis during concurrent manometric and video recording of a 5-ml liquid barium swallow. The tracings from the video images of the fluoroscopic sequence, on the right, show the distribution of the barium column at the times indicated above the individual tracings. Arrows indicate the corresponding time points on the manometric record. In this example, a single peristaltic sequence completely cleared the barium bolus from the esophagus. Pharyngeal injection of barium into the esophagus occurred at the 1.0-second mark. The entry of barium caused distention and a slightly increased intraluminal pressure, indicated by the downward-pointing arrows at 1.0 second. Shortly thereafter, esophageal peristalsis was initiated. During esophageal peristalsis, luminal closure and, hence, the tail of the barium bolus passed each recording site concurrently with the onset of the manometric pressure wave. At 1.5 seconds, the peristaltic contraction had just reached the proximal recording site, and barium was stripped from the esophagus proximal to that point. Similarly, at 4.2 seconds, the peristaltic contraction was beginning at the third recording site, and correspondingly the tail of the barium bolus was located at the third recording site. Finally, after completion of the peristaltic contraction (at 13.8 seconds), all the barium had been cleared into the stomach. (From Kahrilas *et al.* [32].)

esophagus is not seamless. Instead, there is a distinct transitional zone between the striated- and smooth-muscle esophagus, which is characterized by a low peristaltic amplitude, a slight delay in progression, and an increased likelihood of failed transmission at that point [35]. This break in the peristaltic progression becomes evident when peristaltic amplitude and progression are plotted topographically, as in Figure 2.5. Topographic analysis reveals not only the proximal transitional zone but also a

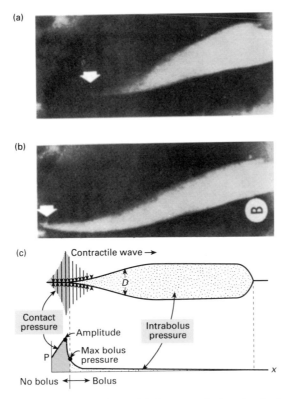

Fig. 2.4 Detailed analysis of the relationship between the intraluminal recording and the bolus transport through a segment of the esophagus. The schematic diagram (c) illustrates the pressure events at the bolus/no bolus interface of the radiographic images (a, b). The density of dots within the schematized esophagus represents the intrabolus pressure, which is greatest at the point of luminal closure. Note that the maximal contact pressure recorded manometrically (c, below) occurs within a closed esophageal lumen that is mechanically isolated from the bolus chamber. (From Brasseur & Dodds [33].)

segmental characteristic of peristaltic progression through the smooth-muscle esophagus: contractions are observed in two distinct segments, followed by contraction of the LES, which is vigorous and persistent, unlike that seen in the adjacent smooth-muscle esophagus [36]. An interesting aspect of topographic analysis is that it provides an explanation for the double-peaked contractile waves often seen in esophageal manometric recordings. A bipeaked contraction can occur in the zone of overlap between adjacent contractile segments if the contractions are not precisely synchronized, resulting in delayed contraction in the distal zone relative to the proximal zone.

Another property of the peristaltic mechanism is deglutitive inhibi-

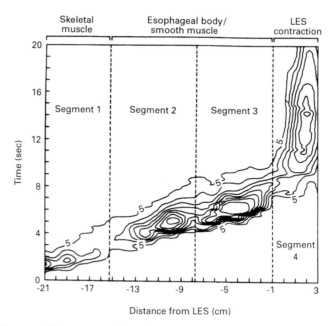

Fig. 2.5 Topographic representation of an esophageal peristaltic wave in normal subjects. The position of the esophagus relative to the LES is indicated on the *x*-axis; time is on the *y*-axis. Isobaric lines are drawn so that the outermost 'ring' is 5 mmHg, the second ring is an isobaric line of 10 mmHg, and each subsequent ring represents a multiple of 20 mmHg. Thus, the innermost island of segment 2 shows the timing and position of a 120-mmHg intraluminal contraction. Note that there are four distinct contractile segments of the esophagus: one in the striated-muscle segment, two in the smooth-muscle body, and finally the LES. Each contractile segment is separated by a pressure trough. (From Clouse & Staiano [36].)

tion. A second swallow, initiated while the earlier peristaltic contraction is still progressing in the striated-muscle esophagus, causes rapid and complete inhibition of the contraction induced by the first swallow [37]. If the first swallow has reached the smooth-muscle esophagus, it may proceed distally for a few seconds after the second swallow, but its peristaltic amplitude diminishes progressively until it disappears [38]. When swallows occur in a series at short intervals, the esophagus remains inhibited and quiescent and the LES remains relaxed. After the last swallow in the series, a normal peristaltic contraction occurs. Closely grouped swallows can, however, alter the amplitude or velocity of the final peristaltic contraction and even render it nonperistaltic. The influence of these swallows can persist for 20–30 seconds after the first swallow, and the effect is sensitive to the size of the bolus, emphasizing the role of afferent feedback [39, 40]. Inhibition of basal LES tone induced by swallowing occurs concurrently with the deglutitive inhibition that tra-

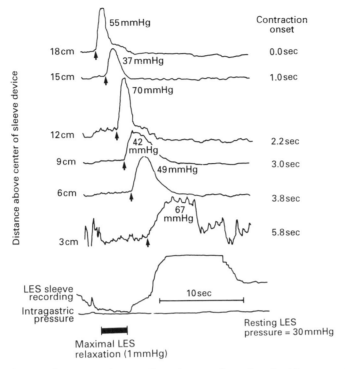

Fig. 2.6 A normal manometric recording of an esophageal peristaltic contraction. LES pressure was recorded by a sleeve transducer that eliminates artifactual relaxation caused by esophageal shortening during swallow. Note that the LES relaxation began early in the swallow, prior to the onset of contraction 18 cm above the LES and nearly concurrently with the pharyngeal contraction. The onset of the pharyngeal contraction is indicated by the slight increase in intraluminal pressure several seconds before onset of the contraction at the recording site 12 cm above the LES. Note that propagation of the peristaltic contraction is defined by the timing of the onset of the pressure complex at each recording site, because this is the event that indicates luminal closure.

verses the smooth-muscle esophagus (Figure 2.6). The LES relaxation commences well before onset of the peristaltic contraction in the proximal esophagus. Deglutitive inhibition can be demonstrated experimentally in the tubular esophagus by creating an artificial high-pressure zone (by balloon distention of the esophageal lumen) and recording the intraluminal pressure between the balloon and the esophageal wall (Figure 2.7). Once the high-pressure zone is established in the normally flaccid tubular esophagus, deglutitive inhibition throughout the length of the esophagus occurs concurrently with the pharyngeal swallow [41].

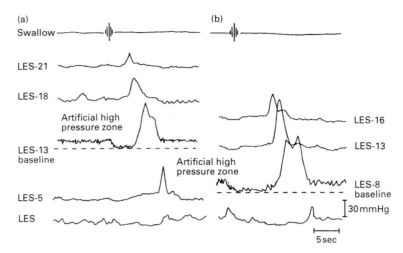

Fig. 2.7 Demonstration of deglutitive inhibition in the tubular esophagus by the creation of an artificial high-pressure zone. The artificial high-pressure zone was created (a) 13 cm above the LES and (b) 8 cm above the LES by inflating a balloon within the esophagus and interposing the manometric sensor between the wall of the esophagus and the balloon. Note that the contraction within the artificial high-pressure zone was inhibited concurrently with the pharyngeal swallow, much the same as with the LES illustrated in Figure 2.6. (From Sifrim *et al.* [41].)

Physiologic control of the esophagus

Distinct physiologic control mechanisms govern the striated and smooth esophageal musculatures. The striated-muscle esophagus receives exclusively excitatory vagal innervation, and the peristaltic contraction of this segment results from the sequential activation of motor units in a craniocaudal sequence. There is convincing evidence [16] that the organization of peristalsis in the striated-muscle esophagus is subject to control from within the swallowing center of the medulla in much the same way as the oropharyngeal musculature is.

Vagal control of the smooth-muscle esophagus is more complex than that of the striated-muscle esophagus. Vagal fibers synapse on neurons of the myenteric plexus rather than directly at neuromuscular junctions, and vagal stimulation can either excite or inhibit the esophageal musculature, depending on which myenteric plexus neurons are activated [42, 43]. Furthermore, although facilitated by vagal fibers, the myenteric plexus neurons are able to organize peristalsis themselves, as indicated by the absence of vagal activity during secondary peristalsis (Figure 2.8) [16, 44]. A second population of vagal efferents is activated with a short latency and probably represents central mediation of deglutitive inhibition [45].

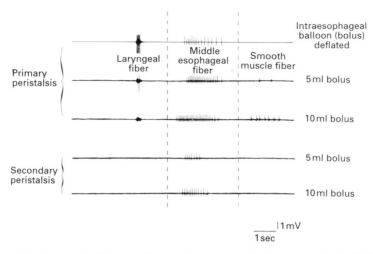

Fig. 2.8 Vagal control of the smooth-muscle esophagus in the unanesthetized baboon, detected by the nerve suture technique. Vagal fibers going to the middle and distal (smooth-muscle) esophagus are cut and then rerouted so that they innervate striated muscle. Once the fibers have innervated the striated muscle, nerve fiber activity can be detected by recording from the striated muscle. Note that the frequency of vagal excitation increased with bolus (balloon) size during primary peristalsis but was completely absent in the smooth-muscle segment during secondary peristalsis, regardless of bolus size. (Modified with permission from Roman & Tieffenbach [44].)

Thus, the activity of neurons in the dorsal motor nucleus of the vagus reflects several properties of primary peristalsis in the smooth-muscle esophagus, including deglutitive inhibition and the speed and vigor of peristaltic contractions.

As mentioned above, the esophagus has an intramural nerve network, the myenteric plexus, located between the longitudinal and circular muscles that can generate peristaltic contractions. Although the relationship between the morphology and function of the nerve plexuses has yet to be determined, it is apparent that there are two main types of effector neurons within the esophageal myenteric plexus (Figure 2.9) [46]. Excitatory neurons mediate contraction of both longitudinal and circular muscle layers via cholinergic receptors. Inhibitory neurons predominantly affect the circular muscle layer via nitric oxide neurons [47–49]. Cholinergic excitation of the excitatory neurons is nicotinic, whereas that of the nitric oxide neurons can be muscarinic as well. Both types of neurons innervate the entire smooth-muscle esophagus, including the LES. The process that mediates LES relaxation is identical to the process that mediates the inhibitory front along the esophagus; indeed, the smooth muscle of the sphincter should be viewed as identical to the

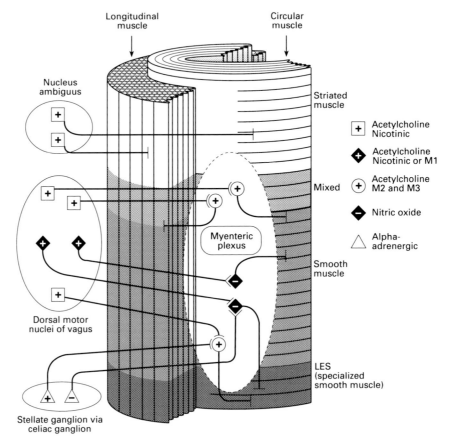

Fig. 2.9 Physiologic control of the esophageal musculature. Control mechanisms of the striated and smooth-muscle segments are distinct. In the striated-muscle segment, muscle fibers are directly innervated by motor neurons in the nucleus ambiguus. In the smooth-muscle segment, the neurons in the myenteric plexus are interposed between medullary motor neurons in the dorsal motor nucleus of the vagus and the smooth-muscle cells. The myenteric plexus contains both excitatory and inhibitory neurons. (From Kahrilas [46].)

adjacent circular muscle, except that it maintains a tonic contraction at rest via a myogenic mechanism [50].

Esophageal motility disorders

As outlined above, the physiologic components of esophageal peristalsis involve the coordinated inhibition and excitation of the circular and longitudinal muscle layers of the esophagus. Thus, pathophysiologic processes can be categorized as dysfunctions of deglutitive inhibition (including sphincter relaxation), or of propagated excitation, or both. Since esophageal motor disorders are not diagnosed histopathologically, diagnosis depends on the definition of these functional aberrations. Even in the unusual circumstance of an esophageal specimen being available, histopathologic examination can be used to define a peristaltic disorder only in the case of achalasia, in which there is a quantifiable decrease in the number of ganglionic cells of the myenteric plexus [51]. Therefore, radiographic or manometric methods are used to evaluate peristaltic function, and the findings are used to characterize the syndrome. Table 2.1 illustrates an attempt to categorize esophageal motility disorders on the basis of assessments of deglutitive inhibition and sequenced excitation. Because clinical manometry and radiology assess function at a muscular rather than a neurophysiologic level, esophageal motor disorders are defined in Table 2.1 in terms of relaxation and contraction characteristics.

There are relatively few well-defined motility disorders and, predictably, the functional characteristics of some disorders overlap. In some situations it can be very difficult to make a definitive diagnosis. In addition, there is considerable debate over the significance of some of the manometric findings in spastic disorders [52]. With these considerations in mind, the following discussion will focus on disease entities with clear diagnostic or therapeutic implications, rather than on manometric phenomena of unproven significance. The exception is gastroesophageal reflux disease (GERD), which, although highly significant, is covered in other chapters.

Table 2.1 Disorders of peristaltic function.

	Relaxation		Contraction	
	Excessive	Inadequate	Excessive	Inadequate
UES	—	Cricopharyngeal bar	—	—
Body	—	Vigorous achalasia Diffuse esophageal spasm	Spastic disorders*	Advanced achalasia Pseudoachalasia Scleroderma Obstruction
LES	GERD	Achalasia Pseudoachalasia	Achalasia Pseudoachalasia Spastic disorders*	GERD Scleroderma

*Spastic disorders include a number of 'minor motor disorders,' such as nutcracker esophagus and hypertensive LES, as well as esophageal spasm.
GERD, gastroesophageal reflux disease; LES, lower esophageal sphincter; UES, upper esophageal sphincter.

Symptoms of esophageal motility disorders

Dysphagia is the fundamental symptom experienced by patients with esophageal motility disorders. Esophageal, as opposed to oropharyngeal, dysphagia is suggested by the absence of associated aspiration, cough, or oral residue. Heartburn, esophagopharyngeal regurgitation, chest pain, odynophagia, and intermittent esophageal obstruction are characteristic of esophageal dysphagia. However, an important limitation of the patient history is that patients with esophageal dysphagia may inaccurately identify the location of the obstruction. For example, with a distal esophageal obstruction caused by an esophageal ring or an esophageal motor disorder, patients often experience the sensation of dysphagia at the level of the neck; patients with this type of obstruction correctly identify the location of the dysfunction only 60% of the time [53]. Therefore, regardless of the patient's perception of the location of the problem, the physician should evaluate the entire esophagus. Swallowing difficulty with both solids and liquids is suggestive of a motor disorder, while difficulty only with solids suggests a mechanical obstruction.

Cricopharyngeal dysfunction can also cause symptoms of dysphagia and regurgitation, most commonly in association with a hypopharyngeal diverticulum or a cricopharyngeal bar. Acquired diverticula occur most commonly in men after the sixth decade of life. The most frequent site of herniation is the midline between the oblique fibers of the inferior pharyngeal constrictor and the cricopharyngeus muscle, corresponding to Killian's dehiscence [54]. The second most frequent site is the lateral slit separating the cricopharyngeus muscle from the fibers of the proximal end of the esophagus, through which the recurrent laryngeal nerve and its accompanying vessels run to supply the larynx [55]. Less common locations include the site of penetration of the inferior thyroid artery into the hypopharynx and the junction of the middle and inferior constrictor muscles [56]. The unifying characteristic of all these locations is that they are sites of potential weakness of the muscular lining of the hypopharynx. This commonality supports the notion that hypopharyngeal diverticula represent a wear-and-tear phenomenon resulting from pulsion forces, rather than a manifestation of a pharyngeal contractile abnormality. Hypopharyngeal diverticula are generally asymptomatic until they become large enough to accommodate and store a substantial amount of food or liquid. In most cases, the symptom is postswallow regurgitation, or even aspiration, of the material within the pharyngeal pouch.

Cricopharyngeal dysfunction

An obvious manifestation of cricopharyngeal dysfunction is the development of a hypopharyngeal diverticulum, the pathogenesis of which has been the subject of much speculation and debate [57]. Diverticula have been hypothesized to result from delayed UES relaxation, failure of relaxation, or premature contraction [58–61]. However, few credible data support any of these hypotheses, and other investigations [62] have demonstrated no manometric abnormalities. Particularly presumptive is use of the term *cricopharyngeal achalasia* to describe a cricopharyngeal bar. This description implies an analogy to achalasia of the cardia, which is caused by postganglionic denervation of the smooth-muscle esophagus and is characterized by esophageal aperistalsis and impaired LES relaxation. No motor abnormality or denervation has been shown to be involved in the pathogenesis of either cricopharyngeal bars or hypopharyngeal diverticula. Furthermore, cricopharyngeal denervation would result in a hypotensive sphincter [21], as distinguished from the hypertensive LES caused by the absence of inhibitory innervation.

A more plausible explanation of hypopharyngeal diverticula is that they result from a restrictive myopathy of the cricopharyngeus muscle. Histologic examination of surgical specimens of cricopharyngeus muscle strips obtained from patients with hypopharyngeal diverticula has shown the presence of muscle fiber degeneration in association with fibroadipose tissue replacement; these structural changes would reduce UES compliance and opening [63]. Although the mechanism of these histologic changes is not known, their occurrence supports the hypothesis that fibrosis of the cricopharyngeus impairs UES opening by reducing sphincter compliance. Thus, although the muscle relaxes normally during a swallow, it cannot distend normally, resulting in the appearance of a cricopharyngeal bar during a barium swallow (Figure 2.10). Diminished sphincter compliance is associated with an increase in hypopharyngeal pressure such that trans-sphincteric flow is maintained through the smaller UES opening. Hypopharyngeal manometric studies have demonstrated that this restricted UES aperture leads to an increased intrabolus pressure above the cricopharyngeus during swallowing (Figure 2.11). The normal sphincter is extremely compliant: the range of the upstream intrabolus pressure varies only from 6 to 18 mmHg as the swallow volume is increased from 2 to 30 ml. However, in patients with cricopharyngeal bars, upstream pressures range from 13 to 68 mmHg for the same range of bolus volumes [64]. The same phenomenon has been

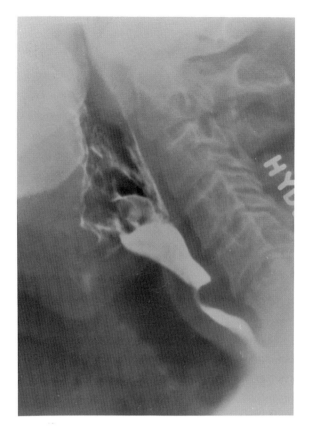

Fig. 2.10 Cricopharyngeal bar in a patient with oropharyngeal dysphagia. The posterior indentation of the barium column is caused by a noncompliant cricopharyngeus muscle. (Courtesy of Richard Gore MD, Northwestern University, Chicago.)

demonstrated in patients with Zenker's diverticulum, suggesting that diverticulum formation is an eventual consequence of the increased stress on the hypopharynx that results from the increased intrabolus pressure [65]. Manometric studies performed without simultaneous fluoroscopy do not allow for this critical distinction between intrabolus pressure and incomplete sphincter relaxation. Intrabolus pressure is recorded from within the bolus in the open hypopharynx, while contractile pressure is recorded from within a closed sphincter segment.

The treatment of hypopharyngeal diverticulum is a cricopharyngeal myotomy with or without a diverticulectomy. Surgical series have reported success with diverticulectomy alone [66], myotomy alone [67, 68], and with both diverticulectomy and myotomy [69]. In all likelihood, there are instances in which a limited procedure would be adequate, but a

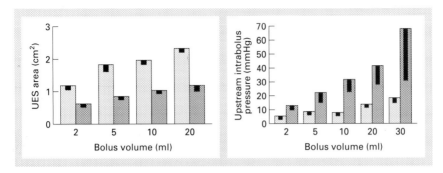

Fig. 2.11 Estimates of the UES cross-sectional area and corresponding upstream intrabolus pressure during swallowing in normal volunteers (light columns) and patients with cricopharyngeal bars (dark columns). In normal volunteers the sphincter is highly compliant, and an increase in the bolus volume is accompanied by an increased cross-sectional area and a minimal increment in intrabolus pressure. Patients with cricopharyngeal bars exhibit a minimal increment in the cross-sectional area of the sphincter together with an increased bolus volume, leading to dramatic increases in intrabolus pressure. Hanging bars indicate standard errors of the mean (SEM). (From Dantas *et al.* [64].)

definitive approach to the problem of pulsion diverticula should involve both diverticulectomy and myotomy. With diverticulectomy alone, there is a risk of recurrence because the underlying stenosis at the level of the cricopharyngeus is not remedied. Similarly, myotomy alone may not solve the problem of food accumulation within the diverticulum, with its attendant regurgitation and aspiration. Small diverticula may, however, disappear spontaneously following myotomy. A recent study [65] found that after diverticulectomy with myotomy, sphincter compliance was restored to normal in five patients, as indicated by normal hypopharyngeal intrabolus pressure during swallowing.

The criteria for performing a cricopharyngeal myotomy should be:
1   the presence of significant dysphagia leading to local discomfort, weight loss, or aspiration;
2   confirmation of UES dysfunction by videoradiography, preferably with intraluminal manometry;
3   the absence of clinically significant gastroesophageal reflux or gastroesophageal regurgitation [70].

These criteria are fulfilled in patients with hypopharyngeal diverticula or symptomatic cricopharyngeal bars, but probably not in many other instances. Although myotomy is a relatively safe procedure that can be performed with only local anesthesia [71], sudden death from aspiration is a reported complication [67, 72, 73], emphasizing the need to assess LES competence preoperatively. The combination of a cricopharyngeal myotomy and LES incompetence is particularly devastating and leads to refractory aspiration. If a myotomy is essential in this circumstance, it should be paired with an antireflux procedure.

Achalasia

Achalasia is the most easily recognized and best-defined motor disorder of the esophagus. First recognized more than 300 years ago, this disorder was initially labeled as cardiospasm, reflecting the observation that it was caused by a functional, rather than an anatomic, obstruction of the esophagus at the cardiac sphincter, with no obstructing lesions evident in autopsy specimens. In 1937, Lendrum [74] proposed that this functional esophageal obstruction resulted from incomplete relaxation of the LES and renamed the disease *achalasia* ('failure to relax'). Achalasia is a rare disease, with an estimated incidence of about 1 per 100 000 population per year [75]. It affects both sexes equally and usually presents in adults. Although achalasia is almost universally idiopathic in North America, it is closely mimicked by the esophageal involvement in Chagas' disease, which is caused by infection with *Trypanosoma cruzi*, an endemic parasite in areas of South America. A key distinction between idiopathic achalasia and achalasia that develops in the late stage of Chagas' disease is the selective involvement of the esophagus in the former condition, compared with multiple organ involvement in Chagas' disease, including cardiomyopathy, megaureter, megaduodenum, and megacolon [76].

Achalasia is characterized by: (i) failure of the LES to relax completely with swallowing, and (ii) aperistalsis of the smooth-muscle esophagus. The resting LES pressure is elevated in about 60% of patients with achalasia. If there are nonperistaltic, spasm-like contractions in the esophageal body, the disease is classified as vigorous achalasia. Achalasia is thought to result from postganglionic denervation of the smooth-muscle esophagus. In a recent morphologic study [51], a diminished number of myenteric ganglionic cells and inflammation within the myenteric plexus were observed in all 42 esophagi resected from patients with advanced achalasia. It is not known whether the disease selectively affects excitatory or inhibitory neurons but, clearly, impairment of inhibitory neurons is an early manifestation of the disease. Using an intraesophageal balloon technique, Sifrim et al. [77] observed impairment of deglutitive relaxation in the esophageal body and the LES in patients with early, nondilated achalasia. It has become increasingly evident that the neurons responsible for deglutitive inhibition (including sphincter relaxation), which were previously characterized as nonadrenergic–noncholinergic, utilize nitric oxide as a neurotransmitter [78]. Nitric oxide synthase has been found to be absent in the gastroesophageal junction in patients with achalasia [78], and animal models of achalasia have been established using nitric oxide inhibitors such as *N*-omega-nitro-L-arginine (L-NNA) [79].

Clinical manifestations of achalasia may include dysphagia, regurgitation, chest pain, weight loss, and aspiration pneumonia. The pattern of dysphagia in patients with achalasia, especially in individuals with a dilated esophagus, is unique. They often sense the passage of material from the esophagus into the stomach and attempt to augment this sensation by drinking a lot while eating or by engaging in various maneuvers, such as straightening the back, raising their arms over their heads, or standing, to increase intraesophageal pressure. Predictably, regurgitation can be problematic when large amounts of food are retained in the dilated esophagus. Classically, patients complain of regurgitant on their bedsheets when sleeping in the supine position, and often by the time they seek medical advice, they have elected to use several pillows or to sleep upright in a chair. Chest pain is a frequent complaint early in the course of the disease; its etiology is unknown. An interesting but rare symptom of achalasia is airway compromise, which results from compression of the trachea by the dilated esophagus [80]. This complication results from a dysfunctional belch reflex caused either by neural degeneration or by the dysfunction of stretch receptors within the esophageal wall caused by the dilated esophagus [81].

Achalasia is diagnosed by a barium swallow X-ray (Figure 2.12) or by esophageal manometry (Figure 2.13). The characteristic X-ray appearance is a dilated intrathoracic esophagus with an air–fluid level. The LES tapers to a point, giving the distal esophagus a beak-like appearance. The beak does not open with swallowing but will open following inhalation of amyl nitrite, a smooth-muscle relaxant [82]. The defining manometric features of achalasia are aperistalsis and incomplete LES relaxation; these features are present in more than 90% of patients who meet the available clinical criteria of achalasia. Other manometric features, such as an increased intraesophageal baseline pressure or isobaric waveforms, provide supportive evidence of achalasia [83]. In a prospective comparison of diagnostic modalities [84], radiologic findings suggested achalasia in only 21 of 33 patients who had received a diagnosis of achalasia based on manometric findings, while endoscopic findings suggested the correct diagnosis in fewer than one-third of patients.

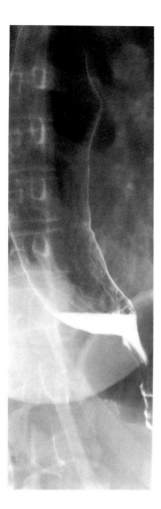

Fig. 2.12 Characteristic barium swallow in a patient with idiopathic achalasia. Note the esophageal dilatation with an air–fluid level and the smooth tapering at the gastroesophageal junction. Radiographic findings can be much more subtle in the early phases of the disease.

It is important to emphasize that neither radiographic nor manometric features are specific for idiopathic achalasia or achalasia associated with Chagas' disease; tumor-related pseudoachalasia accounts for up to 5% of cases of manometrically defined achalasia. Pseudoachalasia is more likely in older patients and when there is an abrupt onset of symptoms and early weight loss [85]. Tumor infiltration (especially carcinoma in the gastric fundus) can completely mimic the functional impairment seen with idiopathic achalasia (see Table 2.1). Because of this potential pitfall, a thorough anatomic examination, including endoscopy, should be part of the diagnostic evaluation of every potential new case of achalasia. An observation during endoscopy that is suggestive of pseudoachalasia is the presence of more than a slight resistance to the passage of the endoscope across the gastroesophageal junction; in idiopathic achalasia, the endo-

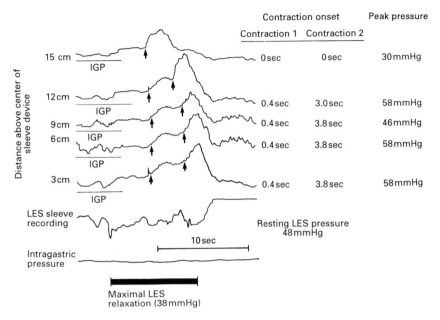

Fig. 2.13 An esophageal manometric recording in a patient with idiopathic achalasia. The resting LES pressure is high and demonstrates minimal deglutitive relaxation. Although there is a propagated contraction in the proximal (striated-muscle) esophagus, there is no propagated contraction in the smooth-muscle esophagus, as indicated by the simultaneous onset of the contraction waves. Finally, the resting intraesophageal pressure is higher than the intragastric pressure (IGP), which is the reverse of the normal situation. Arrows indicate the onset of contraction 1 and contraction 2.

scope should pop through with the application of gentle pressure. If pseudoachalasia is still suspected, an endoscopic biopsy, computed tomography, magnetic resonance imaging, or endoscopic ultrasound should be considered for further evaluation, depending on the circumstances. Regardless of the cause of the achalasia syndrome, the esophageal body exhibits denervation supersensitivity to cholinomimetic agents, which is the basis of the methacholine (Mecholyl) test. Administration of methacholine provokes spasm in the otherwise atonic esophagus in 80–90% of patients [85].

Achalasia is treated by either pharmacologic incapacitation or mechanical disruption of the LES. Medical treatments, on the whole, are not very effective and perhaps are more useful as temporizing maneuvers than as definitive therapies. Smooth-muscle relaxants such as nitrates or nifedipine [86] administered sublingually immediately before eating may provide partial relief. Experimental approaches to therapy for achalasia include the use of nitric oxide agonists [87] and the local injection of botulinum toxin into the sphincter muscle [88]. Disruption of the LES, either surgically (Heller myotomy) or by use of a pneumatic dilator, remains the definitive treatment. The risk of esophageal perforation during pneumatic dilatation ranges from 1 to 5%. The only controlled trial [89] that compared these treatment modalities (conducted by a surgeon) concluded that the surgical approach was somewhat superior.

Pneumatic dilatation of the esophagus is accomplished using inflatable balloon dilators, which achieve a forceful stretching of the LES to a diameter of about 3 cm. This procedure is completely different from the type of dilatation used to treat peptic strictures. Therapy with conventional dilators (up to 56 French) provides only very temporary benefit in patients with achalasia. Pneumatic dilators are positioned across the gastroesophageal junction either radiographically (Rigiflex dilator) or endoscopically (Witzel dilator) and inflated to 6–9 psi (41–62 kPa) for 30–60 seconds. The best predictor of efficacy following a pneumatic dilatation is the postdilatation LES pressure. LES pressures of less than 10 mmHg are associated with prolonged remission; patients with pressures greater than 20 mmHg derive little benefit from the procedure [90]. It is neither unusual nor dangerous to repeat pneumatic dilatation two or three times when the initial result is unsatisfactory. Following pneumatic dilatation, many practitioners routinely examine the esophagus fluoroscopically using water-soluble contrast material to ensure there is no perforation. If any substantial perforation has occurred, surgical repair should be performed quickly. When perforation induced by pneumatic dilatation is recognized and treated promptly, the outcome is comparable to that in patients who undergo elective myotomy [91].

The standard surgical treatment of achalasia is the Heller myotomy, performed via a thoracotomy. Once exposed, the circular muscle layer of the esophagus is cut from the distal esophagus to the proximal stomach. Some surgeons perform an antireflux procedure concurrently with the myotomy, while others reserve this added manipulation for patients with an associated hiatal hernia [92]. Although clearly efficacious, the Heller myotomy is associated with considerable morbidity, which has led most patients to elect pneumatic dilatation as the initial intervention. However, new surgical approaches to achalasia using laparoscopic or thoracoscopic techniques may tip the balance toward selecting surgery as the initial intervention, since these techniques substantially reduce the morbidity. In a recent series [93], 24 patients with achalasia treated either thoracoscopically or laparoscopically had outcomes similar to those of patients who underwent open procedures, but the median hospitalization of the former patients was only 3 days.

Spastic disorders

Abnormal peristalsis can cause dysphagia, typically for both solids and liquids, and chest pain. The pain may mimic angina pectoris. An esophageal cause of chest pain should be considered only after careful consideration of potential cardiopulmonary causes. However, even within the spectrum of esophageal diseases, neither chest pain nor dysphagia is specific for a spastic disorder, as both symptoms are characteristic of other common esophageal disorders, including peptic or infectious esophagitis. A spastic disorder should be considered if symptoms remain unexplained after these more common diagnostic possibilities have been excluded by the appropriate radiographic studies, an endoscopic evaluation, and, in some patients, a therapeutic trial of antisecretory medication.

Unlike with achalasia, the esophagus in a patient with a spastic disorder usually retains its ability to propagate primary peristaltic waves most of the time. Thus, there are no uniform radiographic, manometric, or histopathologic criteria for defining esophageal spastic disorders. Partly because of this, the criteria for diagnosing diffuse esophageal spasm (DES) remain variable and confusing [94]. In an unequivocal case of DES, nonperistaltic, high-amplitude, prolonged contractions are observed on esophageal manometry and are associated with chest pain (Figure 2.14). These unequivocal cases are probably associated with a defect in the neuronal architecture of deglutitive inhibition, placing them along the continuum of vigorous achalasia and achalasia (see Table 2.1) [77]. The LES typically functions normally. Radiographically, DES may appear as a 'corkscrew' esophagus (Figure 2.15). It must be emphasized, however, that neither the tertiary contractions (nonperistaltic, simultaneous esophageal contractions) seen on X-ray nor the simultaneous contractions seen manometrically are pathognomonic of esophageal spasm; both may also be seen in asymptomatic individuals [95].

Manometric abnormalities are prevalent in patients with chest pain or dysphagia [95]. However, manometric findings consistent with achalasia or DES account for only a small minority of these abnormalities. DES is more variably defined than is achalasia, but simultaneous contractions following 30% or more of swallows have not been reported among controls, suggesting that this finding is related to dysphagia or chest pain [96]. Achalasia appears to be present in less than 1% of subjects when

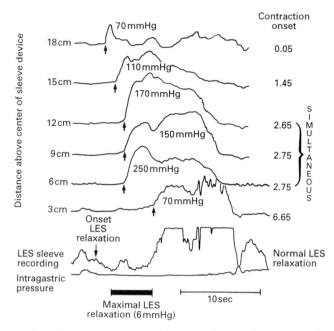

Fig. 2.14 Esophageal manometric recording in a patient with symptomatic DES. Resting LES pressure and deglutitive relaxation are normal. There is a high-amplitude, prolonged, simultaneous contraction in the smooth-muscle esophagus, which is accompanied by pain.

chest pain is the principal symptom. Similarly, DES is found, on average, in 5% or fewer of patients with chest pain. Most manometric findings fall into the category of 'nonspecific disorders,' an umbrella term encompassing manometric abnormalities that are insufficient to establish a diagnosis of achalasia, DES, or typical scleroderma-like esophageal dysfunction [95]. The most common manometric patterns are exaggerated contractions in the esophageal body (increased wave amplitudes, waves of long duration, and multipeaked waves) and a hypertensive LES [97, 98]. An increased wave amplitude ('nutcracker esophagus') is the most commonly detected pattern, accounting for a large proportion of patients with nonspecific disorders (Figure 2.16).

As with achalasia, the simultaneous contractions typical of DES impair bolus transit through the esophagus, potentially explaining the associated dysphagia [99]. However, functional abnormalities associated with nonspecific motor disorders are generally not recognized. Furthermore, long-term observations have shown neither a correlation between the clinical course and manometric findings nor consistent manometric diagnostic criteria over time [95, 100, 101]. Therapeutic trials of smooth-

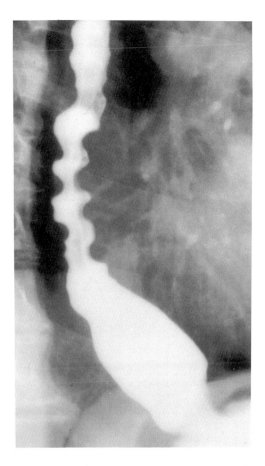

Fig. 2.15 'Corkscrew' esophagus on barium X-ray in a patient with symptomatic DES.

muscle relaxants, tranquilizers, or bougienage have similarly shown no correlation between the modification of manometric findings and the therapeutic response [102–105]. In summary, it is difficult to determine the relevance of nonspecific motility disturbances to either symptoms or function, making their detection of no generalizable value. Of greater clinical importance is the finding that reflux disease often explains the symptoms of esophageal dysfunction, whether nonspecific motor abnormalities are present or not. Bancewicz *et al.* [106] found that intensive antireflux therapy was the most useful approach for a large group of symptomatic patients without a specific motor disorder. Similarly, Achem *et al.* [107] found that antireflux therapy benefited patients with unexplained chest pain, regardless of the presence or absence of nonspecific motor abnormalities.

Ironically, medical therapy for esophageal spasm is similar to therapy

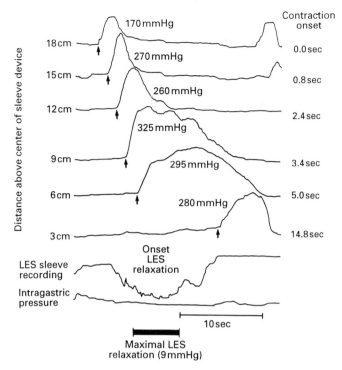

Fig. 2.16 Manometric recording in a patient with a nonspecific motor disorder manifested by extremely hypertensive peristalsis and a hypertensive LES (resting pressure greater than 60 mmHg). Paradoxically, this patient complained of dysphagia that was alleviated with antireflux therapy.

for coronary artery disease, a disorder with which esophageal spasm can be confused. However, despite the dogma that states that patients should be treated with smooth-muscle relaxants, data from controlled studies on the medical treatment of esophageal spasm are limited. There are no long-term outcome studies on the use of smooth-muscle relaxants to treat DES, and the entire basis for this therapy remains at an anecdotal level [83]. Similarly, there are no controlled studies of pneumatic dilatation or myotomy in patients with well-defined DES. In some patients, DES may evolve into achalasia, for which there are defined treatment strategies [108]. At this time, however, therapy for esophageal spastic disorders is typically a trial-and-error experience, reflecting the inhomogeneity of the patient population.

References

1 Arey LB, Tremaine MJ. Muscle content of lower oesophagus of man. *Anat Rec* 1933;**56**:315–20.

2 Meyer GW, Austin RM, Brady CE 3rd, Castell DO. Muscle anatomy of the human esophagus. *J Clin Gastroenterol* 1986;**8**:131–4.

3 Liebermann-Meffert D, Allgower M, Schmid P, Blum AL. Muscular equivalent of the lower esophageal sphincter. *Gastroenterology* 1979;**76**:31–8.

4 Nyhus LM, Baker RJ. *Masters of Surgery*. Boston: Little, Brown & Co, 1984.

5 Mittal RK, Rochester DF, McCallum RW. Electrical and mechanical activity in the human lower esophageal sphincter during diaphragmatic contraction. *J Clin Invest* 1988;**81**:1182–9.

6 Kahrilas PJ. The anatomy and physiology of dysphagia. In: Gelfand DW, Richter JE, eds. *Dysphagia: Diagnosis and Treatment*. New York: Igaku-Shoin Medical Publishers Inc, 1989:15.

7 Christensen J, Rick GA. Nerve cell density in the submucous plexus throughout the gut of cat and opossum. *Gastroenterology* 1985;**89**:1064–9.

8 Higgs B, Kerr FWL, Ellis FH Jr. The experimental production of esophageal achalasia by electrolytic lesions in the medulla. *J Thorac Cardiovasc Surg* 1965;**50**:613–25.

9 Niel JP, Gonella J, Roman C. Localisation par la technique de marquage a la peroxydase des corps cellulaires des neurones ortho et parasympatiques innervant le sphincter oesophagien inferieur du chat. *J Physiol (Paris)* 1980;**76**:591–9.

10 Andrew BL. The nervous control of the cervical oesophagus of the rat during swallowing. *J Physiol (Lond)* 1956;**134**:729–40.

11 Lund WS, Ardran GM. The motor nerve supply of the cricopharyngeal sphincter. *Ann Otol Rhinol Laryngol* 1964;**73**:599–617.

12 Hwang K, Grossman MI, Ivy AC. Nervous control of the cervical esophagus. *Am J Physiol* 1948;**154**:343–57.

13 Floyd K. Cholinesterase activity in sheep oesophageal muscle. *J Anat* 1973;**116**:357–73.

14 Samarasinghe DD. Some observations on the innervation of the striated muscle in the mouse esophagus – an electron microscope study. *J Anat* 1972;**112**:173–84.

15 Abe S. On the histology and the innervation of the esophagus and the first forestomach of the goat. *Arch Histol Jpn* 1959;**16**:109–29.

16 Roman C, Gonella J. Extrinsic control of digestive tract motility. In: Johnson LR, ed. *Physiology of the Gastrointestinal Tract*, 2nd edn. New York: Raven Press, 1987:507–53.

17 Yamamoto T. Histological studies on the innervation of the esophagus in Formosan macaque. *Arch Histol Jpn* 1960;**18**:545–64.

18 Kahrilas PJ, Dodds WJ, Dent J, Logemann JA, Shaker R. Upper esophageal sphincter functions during deglutition. *Gastroenterology* 1988;**95**:52–62.

19 Welch RW, Luckmann K, Ricks PM, Drake ST, Gates GA. Manometry of the normal upper esophageal sphincter and its alterations in laryngectomy. *J Clin Invest* 1979;**63**:1036–41.

20 Kahrilas PJ, Dent J, Dodds WJ, Hogan WJ, Arndorfer RC. A method for continuous monitoring of upper esophageal sphincter pressure. *Dig Dis Sci* 1987;**32**:121–8.

21 Asoh R, Goyal RK. Manometry and electromyography of the upper esophageal sphincter in the opossum. *Gastroenterology* 1978;**74**:514–20.

22 Jacob P, Kahrilas PJ, Herzon G, McLaughlin B. Determinants of upper esophageal sphincter pressure in dogs. *Am J Physiol* 1990;**259**:G245–51.

23 Kahrilas PJ, Dodds WJ, Dent J, Wyman JB, Hogan WJ, Arndorfer RC. Upper esophageal sphincter function during belching. *Gastroenterology* 1986;**91**:133–40.

24 Cook IJ, Dent J, Shannon S, Collins SM. Measurement of upper esophageal sphincter pressure: effect of acute emotional stress. *Gastroenterology* 1987; **93**:526–32.

25 Vanner RG, Pryle BJ, O'Dwyer JP, Reynolds F. Upper oesophageal sphincter pressure and the intravenous induction of anaesthesia. *Anaesthesia* 1992;**47**:371–5.

26 Kahrilas PJ, Dodds WJ, Dent J, Haeberle B, Hogan WJ, Arndorfer RC. The effect of sleep, spontaneous gastroesophageal reflux, and a meal on upper esophageal sphincter pressure in normal human volunteers. *Gastroenterology* 1987;**92**:466–71.

27 Gerhardt DC, Shuck TJ, Bordeaux RA, Winship DH. Human upper esophageal sphincter: response to volume, osmotic, and acid stimuli. *Gastroenterology* 1978;**75**:268–74.

28 Freiman JM, El-Sharkawy TY, Diamant NE. Effect of bilateral vagosympathetic nerve blockade on response of the dog upper esophageal sphincter (UES) to intraesophageal distention and acid. *Gastroenterology* 1981;**81**:78–84.

29 Vakil NB, Kahrilas PJ, Dodds WJ, Vanagunas A. Absence of an upper esophageal sphincter response to acid reflux. *Am J Gastroenterol* 1989;**84**:606–10.

30 Dodds WJ, Stewart ET, Hodges D, Zboralske FF. Movement of the feline esophagus associated with respiration and peristalsis: an evaluation using tantalum markers. *J Clin Invest* 1973;**52**:1–13.

31 Edmundowicz SA, Clouse RE. Shortening of the esophagus in response to swallowing. *Am J Physiol* 1991;**260**:G512–16.

32 Kahrilas PJ, Dodds WJ, Hogan WJ. The effect of peristaltic dysfunction on esophageal volume clearance. *Gastroenterology* 1988;**94**:73–80.

33 Brasseur JG, Dodds WJ. Interpretation of intraluminal manometric measurements in terms of swallowing mechanics. *Dysphagia* 1991;**6**:100–19.

34 Li M, Brasseur JG, Dodds WJ. Analyses of normal and abnormal esophageal transport using computer simulations. *Am J Physiol* 1994;**266**:G525–43.

35 Brasseur JG. Mechanical studies of the esophageal function. *Dysphagia* 1993;**8**:384–6.

36 Clouse RE, Staiano A. Topography of normal and high-amplitude esophageal peristalsis. *Am J Physiol* 1993;**265**:G1098–107.

37 Hellemans J, Vantrappen G, Janssens J. Electromyography of the esophagus. In: Vantrappen G, Hellemans J, eds. *Diseases of the Esophagus*. New York: Springer-Verlag, 1974:270–85.

38 Meyer GW, Gerhardt DC, Castell DO. Human esophageal response to rapid swallowing: muscle refractory period or neural inhibition? *Am J Physiol* 1981;**241**:G129–36.

39 Ask P, Tibbling L. Effect of time interval between swallows on esophageal peristalsis. *Am J Physiol* 1980;**238**:G485–90.

40 Vanek AW, Diamant NE. Responses of the human esophagus to paired swallows. *Gastroenterology* 1987;**92**:643–50.

41 Sifrim D, Janssens J, Vantrappen G. A wave of inhibition precedes primary peristaltic contractions in the human esophagus. *Gastroenterology* 1992;**103**:876–82.

42 Diamant NE, El-Sharkawy TY. Neural control of esophageal peristalsis: a conceptual analysis. *Gastroenterology* 1977;**72**:546–56.

43 Gonella J, Niel JP, Roman C. Vagal control of lower oesophageal motility in the cat. *J Physiol (Lond)* 1977;**273**:647–64.

44 Roman C, Tieffenbach L. Enregistrement de l'activite unitaire des fibres motrices

vagales destinee a l'oesophage du babouin. *J Physiol (Paris)* 1972;**64**:479–506.

45 Gidda JS, Goyal RK. Swallow-evoked action potentials in vagal preganglionic efferents. *J Neurophysiol* 1984;**52**:1169–80.

46 Kahrilas PJ. Functional anatomy and physiology of the esophagus. In: Castell DO, ed. *The Esophagus*, 2nd edn. Boston: Little, Brown and Co, 1995:1–28.

47 Conklin JL, Du C, Murray JA, Bates JN. Characterization and mediation of inhibitory junction potentials from opossum lower esophageal sphincter. *Gastroenterology* 1993;**104**:1439–44.

48 Titrup A, Svane D, Forman A. Nitric oxide mediating NANC inhibition in opossum lower esophageal sphincter. *Am J Physiol* 1991;**260**:G385–9.

49 Yamato S, Spechler SJ, Goyal RK. Role of nitric oxide in esophageal peristalsis in the opossum. *Gastroenterology* 1992;**103**:197–204.

50 Goyal RK, Rattan S. Genesis of basal sphincter pressure: effect of tetrodotoxin on lower esophageal sphincter pressure in opossum in vivo. *Gastroenterology* 1976;**71**:62–7.

51 Goldblum JR, Whyte RI, Orringer MB, Appelman HD. Achalasia: a morphologic study of 42 resected specimens. *Am J Surg Pathol* 1994;**18**:327–37.

52 Kahrilas PJ. Nutcracker esophagus: an idea whose time has gone? *Am J Gastroenterol* 1993;**88**:167–9.

53 Edwards DAW. History and symptoms of esophageal disease. In: Vantrappen G, Hellemans J, eds. *Diseases of the Esophagus*. Berlin: Springer-Verlag, 1974:103–18.

54 Zaino C, Jacobson HG, Lepow H, Ozturk CH. *The Pharyngoesophageal Sphincter*. Springfield, Ill: Charles C Thomas, 1970.

55 Shallow TA. Combined one stage closed method for treatment of pharyngeal diverticula. *Surg Gynecol Obstet* 1936;**62**:624–33.

56 Lahey FH. Pharyngo-esophageal diverticulum: its management and complications. *Ann Surg* 1946;**124**:617–36.

57 Goyal RK. Disorders of the cricopharyngeus muscle. *Otolaryngol Clin North Am* 1984;**17**:115–30.

58 Ardran GM, Kemp FH, Lund WS. The aetiology of the posterior pharyngeal diverticulum: a cineradiographic study. *J Laryngol Otol* 1964;**78**:333–49.

59 Negus VE. The etiology of pharyngeal diverticula. *Bull Johns Hopkins Hosp* 1957;**101**:209–23.

60 Sutherland HD. Cricopharyngeal achalasia. *J Thorac Cardiovasc Surg* 1962;**43**:114–26.

61 Wilson CP. Pharyngeal diverticula, their cause and treatment. *J Laryngol Otol* 1962;**76**:151–80.

62 Knuff TE, Benjamin SB, Castell DO. Pharyngeal (Zenker's) diverticulum: a reappraisal. *Gastroenterology* 1982;**82**:734–6.

63 Cook IJ, Blumbergs P, Cash K, Jamieson GG, Shearman DJ. Structural abnormalities of the cricopharyngeus muscle in patients with pharyngeal (Zenker's) diverticulum. *J Gastroenterol Hepatol* 1992;**7**:556–62.

64 Dantas RO, Cook IJ, Dodds WJ, Kern MK, Lang IM, Brasseur JG. Biomechanics of cricopharyngeal bars. *Gastroenterology* 1990;**99**:1269–74.

65 Cook IJ, Gabb M, Panagopoulos V *et al.* Pharyngeal (Zenker's) diverticulum is a disorder of upper esophageal sphincter opening. *Gastroenterology* 1992;**103**:1229–35.

66 Clagett OT, Payne WS. Surgical treatment for pulsion diverticula of the hypopharynx: one-stage resection in 478 cases. *Dis Chest* 1960;**37**:257–61.

67 Blakeley WR, Garety EJ, Smith DE. Section of the circopharyngeus muscle for dysphagia. *Arch Surg* 1968;**96**:745–62.

68 Van Overbeek JJM, Betlem HC. Cricopharyngeal myotomy in pharyngeal paralysis: cineradiographic and manometric indications. *Ann Otol Rhinol Laryngol* 1979;**88**:596–602.

69 Ellis FH Jr, Schlegel JF, Lynch VP, Payne WS. Cricopharyngeal myotomy for pharyngo-esophageal diverticulum. *Ann Surg* 1969;**170**:340–9.

70 Hurwitz AL, Duranceau A, Haddad JK. Oropharyngeal dysphagia. In: Smith LE, ed. *Major Problems in Internal Medicine. Volume XVI: Disorders of Esophageal Motility.* Philadelphia: WB Saunders Co, 1979:67–84.

71 Hiebert CA. Surgery for cricopharyngeal dysfunction under local anesthesia. *Am J Surg* 1976;**131**:423–7.

72 Akl BF, Blakeley WR. Late assessment of results of cricopharyngeal myotomy for cervical dysphagia. *Am J Surg* 1974;**128**:818–22.

73 Mitchell RL, Armanini GB. Cricopharyngeal myotomy: treatment of dysphagia. *Ann Surg* 1975;**181**:262–6.

74 Lendrum FC. Anatomic features of the cardiac orifice of the stomach with special reference to cardiospasm. *Arch Intern Med* 1937;**59**:474.

75 Mayberry JF, Atkinson M. Studies of incidence and prevalence of achalasia in the Nottingham area. *Q J Med* 1985;**56**:451–6.

76 Koberle F. Chagas' disease and Chagas' syndromes: the pathology of American trypanosomiasis. *Adv Parasitol* 1968;**6**:63–116.

77 Sifrim D, Janssens J, Vantrappen G. Failing deglutitive inhibition in primary esophageal motility disorders. *Gastroenterology* 1994;**106**:875–82.

78 Mearin F, Mourelle M, Guarner F, Salas A, Moncada S, Malagelada J-R. Absence of nitric oxide synthase in the gastroesophageal junction of patients with achalasia. *Gastroenterology* 1993;**104**:A550.

79 Helm JF, Layman RD, Eckert MD. Effect of chronic administration of N-omega-nitro-L-arginine (LNNA) on the opossum esophagus and lower esophageal sphincter (LES) resembles achalasia. *Gastroenterology* 1992;**103**:1375.

80 Panzini L, Traube M. Stridor from tracheal obstruction in a patient with achalasia. *Am J Gastroenterol* 1993;**88**:1097–100.

81 Massey BT, Hogan WJ, Dodds WJ, Dantas RO. Alteration of the upper esophageal sphincter belch reflex in patients with achalasia. *Gastroenterology* 1992;**103**:1574–9.

82 Dodds WJ, Stewart ET, Kishk SM, Kahrilas PJ, Hogan WJ. Radiologic amyl nitrite test for distinguishing pseudoachalasia from idiopathic achalasia. *Am J Roentgenol* 1986;**146**:21–3.

83 McCord GS, Staiano A, Clouse RE. Achalasia, diffuse esophageal spasm and non-specific motor disorders. *Baillières Clin Gastroenterol* 1991;**5**:307–35.

84 Howard PJ, Maher L, Pryde A, Cameron EW, Heading RC. Five year prospective study of the incidence, clinical features, and diagnosis of achalasia in Edinburgh. *Gut* 1992;**33**:1011–15.

85 Kahrilas PJ, Kishk SM, Helm JF, Dodds WJ, Harig JM, Hogan WJ. Comparison of pseudoachalasia and achalasia. *Am J Med* 1987;**82**:439–46.

86 Bortolotti M, Labo G. Clinical and manometric effects of nifedipine in patients with esophageal achalasia. *Gastroenterology* 1981;**80**:39–44.

87 Marzio L, Cennamo L, DeLaurentiis MF, Grossi L. Cimetropium bromide reduces esophageal lower sphincter pressure and transit time in patients affected by primary achalasia. *Gastroenterology* 1993;**104**:A547.

88 Pasricha PJ, Ravich WJ, Hendrix TR, Sostre S, Jones B, Kalloo AN. Treatment of achalasia with intrasphincteric injection of botulinum toxin: a pilot trial. *Ann Intern Med* 1994;**121**:590–1.

89 Csendes A, Braghetto I, Henriquez A, Cortes C. Late results of a prospective randomised study comparing forceful dilatation and oesophagomyotomy in patients with achalasia. *Gut* 1989;**30**:299–304.

90 Eckardt VF, Aignherr C, Bernhard G. Predictors of outcome in patients with achalasia treated by pneumatic dilation. *Gastroenterology* 1992;**103**:1732–8.

91 Schwartz HM, Cahow CE, Traube M. Outcome after perforation sustained during pneumatic dilatation for achalasia. *Dig Dis Sci* 1993;**38**:1409–13.

92 Cuschieri A. Endoscopic oesophageal myotomy for specific motility disorders and non-cardiac chest pain. *Endosc Surg Allied Technol* 1993;**1**:280–7.

93 Pellegrini CA, Leichter R, Patti M, Somberg K, Ostroff JW, Way L. Thoracoscopic esophageal myotomy in the treatment of achalasia. *Ann Thorac Surg* 1993;**56**:680–2.

94 Richter JE, Castell DO. Diffuse esophageal spasm: a reappraisal. *Ann Intern Med* 1984;**100**:242–5.

95 Kahrilas PJ, Clouse RE, Hogan WJ. American Gastroenterological Association technical review on the clinical use of esophageal manometry. *Gastroenterology* 1994;**107**:1865–84.

96 Clouse RE, Staiano A. Manometric patterns using esophageal body and lower sphincter characteristics: findings in 1013 patients. *Dig Dis Sci* 1992;**37**:289–96.

97 Benjamin SB, Gerhardt DC, Castell DO. High amplitude, peristaltic esophageal contractions associated with chest pain and/or dysphagia. *Gastroenterology* 1979;**77**:478–83.

98 Traube M, Albibi R, McCallum RW. High-amplitude peristaltic esophageal contractions associated with chest pain. *JAMA* 1983;**250**:2655–9.

99 Massey BT, Dodds WJ, Hogan WJ, Brasseur JG, Helm JF. Abnormal esophageal motility: an analysis of concurrent radiographic and manometric findings. *Gastroenterology* 1991;**101**:344–54.

100 Achem SR, Crittenden J, Kolts B, Burton L. Long-term clinical and manometric follow-up of patients with nonspecific esophageal motor disorders. *Am J Gastroenterol* 1992;**87**:825–30.

101 Swift GL, Alban-Davies H, McKirdy H, Lowndes R, Lewis D, Rhodes J. A long-term clinical review of patients with oesophageal chest pain. *Q J Med* 1991;**81**:937–44.

102 Richter JE, Dalton CB, Bradley LA, Castell DO. Oral nifedipine in the treatment of noncardiac chest pain in patients with the nutcracker esophagus. *Gastroenterology* 1987;**93**:21–8.

103 Clouse RE, Lustman PJ, Eckert TC, Ferney DM, Griffith LS. Low-dose trazodone for symptomatic patients with esophageal contraction abnormalities: a double-blind, placebo-controlled trial. *Gastroenterology* 1987;**92**:1027–36.

104 Cattau EL Jr, Castell DO, Johnson DA *et al.* Diltiazem therapy for symptoms associated with nutcracker esophagus. *Am J Gastroenterol* 1991;**86**:272–6.

105 Winters C, Artnak EJ, Benjamin SB, Castell DO. Esophageal bougienage in symptomatic patients with the nutcracker esophagus: a primary esophageal motility disorder. *JAMA* 1984;**252**:363–6.

106 Bancewicz J, Osugi H, Marples M. Clinical implications of abnormal oesophageal motility. *Br J Surg* 1987;**74**:416–19.

107 Achem SR, Kolts BE, Wears R, Burton L, Richter JE. Chest pain associated with nutcracker esophagus: a preliminary study of the role of gastroesophageal reflux. *Am J Gastroenterol* 1993;**88**:187–92.

108 Vantrappen G, Janssens J, Hellemans J, Coremans G. Achalasia, diffuse esophageal spasm and related motility disorders. *Gastroenterology* 1979;**76**:450–7.

Gastroesophageal Reflux Disease: Pathogenesis and Diagnosis

André J.P.M. Smout

Our knowledge of the pathophysiologic processes that lead to gastro-esophageal reflux disease (GERD) has deepened considerably during the past decade, owing to new investigational techniques such as prolonged lower esophageal sphincter (LES) manometry and 24-hour esophageal pH and pressure monitoring. Indeed, some of these techniques have become important diagnostic tools.

The lack of a uniform definition for GERD is a problem encountered in studies of pathophysiology and diagnosis. Some investigators have defined the disease on the basis of macroscopic or microscopic signs of esophagitis, while others have placed emphasis on symptoms. Still others have used esophageal acid exposure as the most important diagnostic criterion. These differences should be borne in mind when reviewing the literature.

Pathogenesis

The lower esophageal sphincter

Beyond any doubt, the key factor in the pathogenesis of GERD is dis-ordered function of the LES. This sphincter is characterized anatomically and manometrically as a 3-cm zone of specialized muscle that maintains a tonic activity. The end-expiratory pressure in the sphincter is 8–20 mmHg above the end-expiratory gastric pressure. The LES is kept in place by the phrenoesophageal ligament, which forms a sheath around the esophagus, anchoring its most distal end to the diaphragm. During respiratory movements, however, the LES slides in and out of the esophageal hiatus in the diaphragm. As will be discussed, the right crus of this hiatus, in particular, contributes to the antireflux barrier [1].

In contrast to what many pathophysiologic studies seem to suggest, there is considerable minute-to-minute variation in LES pressure. Pro-longed manometry with a sleeve sensor shows large fluctuations in LES pressure related to the interdigestive migrating motor complex (MMC), with the pressure being lowest during phase I (motor quiescence) and highest during phase III (the activity front) of the MMC [2, 3]. This participation of the LES in the MMC has been thought to prevent reflux during late phase II and phase III [2]. However, other investigators have reported that in the fasting state, reflux episodes are significantly more frequent during phase III in the antrum. As many as 95% of nocturnal reflux episodes are associated with interdigestive gastric motor activity [4]. It is not known as yet whether impaired LES involvement in the MMC plays a pathogenic role in GERD.

Before the discovery of the dynamics of LES function, a chronically decreased basal LES pressure was considered to be the most important factor in the pathogenesis of GERD. Later observations [5] revealed a considerable overlap in LES pressure between patients with GERD and healthy subjects. There is little controversy over the fact that the LES pressure is significantly reduced in patients with severe or complicated reflux disease, such as grade IV esophagitis, although in milder forms of GERD basal pressure is often found to be normal [5–7].

Controversy still exists as to whether lowered LES tone is the cause or result of chronic reflux. In laboratory animals, the induction of esophagitis leads to a decline in LES pressure, suggesting that the hypotension of the LES associated with GERD may be secondary to the mucosal inflammation [8]. However, clinical studies [7, 9, 10] have shown that healing of reflux esophagitis is not associated with a significant improvement in LES pressure. These clinical observations do not disprove the hypothesis that LES malfunction in GERD is secondary to the inflammation, since the epithelial damage may have been irreversible.

Studies using prolonged manometric monitoring of the LES have led to completely new concepts in the pathophysiology of GERD. In GERD patients with a normal LES pressure, spontaneous transient relaxations of the LES (TLESRs) were found to be the most prevalent mechanism of gastroesophageal reflux [11]. These 'inappropriate' relaxations are defined as a decrease in LES pressure to the level of gastric pressure, lasting at least 5 seconds and not preceded by a swallow (Figure 3.1). The proportion of reflux episodes resulting from TLESRs decreases with increasing severity of reflux disease. In healthy volunteers and patients without endoscopic evidence of esophagitis, reflux occurs exclusively during TLESRs, whereas in patients with erosive esophagitis, about two-thirds of reflux episodes occur by this mechanism [6, 11–13]. In both healthy subjects and patients with GERD, gastric retention has been

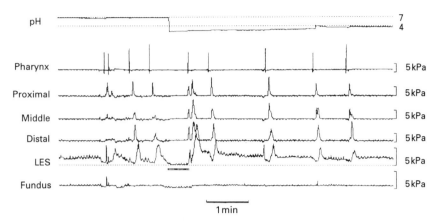

Fig. 3.1 Spontaneous transient LES relaxation (indicated by double horizontal line), followed by gastroesophageal reflux. Recording from ambulatory subject, using perfused sleeve sensor in LES. (With the kind permission of B.L.A.M. Weusten, Utrecht.)

shown to increase the frequency of transient relaxations. This phenomenon may form the basis for the postprandial increase in gastroesophageal reflux seen in health and in disease [14].

The crural diaphragm and hiatal hernia

The association between GERD and hiatal hernia has been described in all clinical textbooks. This relationship is not a direct one. In a series [15] of patients evaluated endoscopically because of dyspeptic symptoms, 42% of those with a hiatal hernia did not have esophagitis. Conversely, only 63% of patients with endoscopically confirmed reflux esophagitis had a hiatal hernia.

Ambulatory esophageal pH studies have demonstrated [16] a higher frequency of gastroesophageal reflux episodes in GERD patients who have a hiatal hernia than in those who do not. It could be hypothesized, therefore, that a hiatal hernia predisposes to gastroesophageal reflux by weakening the LES. However, early manometric observations [17] indicated that basal LES pressure is not decreased in GERD patients as a result of the presence of a hiatal hernia.

More recent investigations have pointed out the role of the crural diaphragm, which strengthens the LES in the absence of a hiatal hernia. With each inspiration the crural diaphragm contracts, thereby contributing to the barrier function of the LES, at moments when reflux would be facilitated by an increase in abdominal pressure and a decrease in intrathoracic pressure [1]. Manometrically, this contribution can be recognized as phasic pressure oscillations superimposed on the tonic LES pressure. After esophagogastrectomy, a high-pressure zone with phasic oscillations can still be found at the level of the diaphragm. This high-pressure zone, due to the diaphragmatic crura, partially relaxes in response to swallowing and contracts in response to increased intra-abdominal pressure [18]. In patients with hiatal hernia, the position of the diaphragm distal to the LES counteracts rather than reinforces normal LES function. A study [19] using videofluoroscopy combined with manometry showed that complete esophageal emptying of swallowed barium occurred less frequently in patients with a hiatal hernia than in those without; in particular, patients in whom the hiatal hernia does not reduce between swallows have incomplete esophageal emptying. In these patients, early retrograde flow from the hiatal sac to the esophagus was observed immediately after LES relaxation. Esophageal clearance of the refluxed material was found to be more disturbed in patients with non-reducing hiatal hernia than in those without [19].

Esophageal clearance

About 50% of patients with reflux disease have prolonged acid clearance times, both in the controlled setting of the acid clearance test and in the noncontrolled but more physiologic setting of ambulatory pH monitoring. Under normal circumstances, esophageal acid clearance is a two-step process. Most of the refluxed volume is cleared rapidly, by one or two peristaltic contractions. The remaining refluxate is neutralized more slowly by swallowed saliva [20, 21]. Thus, both abnormal esophageal peristalsis and abnormal saliva production could play pathogenic roles in GERD. An increased incidence of weak and failed peristaltic contractions has been reported repeatedly in patients with esophagitis. The prevalence of peristaltic dysfunction was found to increase with increasing severity of esophagitis: 25% of individuals with mild esophagitis, compared with 50% of those with severe esophagitis, have peristaltic dysfunction [5]. In patients with low-grade esophagitis, the esophageal motor response to reflux may be normal, while patients with high-grade esophagitis have abnormal responses [22, 23]. A contributing factor to abnormal peristalsis in reflux disease is parasympathetic nerve dysfunction, which correlates well with parameters of esophageal transit and peristalsis [24].

There is still some debate as to whether the abnormal peristalsis found in patients with GERD is a primary abnormality or the consequence of repeated acid injury. Several studies have addressed this question by comparing esophageal contractile activity and LES function before and after healing of esophagitis. In none of the studies reported thus far [7, 10, 25, 26] has healing of esophagitis resulted in improvement in esophageal peristalsis. Recently, however, the aboral traction force generated by graded intraluminal distention was found to improve after healing of esophagitis [26].

At night, esophageal acid clearance is prolonged. Normally, reflux occurring during sleep is associated with arousal and an increased swallowing rate. When arousal does not occur, clearance times are markedly increased, leading to damage to the esophageal mucosa [27, 28].

There is little evidence that impaired salivary production or abnormal composition of the saliva plays an important role in the pathogenesis of reflux esophagitis [29]. Rather, both in healthy controls and in patients with reflux esophagitis, saliva flow increases two- to fourfold when heartburn is induced by esophageal acid perfusion [30]. When acid infusion does not lead to heartburn, salivary flow is affected to a lesser extent [30]. The increased salivary flow accompanying heartburn may act as an endogenous antacid, which serves as a protective response to symptomatic gastroesophageal reflux. When increased saliva flow in response to heartburn (or another gastrointestinal symptom) is perceived by the patient, it is referred to as 'water brash'.

Resistance of esophageal mucosa

The correlation between esophageal acid exposure, as measured by 24-hour pH monitoring, and the severity of reflux esophagitis is poor [31–33]. It is, therefore, thought that abnormalities in the defensive capacity of the esophageal mucosa play a role in the pathogenesis of reflux esophagitis.

Esophageal epithelial cells have at least three ion exchangers that regulate intracellular pH in response to acidification or alkalinization [34]. In the rabbit, serosal bicarbonate ions help protect the esophagus against acid-induced damage by buffering hydrogen ions within the intracellular compartment of the extracellular space [35]. It is not known whether this mechanism is present in humans. Intrinsic bicarbonate secretion from submucous glands in the esophageal mucosa has been identified in some mammals, including humans. These glands have been shown to produce up to two-thirds of the bicarbonate measured in the esophagi of healthy subjects [36]. It is now clear that esophageal bicarbonate secretion is responsible for episodes of alkalinization of the esophagus as observed during pH monitoring [37].

In addition to these factors, variations in the blood supply to the esophagus appear to affect maintenance of esophageal mucosal integrity. It has been shown experimentally [38] that the esophageal blood supply can increase in response to a threat of tissue injury from exposure to luminal acid.

Abnormal composition of refluxate

Patients with GERD do not have a significant increase in basal, meal-stimulated, or maximal gastric acid or pepsin secretion, and the severity of reflux esophagitis is not related to gastric acid output [39]. These observations contradict the notion that GERD is due to abnormal acid secretion and are not in accord with the most widely used therapeutic approach to GERD, which targets the parietal cell. Bile salts can cause esophageal mucosal injury independently of acid, as well as enhance the damaging effect of the hydrogen ion [40]. Trypsin also is capable of inducing esophageal injury, in a dose-dependent manner [41]. The available evidence would suggest, however, that in patients with an intact stomach, reflux of duodenal contents is not a significant pathophysiologic factor. Bile acids and trypsin can reach the esophagus, but their presence reflects the presence of gastric contents. The concentrations of bile acids and trypsin in the esophagus are probably insufficient to cause significant damage [42, 43]. Esophageal bile acid concentrations are not different between healthy subjects, patients with esophagitis, and patients with Barrett's esophagus [42].

Delayed gastric emptying

It has been reported [44] that 41% of patients with GERD have delayed gastric emptying of solid–liquid meals. This observation supports the hypothesis that delayed gastric emptying facilitates reflux by means of larger postprandial gastric volumes and an increased incidence and duration of TLESRs induced by gastric distention [14]. It should be noted, however, that there is no evidence for this sequence of events. In fact, more recent studies [45, 46] have shown that gastric emptying in patients with GERD is often normal or even rapid. Thus, the available data suggest that delayed gastric emptying is unlikely to be a major factor in the pathogenesis of GERD. Nevertheless, it may not be wise to apply this general statement to individual patients, since markedly delayed gastric emptying is encountered on occasion.

Diagnosis

Which test to perform?

The manifestations of GERD are pluriform and variable. Many but not all patients have macroscopically identifiable lesions of the esophageal mucosa. Many patients with GERD have symptoms considered typical of reflux, such as heartburn and acid regurgitation, while others have atypical symptoms, such as angina-like chest pain, wheezing, and hoarseness, or are asymptomatic. In patients with severe reflux symptoms, esophageal acid exposure can be within the normal range. Even esophagitis is occasionally seen in patients with physiologic reflux. These observations make clear that in GERD no single test can provide information on all aspects of the disease. The selection of the diagnostic test(s) depends on the question(s) one wishes to address. In clinical practice, only those tests should be ordered that have outcomes likely to influence the management.

Symptoms

The classic symptoms of GERD are heartburn and regurgitation, the latter defined as an involuntary retrograde delivery of acidic gastric contents to the mouth. These symptoms appear to correlate poorly with esophageal acid exposure [33, 47]. When heartburn or regurgitation clearly dominates the patient's complaints, they have a high specificity (89% and 95%, respectively) but a low sensitivity (38% and 6%, respectively) for gastro-esophageal reflux, defined as excessive acid exposure [47, 48]. In one-third of patients with proven GERD, the history-taking reveals such inconclusive symptoms that no preliminary determination about the presence or absence of GERD can be made [47]. Although statistically significant differences in esophageal acid exposure (time with pH $\leqslant$ 4) have been reported in reflux patients with mild versus severe reflux symptoms, the overlap between the two groups is considerable [32]. Even patients with Barrett's esophagus have a frequency and severity of reflux symptoms similar to those of GERD patients with normal esophageal mucosa [49]. Thus, although symptoms usually provide the impetus for patients to consult their physicians, they are unreliable tools for assessing esophageal acid exposure and mucosal damage. This should not detract from the value, in many cases, of symptoms as a gauge to treatment.

Endoscopy

Fiberoptic endoscopy is the most valuable technique for assessing acid-induced damage to the esophageal mucosa and its complications. Low-grade esophagitis can easily be missed on radiographic examination (barium esophagogram). Esophageal erosions and exudative lesions as observed endoscopically correlate well with histologic evidence of inflammation. Diffuse erythema, edema, mucosal friability, and non-fibrin-covered erythematous lesions are rather nonspecific markers of GERD [48].

It is astonishing that more than 40 different systems of classification of esophagitis have been described in the literature. This absence of uniformity precludes meaningful comparisons of the results of published studies on reflux esophagitis and its treatment. It is hoped that a consensus will be reached on a universal grading system.

The Savary–Miller esophagitis grading scheme, first described in 1978 and recently refined by Ollyo et al. [50], is the most widely used classification. This endoscopic grading system is summarized in Table 3.1. In older classification systems, the presence of Barrett's metaplasia can automatically lead to the classification of high-grade esophagitis; it is now felt that the presence and extent of metaplasia should be described separately from the presence and extent of esophagitis. Usually, reflux esophagitis can be differentiated easily from other causes of esophagitis, such as infection, radiation, and ingestion of caustic agents.

The endoscopic diagnosis of an axial hiatus hernia requires that the squamocolumnar junction (Z-line) be located more than 2 cm above the

Table 3.1 Savary–Miller–Ollyo endoscopic grading system. (Adapted from Ollyo et al. [50].)

Grade I	Single erosion or exudative lesion, on only one longitudinal fold
Grade II	Multiple erosions or exudative lesions, involving more than one longitudinal fold
Grade III	Circular erosive or exudative lesions, or both
Grade IV	Ulcer(s), stricture(s), or short esophagus, singly or in combination
Grade V	Barrett's epithelium, isolated or in association with grade I–IV lesions

diaphragmatic impression. An axial hiatus hernia should be identified during the introduction of the endoscope, before inflation of the stomach reduces its size. The endoscopic diagnosis of Barrett's esophagus requires the presence of a Z-line 2–3 cm proximal to the esophagogastric junction. Islands of squamous epithelium may be present in the Barrett's segment, and islands of columnar epithelium may be present above the squamo-columnar junction.

Histologic examination of biopsies taken in cases of suspected esophagitis may occasionally be helpful, but early microscopic signs of inflammation, such as thickening of the squamous layer and lengthening of the papillae, can also be found in normal subjects [51]. In most patients in whom Barrett's epithelium is seen endoscopically, histologic evaluation of biopsy specimens can confirm not only the presence of Barrett's epithelium but also the type of Barrett's metaplasia and the degree of dysplasia. This information is relevant because intestinal-type Barrett's epithelium carries an increased risk of development of adenocarcinoma.

Ambulatory pH monitoring

Ambulatory 24-hour monitoring of esophageal pH has become an important clinical tool. Some users of the technique, however, continue to attempt to answer questions that cannot be resolved on the basis of pH monitoring. These researchers may have been encouraged by studies that apparently aimed to evaluate the sensitivity and specificity of esophageal pH monitoring in the diagnosis of esophagitis and reflux symptoms. As has been pointed out, GERD is associated with a wide spectrum of related but separate manifestations, and ambulatory 24-hour esophageal pH monitoring may not be the most appropriate test for certain manifestations of GERD. For example, if a practitioner wishes to obtain information about erosive esophagitis, endoscopy would be more appropriate than pH monitoring.

In the analysis of esophageal pH profiles, many variables concerning acid reflux can be calculated. Currently, the cutoff pH value of 4 is widely used to identify reflux episodes. The uniform use of this cutoff value permits comparison between results from different centers, but other threshold values also offer advantages. In the early postprandial period, for example, intragastric contents may have a pH value greater than 4 and episodes of gastroesophageal reflux may go undetected if the usual criterion of a pH less than 4 is applied (Figure 3.2).

It is now generally accepted that the percentage of time with esophageal pH less than 4 is the best overall parameter for gastroesophageal

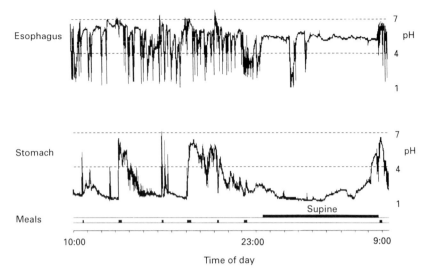

Fig. 3.2 Combined intragastric and intraesophageal pH monitoring in a patient with pathologic reflux. After some meals, the intragastric pH is greater than 4 for up to several hours, precluding detection of gastroesophageal reflux if a criterion of an intraesophageal pH of less than 4 is used.

reflux and that separate analyses of daytime and nighttime episodes should be performed. All reflux parameters based on the identification of individual reflux episodes (such as number and duration of reflux episodes) have the disadvantage that there are different methods of defining the beginning and endpoints of reflux episodes. Differences in computer algorithms used in the automated detection of reflux episodes can lead to considerable differences in results.

Various studies have been performed to establish normal values for esophageal pH, with variable results. The set of normal values described in the pioneer study by Johnson and DeMeester [52] has been criticized for some methodological shortcomings [53]. However, as shown in Table 3.2,

Table 3.2 Normal values (upper limits of normal) in ambulatory esophageal pH monitoring.

	Johnson & DeMeester [52]	Richter *et al.* [54]
% Time pH < 4, total	4.2	5.78
% Time pH < 4, upright	6.3	8.15
% Time pH < 4, supine	1.2	3.45
Reflux episodes, total (*n*)	50	46
Episodes > 5 min (*n*)	3	4
Longest episode (min)	9.2	18.45

their findings do not deviate significantly from the findings of modern, large-scale studies [54]. Some studies [53, 54] have shown an increase in reflux with age, especially in the supine period. This age dependency is usually not taken into account when interpreting clinical pH studies.

Twenty-four-hour esophageal pH monitoring is particularly useful when esophagitis is absent and there is a question of whether symptoms are due to reflux. Several published techniques have attempted to quantify the relationship between reflux events and the symptoms under investigation. Establishing a correlation is an important aspect of the analysis of 24-hour pH studies, but it should be remembered that the contemporaneous occurrence of two events cannot be taken as proof of a cause-and-effect link; both events could be the result of a third event, the true cause [55].

In analyzing the association between chest pain episodes and gastro-esophageal reflux, different research groups have used different time windows. In a study [56] using time windows of various onset and duration, it was concluded that the optimal time window for symptom analysis with 24-hour pH monitoring begins 2 minutes before symptom onset and ends with the onset of pain.

The 'symptom index' (SI), first described in 1988, is defined as the percentage of reflux episodes associated with a fall in pH [57]. The SI also has been described as a 'symptom–reflux association' [33]. While simple and easy to understand, this index has important disadvantages. It does not take into account the number of reflux episodes. The higher the number of reflux episodes, the greater the likelihood of a chance simul-taneous occurrence of symptoms and reflux. The optimal cutoff value for normal versus abnormal findings is not known. Based on receiver oper-ating characteristic analysis, there is evidence [58] to suggest that an SI of 50% or more has the highest specificity and sensitivity in patients with heartburn. In patients with chest pain, however, no acceptable threshold has been found [58].

Recently, our group [59] proposed a simple method to calculate the probability that gastroesophageal reflux episodes and symptoms are related. In this method, the 24-hour pH signal is divided into consecutive 2-minute periods. These periods and the 2-minute intervals preceding the onset of symptoms are evaluated for the occurrence of reflux. Results of the evaluation are then placed in a 4 × 4 contingency table (Figure 3.3). Subsequently, Fisher's exact test is applied to calculate the probability (P value) that reflux and symptom episodes are unrelated. Finally, the symptom association probability (SAP) is calculated as $(1.0 - P) \times 100\%$.

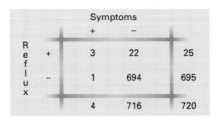

Fig. 3.3 Example of a contingency table containing the number of symptomatic reflux-positive 2-minute periods (3), the number of asymptomatic reflux-positive periods (22), and the symptomatic and asymptomatic 2-minute periods without reflux (1 and 694, respectively). Fisher's exact test yields a P value of 0.0001. The symptom association probability is 99.99%.

With this method, the false-positive and false-negative results that can occur with the SI can be avoided; the former in cases of small numbers of symptom episodes and the latter in cases of large numbers.

Some investigators have suggested that the time period when pH is greater than 7 during 24-hour esophageal pH monitoring would be a good indicator of 'alkaline' reflux, i.e., reflux of duodenal contents through the stomach into the esophagus. More recent observations have made clear, however, that in patients with an intact stomach, duodenal components are present in the refluxate only in very low concentrations [37, 43]. Periods of esophageal alkalinization are almost invariably due to salivation or bicarbonate production by esophageal glands [36, 37]. High pH values also may be due to oxygen sensitivity of antimony electrodes [60]. Consequently, the term 'alkaline reflux' is a misnomer and episodes of alkaline esophageal pH should not be analyzed in clinical studies.

Special forms of esophageal pH monitoring may be useful in selected cases. Combined intragastric and intraesophageal pH monitoring may be of value in patients whose symptoms or esophagitis do not respond adequately to acid-inhibitory treatment. In these cases, combined monitoring will show either that the symptoms are not acid related or that the dose of the antisecretory drug provides inadequate suppression of gastric acid production.

Combined ambulatory esophageal manometry and pHmetry may be of diagnostic value in patients with chronic unexplained cough. When coughing spells, easily recognized in the manometric signal, are preceded by reflux, acid reflux is likely to be a pathogenic factor [61]. In patients with suspected rumination syndrome, simultaneous intragastric pressure monitoring and intraesophageal pH monitoring may be required to establish the diagnosis unequivocally [62]. In these patients, postprandial

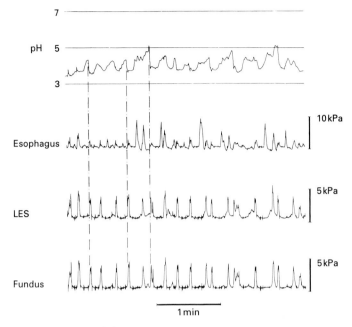

Fig. 3.4 Rumination in an adult patient presenting with reflux symptoms. Combined esophagogastric pressure and pH recordings show that most postprandial reflux episodes are preceded by intragastric pressure spikes, caused by abdominal straining. Note that in this example intraesophageal pH fluctuates around 4 as a consequence of a very high frequency of reflux episodes.

reflux is wilfully induced by contractions of the abdominal wall muscles and the diaphragm, leading to intra-abdominal pressure spikes (Figure 3.4).

Acid perfusion test

In this test, first described in 1958, a hydrochloric acid solution is perfused into the esophagus, with the patient in an upright or supine position. Alternating infusions of acid and saline are administered in a single-blinded fashion and the patient is instructed to report his or her symptoms. The test is positive when reproduction of the patient's symptoms occurs only during acid perfusion.

With the advent of ambulatory esophageal pH monitoring, the need for the acid perfusion test has declined rapidly. Owing to the relatively short observation period, the test is less sensitive than ambulatory monitoring. In patients with noncardiac chest pain, the yield of the acid perfusion test was lower than that of 24-hour pH monitoring [63].

Scintigraphy

Theoretically, scintigraphic assessment of gastroesophageal reflux, using a radiolabeled test meal and a gamma camera, can provide information that complements the findings on pH monitoring. For example, scintigraphy is more sensitive for detecting reflux during the first postprandial hour(s), when intragastric contents often have a nonacidic pH. The results of a radionuclide reflux scan can be quantified as the number of reflux episodes and the percentage of radioactivity that appears cephalad to the LES. However, the short duration of the imaging limits the value of gastroesophageal scintigraphy [64]. The specificity of the technique appears to be satisfactory, but the sensitivity does not exceed 60% [64]. The use of scintigraphy in GERD has not yet gained much popularity.

Esophageal manometry

In most patients with suspected GERD, esophageal manometry is not part of the diagnostic workup. This approach probably is sensible since GERD is not associated with specific manometric abnormalities. The basal tone of the LES, measured by means of a stationary or a rapid pull-through technique, or by prolonged monitoring with a sleeve sensor, correlates rather poorly with other, more directly relevant markers of GERD [65]. Analysis of the incidence of TLESRs, although of considerable pathophysiologic significance, has not yet been shown to be clinically useful.

Manometry not only provides information about LES function, but also enables assessment of the motor function of the esophageal body. Parameters such as contraction amplitude, duration, and propagation yield data on the clearing capacity of the tubular esophagus. Peristaltic dysfunction has been shown to be increasingly prevalent with increasing severity of peptic esophagitis [5]. However, the clinical relevance of such information is generally felt to be limited.

Most clinicians would agree that esophageal manometry is indicated in patients with GERD in whom surgery is considered. In these patients, the presence of severe esophageal motor disorders, such as achalasia and disorders associated with systemic sclerosis, should be ruled out. Unbelievable as it may seem, tertiary referral centers occasionally see patients with achalasia in whom antireflux surgery has been performed, obviously without adequate prior workup. In patients with severe peristaltic dysfunction, fundoplication should perhaps not be carried out at all; when performed, the fundic wrap should be made 'floppy' to prevent post-operative dysphagia.

Conclusion

The pathogenesis of GERD is multifactorial. Different mechanisms may be involved in different patients. Motility factors appear to be of primary importance. The key motor abnormalities are defective LES function and impairment of the contribution of the crural diaphragm to the esophagogastric high-pressure zone.

Since GERD is a pluriform disease, no single diagnostic test is sufficient to evaluate the patient. Consequently, multiple tests may be required to characterize an individual patient's condition adequately. However, not all aspects of the disease may need full characterization in all patients. Twenty-four-hour pH monitoring is an important new tool in the workup of patients with suspected GERD. Its use is indicated in patients without esophagitis, those with equivocal symptoms, poor responders to treatment, and patients in whom antireflux surgery is considered. It is remarkable that the factors that appear to be most important in the pathophysiology of GERD are not identical to those considered most relevant in the diagnostic workup.

References

1 Mittal RK, Rochester DF, McCallum RW. Effect of the diaphragmatic contraction on lower esophageal sphincter pressure in man. *Gut* 1987;**28**:1564–8.

2 Dent J, Dodds WJ, Sekiguchi T, Hogan WJ, Arndorfer RC. Interdigestive phasic contractions of the human lower esophageal sphincter. *Gastroenterology* 1983;**84**:453–60.

3 Smout AJPM, Bogaard JW, van Hattum J, Akkermans LMA. Effects of cimetidine and ranitidine on interdigestive and postprandial lower esophageal sphincter pressures and plasma gastrin levels in normal subjects. *Gastroenterology* 1985;**88**:557–63.

4 Gill RC, Kellow JE, Wingate DL. Gastro-oesophageal reflux and the migrating motor complex. *Gut* 1987;**28**:929–34.

5 Kahrilas PJ, Dodds WJ, Hogan WJ, Kern M, Arndorfer RC, Reece A. Esophageal peristaltic dysfunction in peptic esophagitis. *Gastroenterology* 1986;**91**:897–904.

6 Dent J, Holloway RH, Toouli J, Dodds WJ. Mechanisms of lower oesophageal sphincter incompetence in patients with symptomatic gastroesophageal reflux. *Gut* 1988;**29**:1020–8.

7 Timmer R, Breumelhof R, Nadorp JHSM, Smout AJPM. Oesophageal motility and gastro-oesophageal reflux before and after healing of reflux oesophagitis: a study using 24-hour ambulatory pH and pressure monitoring. *Gut* 1994;**35**:1519–22.

8 Eastwood GL, Castell DO, Higgs RH. Experimental esophagitis in cats impairs lower esophageal sphincter pressure. *Gastroenterology* 1975;**69**:146–53.

9 Katz PO, Knuff TE, Benjamin SB, Castell DO. Abnormal esophageal pressures in reflux esophagitis: cause or effect? *Am J Gastroenterol* 1986;**81**:744–6.

10 Eckardt VF. Does healing of esophagitis improve esophageal motor function? *Dig Dis Sci* 1988;**33**:161–5.

11 Dodds WJ, Dent J, Hogan WJ *et al.* Mechanisms of gastroesophageal reflux in patients with reflux esophagitis. *N Engl J Med* 1982;**307**:1547–52.

12 Mittal RK, McCallum RW. Characteristics and frequency of transient relaxation of the lower esophageal sphincter in patients with reflux esophagitis. *Gastroenterology* 1988;**95**:593–9.

13 Schoeman MN, Tippett MD, Akkermans LMA, Dent J, Holloway RH. Mechanisms of gastroesophageal reflux in ambulant healthy human subjects. *Gastroenterology* 1995;**108**:83–91.

14 Holloway RH, Hongo M, Berger K, McCallum RW. Gastric distention: a mechanism for postprandial gastroesophageal reflux. *Gastroenterology* 1985;**89**:779–84.

15 Berstad A, Weberg R, Larsen IF, Hoel B, Hauer-Jensen M. Relationship of hiatus hernia to reflux oesophagitis: a prospective study of coincidence, using endoscopy. *Scand J Gastroenterol* 1986;**21**:55–8.

16 DeMeester TR, Lafontaine E, Joelsson BE *et al.* Relationship of a hiatal hernia to the function of the body of the esophagus and the gastroesophageal junction. *J Thorac Cardiovasc Surg* 1981;**82**:547–58.

17 Cohen S, Harris LD. Does hiatus hernia affect competence of the esophageal sphincter? *N Engl J Med* 1971;**284**:1053–6.

18 Klein WA, Parkman HP, Dempsey DT, Fisher RS. Sphincterlike thoracoabdominal high pressure zone after esophagogastrectomy. *Gastroenterology* 1993;**105**:1362–9.

19 Sloan S, Kahrilas P. Impairment of esophageal emptying with hiatal hernia. *Gastroenterology* 1991;**100**:596–605.

20 Helm JF, Dodds WJ, Pelc LR, Palmer DW, Hogan WJ, Teeter BC. Effect of esophageal emptying and saliva on clearance of acid from the esophagus. *N Engl J Med* 1984;**310**:284–8.

21 Shaker R, Kahrilas PJ, Dodds WJ, Hogan WJ. Oesophageal clearance of small amounts of equal or less than one millilitre of acid. *Gut* 1992;**33**:7–10.

22 Timmer R, Breumelhof R, Nadorp JHSM, Smout AJPM. The oesophageal motor response to reflux is not impaired in reflux oesophagitis. *Gut* 1993;**34**:317–20.

23 Timmer R, Breumelhof R, Nadorp JHSM, Smout AJPM. Ambulatory esophageal pressure and pH monitoring in patients with high-grade reflux esophagitis. *Dig Dis Sci* 1994;**39**:2084–9.

24 Cunningham KM, Horowitz M, Riddell PS *et al.* Relations among autonomic nerve dysfunction, oesophageal motility, and gastric emptying in gastro-oesophageal reflux disease. *Gut* 1991;**32**:1436–40.

25 Allen ML, McIntosh DL, Robinson MG. Healing or amelioration of esophagitis does not result in increased lower esophageal sphincter or esophageal contractile pressure. *Am J Gastroenterol* 1990;**85**:1331–4.

26 Williams D, Thompson DG, Heggie L, O'Hanrahan T, Bancewicz J. Esophageal clearance function following treatment of esophagitis. *Gastroenterology* 1994;**106**:108–16.

27 Orr WC, Johnson LF, Robinson MG. Effect of sleep on swallowing, esophageal peristalsis, and acid clearance. *Gastroenterology* 1984;**86**:814–19.

28 Sondheimer JM. Clearance of spontaneous gastroesophageal reflux in awake and sleeping infants. *Gastroenterology* 1989;**97**:821–6.

29 Sonnenberg A, Steinkamp U, Weise A *et al.* Salivary secretion in reflux esophagitis. *Gastroenterology* 1982;**83**:889–95.

30 Helm JF, Dodds WJ, Hogan WJ. Salivary response to esophageal acid in normal subjects and patients with reflux esophagitis. *Gastroenterology* 1987;**93**:1393–7.

31 Schindlbeck NE, Heinrich C, Konig A, Dendorfer A, Pace F, Müller-Lissner SA. Optimal thresholds, sensitivity, and specificity of long-term pH-metry for the detection of gastroesophageal reflux disease. *Gastroenterology* 1987;**93**:85–90.

32 Mattioli S, Pilotti V, Spangaro M *et al.* Reliability of 24-hour home esophageal pH monitoring in diagnosis of gastroesophageal reflux. *Dig Dis Sci* 1989;**34**:71–8.

33 Howard PJ, Maher L, Pryde A, Heading RC. Symptomatic gastro-oesophageal reflux, abnormal oesophageal acid exposure, and mucosal acid sensitivity are three separate, though related, aspects of gastro-oesophageal reflux disease. *Gut* 1991;**32**:128–32.

34 Tobey NA, Reddy SP, Khalbuss WE, Silvers SM, Cragoe EJ Jr, Orlando RC. Na^+-dependent and -independent Cl^-/HCO_3^- exchangers in cultured esophageal epithelial cells. *Gastroenterology* 1993;**104**:185–95.

35 Tobey NA, Powell DW, Schreiner VJ, Orlando RC. Serosal bicarbonate protects against acid injury to rabbit esophagus. *Gastroenterology* 1989;**96**:1466–77.

36 Brown CM, Snowdon CF, Slee B, Sandle LN, Rees WDW. Measurement of bicarbonate output from the intact human oesophagus. *Gut* 1993;**34**:872–80.

37 Singh S, Bradley LA, Richter JE. Determinants of oesophageal 'alkaline' pH environment in controls and patients with gastro-oesophageal reflux disease. *Gut* 1993;**34**:309–16.

38 Hollwarth ME, Smith M, Kvietys PR, Granger DN. Esophageal blood flow in the cat. *Gastroenterology* 1986;**90**:622–7.

39 Hirschowitz BI. A critical analysis, with appropriate controls, of gastric and pepsin secretion in clinical esophagitis. *Gastroenterology* 1991;**101**:1149–58.

40 Hopwood D, Bateson MC, Milne G, Bouchier IAD. Effects of bile acids and hydrogen ion on the fine structure of oesophageal epithelium. *Gut* 1981; **22**:306–11.

41 Lillemoe KD, Johnson LF, Harmon JW. Alkaline esophagitis: a comparison of the ability of components of the gastroduodenal contents to injure the rabbit esophagus. *Gastroenterology* 1983;**85**:621–8.

42 Gotley DC, Morgan AP, Ball D, Owen RW, Cooper MJ. Composition of gastro-oesophageal refluxate. *Gut* 1991;**32**:1093–9.

43 Mittal RK, Reuben A, Whitney JO, McCallum RW. Do bile acids reflux into the esophagus? A study of normal subjects and patients with gastroesophageal reflux disease. *Gastroenterology* 1987;**92**:371–5.

44 McCallum RW, Berkowitz DM, Lerner E. Gastric emptying in patients with gastroesophageal reflux. *Gastroenterology* 1981;**80**:285–91.

45 Johnson DA, Winters C, Drane WE *et al.* Solid-phase gastric emptying in patients with Barrett's esophagus. *Dig Dis Sci* 1986;**31**:1217–20.

46 Shay SS, Eggli D, McDonald C, Johnson LF. Gastric emptying of solid food in patients with gastroesophageal reflux. *Gastroenterology* 1987;**92**:459–65.

47 Klauser AG, Schindlbeck NE, Müller-Lissner SA. Symptoms in gastro-oesophageal reflux disease. *Lancet* 1990; **335**:205–8.

48 Johnsson F, Joelsson B, Gudmundsson K, Greiff L. Symptoms and endoscopic findings in the diagnosis of gastroesophageal reflux disease. *Scand J Gastroenterol* 1987;**22**:714–18.

49 Winters C Jr, Spurling TJ, Chobanian SJ *et al.* Barrett's esophagus: a prevalent, occult complication of gastroesophageal reflux disease. *Gastroenterology* 1987;**92**:118–24.

50 Ollyo JB, Fontolliet C, Brossard E, Lang F. Savary's new endoscopic classification of reflux esophagitis. *Acta Endosc* 1992;**22**:307–20.

51 Funch-Jensen P, Kock K, Christensen LA *et al.* Microscopic appearance of the esophageal mucosa in a consecutive series of patients submitted to upper endoscopy: correlation with gastroesophageal reflux symptoms and macroscopic findings. *Scand J Gastroenterol* 1986;**21**:65–9.

52 Johnson LF, DeMeester TR. Twenty-four-hour pH monitoring of the distal esophagus. *Am J Gastroenterol* 1974;**62**:325–32.

53 Smout AJPM, Breedijk M, van der Zouw C, Akkermans LMA. Physiological gastroesophageal reflux and esophageal motor activity studied with a new system for 24-hour recording and automated analysis. *Dig Dis Sci* 1989;**34**:372–8.

54 Richter JE, Bradley LA, DeMeester TR, Wu WC. Normal 24-hour ambulatory esophageal pH values: influence of study center, pH electrode, age, and gender. *Dig Dis Sci* 1992;**37**:849–56.

55 Orr WC. The physiology and philosophy of cause and effect. *Gastroenterology* 1994;**107**:1898–901.

56 Lam HGT, Breumelhof R, Roelofs JMM, van Berge Henegouwen GP, Smout AJPM. What is the optimal time window in symptom analysis of 24-hour esophageal pressure and pH data? *Dig Dis Sci* 1994;**39**:402–9.

57 Wiener GJ, Richter JE, Cooper JB, Wu WC, Castell DO. The symptom index: a clinically important parameter of ambulatory 24-hour esophageal pH monitoring. *Am J Gastroenterol* 1988;**83**:358–61.

58 Singh S, Richter JE, Bradley LA, Haile JM. The symptom index: differential usefulness in suspected acid-related complaints of heartburn and chest pain. *Dig Dis Sci* 1993;**38**:1402–8.

59 Weusten BLAM, Roelofs JMM, Akkermans LMA, van Berge Henegouwen GP, Smout AJPM. The symptom-association probability: an improved method for symptom analysis of 24-hour esophageal pH data. *Gastroenterology* 1994;**107**:1741–5.

60 Sjoberg F, Gustafsson U, Tibbling L. Alkaline oesophageal reflux: an artifact due to oxygen corrosion of antimony pH electrodes. *Scand J Gastroenterol* 1992;**27**:1084–8.

61 Paterson WG, Murat BW. Combined ambulatory esophageal manometry and dual-probe pH-metry in evaluation of patients with chronic unexplained cough. *Dig Dis Sci* 1994;**39**:1117–25.

62 Amarnath RP, Abell TL, Malagelada J-R. The rumination syndrome in adults: a characteristic manometric pattern. *Ann Intern Med* 1986;**105**:513–18.

63 Hewson EG, Sinclair JW, Dalton CB, Richter JE. Twenty-four-hour esophageal pH monitoring: the most useful test for evaluating noncardiac chest pain. *Am J Med* 1991;**90**:576–83.

64 Jenkins AF, Cowan RJ, Richter JE. Gastroesophageal scintigraphy: is it a sensitive screening test for gastroesophageal reflux disease? *J Clin Gastroenterol* 1985;**7**:127–31.

65 Pope CE II. Is determination of LES pressure clinically useful? *Dig Dis Sci* 1981;**26**:1025–7.

« 4 »

Gastroesophageal Reflux Disease:
Acute and Chronic Treatment

Robert S. Fisher

Introduction

Gastroesophageal reflux disease (GERD) is a ubiquitous problem encountered by physicians in all specialties. Nebel *et al.* [1] in 1976 reported that 36% of healthy hospital workers experienced reflux symptoms at least once a month. This high prevalence of symptomatic GERD has been confirmed in Gallup surveys conducted in the US (1988 and 1995) [2, 3] and in a multicenter study completed in England and Scotland by Jones *et al.* (1990) [4].

GERD is a significant clinical problem not only because of a wide range of associated symptoms, atypical as well as classic — including heartburn, regurgitation, dysphagia, chest pain, wheezing, nocturnal coughing, hoarseness, sore throat, abdominal bloating and nausea — but also because of complications such as stricture, bleeding, Barrett's esophagus, and adenocarcinoma of the distal esophagus.

Once a diagnosis of GERD is established, treatment based on a sound understanding of underlying pathogenic mechanisms is effective in relieving symptoms, healing esophagitis, and minimizing complications. In this chapter, a four-phase stepped approach to acute treatment is reviewed; empiric treatment by physicians without diagnostic studies is discussed; and the available choices for long-term maintenance therapy are outlined.

A stepped approach to antireflux treatment

Most gastroenterologists have adopted a stepped approach to the treatment of patients with GERD (Figure 4.1). This approach comprises four phases: nonsystemic treatment (phase I), use of systemic agents (phase II), medical treatment of refractory GERD (phase III), and antireflux surgery (phase IV).

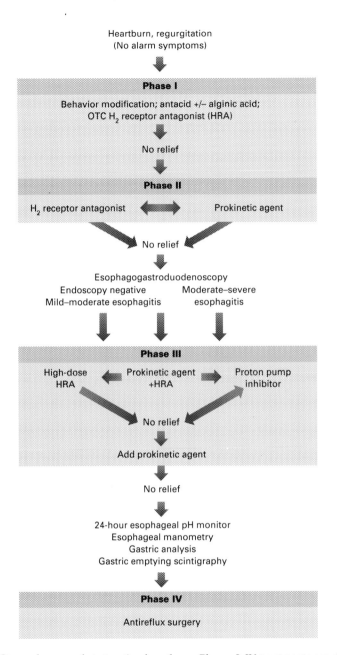

Fig. 4.1 Stepped approach to treating heartburn. Phases I–IV treatments are shown. The place of empiric therapy is indicated. Suggested timing for diagnostic tests is indicated.

Nonsystemic treatment (phase I)

The first step in treating GERD is to institute some simple lifestyle or behavioral modifications (Table 4.1). These measures include: alterations in eating habits, including dietary restrictions and weight loss; postural changes during sleep; changes in medications, if possible; and refraining from cigarette smoking.

Table 4.1 Lifestyle (behavioral) modifications in GERD.

- Alter eating habits
  Small meals
  Do not lie down after eating
  Avoid nocturnal snacks
- Dietary changes
  Avoid fatty foods
  Limit intake of chocolate, onions, peppermint, and alcohol
  Reduce intake of citrus fruit, coffee, and tomato-based products
- Weight reduction
- Postural changes during sleep
- Adjust concurrent medications
- Refrain from cigarette smoking

Gastric distention has been implicated as an aggravating factor in GERD [5, 6]. Therefore, large meals should be avoided and small frequent meals encouraged. Lying down after eating as well as snacking at night should be discouraged. Patients do not have to follow a bland diet but should avoid foods that cause heartburn. Foods with a high fat content, chocolate (rich in fat and xanthines), and carminatives (such as peppermint) may aggravate heartburn by decreasing lower esophageal sphincter (LES) pressure [7] (Table 4.2). Other foods, such as citrus fruits, tomato-based products, and coffee, may increase heartburn by a direct irritating effect on a sensitive esophageal mucosa [7]. Many of these foods would also be avoided on a weight reduction program.

Avoiding complete recumbency during sleep is important both to decrease the number of reflux episodes and to improve esophageal clearance when reflux has occurred [8, 9]. The trunk of the body is best elevated during sleep by placing blocks (bricks, cinder blocks, or customized wooden blocks) under the head of the bed frame, by using a wedge-shaped bolster, or by employing a mechanical hospital bed and placing the patient in a reverse Trendelenburg position.

Certain medications aggravate heartburn by reducing LES pressure [7].

Table 4.2 Foods and medications that predispose to gastroesophageal reflux.

Mechanism	Decrease in LES pressure	Direct irritant of esophagus
Foods	Fatty foods Chocolate Carminatives (e.g., peppermint) Alcohol	Citrus fruit Tomato-based products ? Coffee

Medications	Anticholinergics
	Benzodiazepines
	Beta-adrenergic agonists
	Calcium channel blockers
	Opioids
	Progesterone-containing
	  medications
	Xanthines
		Aspirin and other nonsteroidal
		  anti-inflammatory drugs
		Iron and potassium preparations
		Quinidine derivatives
		Tetracycline derivatives

These include: xanthines such as theophylline; anticholinergic agents, including propantheline, dicyclomine, and tricyclic antidepressants; narcotic analgesics; calcium channel blockers, such as nifedipine, verapamil, and diltiazem; benzodiazepines; beta-adrenergic agonists; and progesterone-containing oral contraceptives (Table 4.2). Other medications, including tetracycline and its derivatives, quinidine preparations, aspirin and other nonsteroidal anti-inflammatory drugs, and both iron and potassium preparations, may injure the esophageal mucosa directly and produce 'pill esophagitis' [7]. Most patients with pill esophagitis will complain of odynophagia as well as heartburn, chest pain, and dysphagia. If at all possible, use of medications that aggravate GERD, whether by increasing reflux of gastric contents or by irritating the esophageal mucosa directly, should be reduced in patients with symptomatic GERD.

For many years, antacids were the mainstay of therapy for patients with symptomatic GERD. Even in 1996, antacids remain the agent of choice when patients self-medicate for heartburn because they provide rapid relief, presumably by neutralizing gastric and esophageal acidity. Some investigators have suggested, however, that heartburn is relieved not by acid neutralization, but by the primary esophageal peristaltic wave stimulated by swallowing antacids, which rapidly clears the esophagus of refluxate. Alginic acid has been added to antacids in an attempt to improve efficacy. Antacid/alginic acid combinations produce a hydrophobic viscous 'raft' that floats on the liquid meniscus within the stomach. Whether this viscous layer selectively delivers antacid into the esophagus during reflux episodes or acts as a mechanical barrier to diminish reflux, or both, has not been clearly determined [8, 10, 11]. Antacid/alginic acid combinations are available in liquid and tablet forms.

Another 'nonsystemic' agent sometimes employed in phase I therapy is sucralfate [12–14]. Sucralfate has a multifaceted mode of action: (i) it binds to exposed protein, providing a protective mechanical barrier against back-diffusion of acid and mucosal exposure to the potentially toxic refluxate; (ii) it binds to bile acids and pepsin; and (iii) it releases endogenous prostaglandins, which may be protective in the upper gastrointestinal (GI) tract. The clinical efficacy of sucralfate in acute GERD has not been firmly established, although some studies have suggested symptomatic relief and mucosal healing of esophagitis. Sucralfate is available in both tablet and suspension preparations.

Recently, over-the-counter (OTC) histamine-2 receptor antagonists (HRAs) have become available in many parts of the world. OTC HRAs are in subprescription doses and are not truly nonsystemic.

Use of systemic agent to treat GERD (phase II)

Although many patients with GERD respond adequately to nonsystemic treatment, the majority of those who seek physician care for symptomatic GERD have already implemented and failed to respond to most of the lifestyle changes as well as the nonsystemic agents outlined above. HRAs have been the cornerstone of medical treatment for GERD. By decreasing acid output and the volume of parietal cell secretions, HRAs raise the pH of gastric contents. Four HRAs are currently available in North America: cimetidine [15–17], ranitidine [18, 19], famotidine [20], and nizatidine [21, 22] (Table 4.3). Although numerous studies have demonstrated the safety and efficacy of the HRAs in diminishing the symptoms of GERD, about 25–40% of patients may not experience symptomatic relief [23, 24]. Some 40–60% of GERD patients with reflux esophagitis will not experience full mucosal healing with standard doses of HRAs [25–30]. Symptomatic relief of GERD requires greater suppression of acid secretion than is required for patients with a duodenal or gastric ulcer [31]. Therefore, twice-daily dosing with the HRAs is recommended. To achieve consistent healing of reflux esophagitis (>70% at 12 weeks), even greater acid suppression is often necessary, requiring yet higher doses of HRA [19, 31].

As a group, the HRAs are among the safest drugs currently in use to treat any disorder. Nevertheless, a few side effects have been reported. Cimetidine, by virtue of its imidazole ring, may affect the hepatic cytochrome P450 (CYP) mixed-function oxidase system and alter the

Table 4.3 Duration of action and dosing of HRA in GERD.

Agent	Duration of action of single hs dose (hour)	Recommended dosage for symptom relief	Recommended dosage for healing of esophagitis
Cimetidine	6–8	300 mg qid 400 mg bid	800 mg bid 400 mg qid
Ranitidine	8–12	150 mg bid	150 mg qid
Famotidine	10–12	20 mg bid	20–40 mg bid
Nizatidine	10–12	150 mg bid	150 mg bid

hs, at bedtime.

metabolism of some coadministered pharmaceutical agents. In addition, cimetidine in high doses has been reported to cause gynecomastia, impotence, and mental confusion. High doses of ranitidine have been associated with mild, transient elevations in hepatic transaminases. Famotidine has been reported to have a deleterious effect on cardiac output. Nizatidine has received relatively infrequent use compared with the other HRAs, and therefore little has been written about its side effects. Overall, few clinically significant side effects have been reported with the HRAs.

Despite their safety record and symptomatic efficacy in most patients, several observations have caused some gastroenterologists to question not only the routine first-line use of HRAs in GERD, but also their long-term use for maintenance.

1 At standard twice-daily dosing of HRAs, partial symptomatic relief and nonhealing of esophageal erosions may occur in up to 20% and 50%, respectively, of patients with symptomatic reflux esophagitis [15–30].

2 Increased dosing with HRAs, which is often required to achieve healing, can be expensive.

3 Questions have arisen about the effect of long-term gastric acid suppression on the bacterial flora of the stomach [32, 33].

Some investigators have proposed a relationship between chronic acid suppression and adenocarcinoma in the distal esophagus and proximal stomach [34], which has increased fivefold over the past 25 years [35]. Before this increase can be attributed to acid suppression and bacterial overgrowth, much more information will be required.

A prokinetic drug that reduces gastroesophageal reflux and decreases the contact time between the potentially toxic gastric refluxate and the esophageal mucosa by stimulating distal esophageal contractions, by improving esophageal clearance, and by avoiding gastric distention is an attractive alternative. A prokinetic drug might be especially useful when heartburn is accompanied by no, or mild, esophagitis or by symptoms such as regurgitation, excessive nocturnal choking, coughing, wheezing, nausea, or abdominal bloating with distention, suggestive of a diffuse motility disturbance. Four prokinetic agents are listed in Table 4.4.

Cisapride, a prokinetic agent associated with few serious side effects, might be considered as first-line systemic treatment in some routine cases. Cisapride acts by selectively activating 5-hydroxytryptamine (5-HT, or serotoninergic) receptors and thereby releasing acetylcholine from the myenteric plexus throughout most regions of the luminal GI tract [36–39]. It increases LES pressure; stimulates contractions in the esophagus, stomach, small intestine, colon, and gallbladder; and improves antro-duodenal coordination across the pylorus. In contrast to other available prokinetic agents, cisapride is a panprokinetic agent, acting throughout the GI tract. Recent studies have demonstrated that cisapride diminishes heartburn and promotes healing in many patients with symptomatic GERD and esophagitis [36–40]. Two multicenter, placebo-controlled trials in the USA and Canada formed the basis for the US Food and Drug Administration (FDA) approval of cisapride to treat nocturnal heartburn [41, 42].

Side effects reported with cisapride include diarrhea, cramping abdominal discomfort, constipation, and headache. Cisapride is metab-olized mainly by the CYP 3A4 isoenzyme. Coadministration of cisapride with drugs that inhibit this isoenzyme may result in high plasma levels of cisapride and produce cardiac arrhythmias, including ventricular tachy-cardia, ventricular fibrillation, torsades de pointes, and prolongation of the QT interval. As a result, cisapride is contraindicated in patients taking ketoconazole, itraconazole, miconazole, troleandomycin, erythromycin, fluconazole, or clarithromycin [43].

Medical treatment for refractory GERD (phase III)

When reflux symptoms fail to resolve or when esophagitis does not heal in response to phase II treatment with an HRA or with cisapride, there are three options:
1   to use a combination of regular-dose HRA with a prokinetic agent;
2   to increase the dose or the dosing frequency of the HRA (see Table 4.3);
3   to use a proton pump inhibitor (PPI) such as omeprazole or lanso-prazole.

Table 4.4 Effects of prokinetic drugs for GERD.

Agent	Elimination half-life (hour)	Dosage	Esophageal contraction	LES pressure	Gastric emptying
Bethanechol	1*	Up to 25 mg qid†	Increased	Increased	No effect
Metoclopramide	4–6	FDA: 10–15 mg qid HPB: 5–10 mg qid	Increased	Increased	Accelerated
Cisapride	7–10	FDA: 10–20 mg qid HPB: 5–10 mg qid *or* 20 mg bid	Increased	Increased	Accelerated
Domperidone	7.5	FDA:† HPB: 10–20 mg qid	No effect	Increased	Accelerated

* Usual duration of action.
† Not FDA approved for GERD.
FDA, US Food and Drug Administration (dosage information obtained from *Physicians' Desk Reference*, 47th edn. Montvale, NJ: Medical Economics Data, 1995); HPB, Health Protection Branch (dosage information obtained from *Compendium of Pharmaceuticals and Specialties*, 28th edn. Ottawa, Ontario: Canadian Pharmaceutical Association, 1993).

If high-dose HRA or a PPI is ineffective, a prokinetic agent may be added.

When reflux symptoms are refractory to an HRA or to cisapride alone, a reasonable option is to administer combination therapy with a regular-dose HRA and a prokinetic agent. Several studies [44, 45] have demonstrated better results with combination therapy than with an HRA alone.

Reflux disease refractory to standard doses of HRAs or to combination therapy may be due to gastric acid hypersecretion characterized by a basal acid output (BAO) greater than 10 mEq/hour [23, 31, 46]. Failure to reduce BAO to less than 1 mEq/hour may result in persistent heartburn or failure to heal esophagitis. More effective suppression of acid secretion, with consequent symptomatic relief and healing of esophagitis, has been reported with increased dosages and increased frequency of dosing of HRAs. For example, enhanced efficacy has been reported with 300 mg twice a day (bid) of ranitidine and nizatidine and 40 mg bid of famotidine, as well as with greater dosing frequency of ranitidine (150–300 mg four times a day (qid)) [19–21, 47].

A third option in patients with refractory GERD is to use a PPI such as omeprazole or, more recently, lansoprazole, at doses of 20 or 30 mg, respectively, once or twice daily [25–27, 48–50]. PPIs are a particularly attractive alternative for patients whose symptoms do not respond satisfactorily to an HRA, a prokinetic agent, or combination therapy, and for patients with moderate to severe (grades III and IV) esophagitis. Both omeprazole and lansoprazole are substituted benzimidazoles which inhibit the proton pump (hydrogen/potassium ion adenosine triphosphatase (ATPase) enzyme) within the parietal cells of the stomach by noncompetitive irreversible antagonism. This enzyme is the final common step in the acid secretory pathway. Controlled trials (25–27, 48–50] assessing PPIs have shown earlier improvement in reflux symptoms and greater endoscopic healing of reflux esophagitis when compared to conventional doses of HRAs. PPIs are particularly effective in patients refractory to HRA treatment and in those with severe or complicated mucosal lesions, as manifested by grade III or IV esophagitis, benign esophageal stricture, confluent distal erosions, or deep ulcerations in an underlying Barrett's epithelium. The enhanced clinical efficacy of PPIs over HRAs is related directly to a greater degree of acid suppression [51]. Omeprazole and lansoprazole appear to be equally effective in achieving potent acid suppression. Differences between the two PPIs include a more rapid onset of action and an absence of effect on CYP with lansoprazole. More extensive experience will determine whether these differences or other as yet unrecognized differences will separate these agents clinically.

Suppression of gastric acid secretion can be a two-edged sword, however. Lansoprazole has been available only for a short time; thus, most of the available literature on PPIs concerns omeprazole. Omeprazole can render patients hypochlorhydric or even achlorhydric, and it would not be surprising if bacterial proliferation in the proximal GI tract were to occur, as has been observed with antacids and HRA [32, 33]. In addition, increased release of gastrin from antral G cells has been reported [52–54]. There may be adverse long-term consequences of the short-term use of omeprazole. After administration of omeprazole for 8–12 weeks, recurrences of symptoms or esophagitis have been reported in up to 60% of patients at 4 months and 82% at 6 months [48]. While some investigators have attributed the high recurrence rates to a selection bias toward refractory patients, others [55, 56] have suggested that omeprazole may induce parietal cell hyperplasia with consequent rebound acid hypersecretion.

The FDA indication for omeprazole has been short-term (4–12 weeks) use in treating refractory heartburn or in healing moderate to severe endoscopic reflux esophagitis. Recently, the FDA approved long-term use of omeprazole for refractory GERD symptoms and severe esophagitis. The FDA indication for lansoprazole is for up to 16 weeks' use for relief of reflux symptoms and healing of erosive esophagitis.

When patients do not respond to regular-dose HRA plus a prokinetic agent, or to high-dose HRA or a PPI alone, another option is to add a prokinetic agent to the high-dose HRA or the PPI. For reasons stated earlier, cisapride is the prokinetic agent of first choice. Studies [44, 45] suggest that cisapride in combination with cimetidine or ranitidine improves the symptomatic and healing responses in patients with GERD, compared to HRA alone.

Because of their side-effect profiles, metoclopramide and bethanechol are usually reserved in phase III therapy, for patients who have not responded to acid-suppressive therapy, with an HRA or PPI, in combination with cisapride. Metoclopramide is a dopamine antagonist that also augments the effect of acetylcholine at cholinergic receptors within the enteric nervous system [57, 58]. It increases LES pressure, improves esophageal clearance, decreases gastroesophageal reflux, and accelerates stomach emptying [59–62]. At a dose of 10 mg 30 minutes before meals and at bedtime, metoclopramide has been reported to improve reflux symptoms better than placebo, and as well as HRA [63–66]. Healing of esophagitis has not been demonstrated convincingly with metoclopramide alone, but when used in conjunction with an HRA such as cimetidine, healing rates were accelerated compared with cimetidine alone [67]. The use of metoclopramide has been limited by its safety profile. About 20–40% of patients experience lethargy, stupor, somnolence, agitation, akathisia, galactorrhea, extrapyramidal reactions sometimes simulating Parkinson's disease, or tardive dyskinesia [68]. These side effects are dose related and almost always reversible.

Bethanechol, a cholinomimetic agent, increases the amplitudes of the resting LES pressure and esophageal contractions [69–71]. Another potentially salutary effect is increased secretion of saliva, which contains bicarbonate. Several studies [72, 73] in children and adults have demonstrated improvement of GERD symptoms and healing of esophagitis in patients treated with bethanechol alone or in conjunction with an HRA. The adult recommended dosage of bethanechol, 25 mg 0.5 hours before meals and at bedtime, has been associated with bladder spasm, urinary frequency, abdominal cramps, blurred vision, or wheezing [74].

Domperidone, a peripheral dopamine antagonist, stimulates the upper GI tract in a similar pattern to metoclopramide. Trials [75–78] evaluating the clinical efficacy of domperidone in GERD have produced inconsistent results. Domperidone does not readily cross the blood–brain barrier, and thus has few central nervous system side effects. As with metoclopramide, domperidone is associated with hyperprolactinemia, resulting in breast enlargement, nipple tenderness, galactorrhea, and amenorrhea in some women. Domperidone has been approved for clinical use in Canada and Europe, but is not yet available in the USA.

Published studies assessing combination therapy of a prokinetic agent with a PPI for acute treatment of GERD are very limited. There are no studies showing that single-agent therapy with a prokinetic agent at any dosage is effective in cases of GERD refractory to HRA or PPI.

Antireflux surgery (phase IV)

Safe and effective surgical procedures that may be considered for patients with severe or refractory GERD include Nissen fundoplication [79], the Hill posterior gastropexy, the Belsey Mark IV gastropexy, and variations of these classic procedures [80, 81]. In each of these techniques, the distal esophagus is anchored below the diaphragm by wrapping the gastric fundus around the abdominal portion of the esophagus and suturing it in place. The procedures differ from each other in surgical approach and extent of the fundal wrap. In a 2-year study, Spechler and associates [82] suggested that antireflux surgery was more effective in controlling reflux symptoms and healing esophagitis long term than medical treatment (comprising lifestyle modifications, antacids, standard-dose HRA, and, in some patients, metoclopramide and sucralfate). This study did not employ high-dose HRAs, PPIs, or cisapride. The investigators stressed, however, that both a well-documented diagnosis and a surgeon skilled at antireflux procedures are essential for a successful outcome.

Antireflux surgery is indicated if benign esophageal strictures, deep esophageal ulcers, or severe erosive esophagitis do not respond to or are not prevented by medical treatment. When gastroesophageal reflux is documented in patients with recurrent asthma or pneumonia that cannot be controlled despite specific treatment of the pulmonary disorder and a vigorous medical antireflux regimen, surgical treatment should be considered. Antireflux surgery is also a therapeutic option in: (i) GERD patients with intractable symptoms and documented reflux; and (ii) young individuals whose symptoms require extensive, inconvenient lifestyle modifications and multiple or potentially expensive medications. Although Barrett's epithelium does not revert to a normal stratified squamous epithelium after either vigorous medical or surgical antireflux treatment, surgery is sometimes employed in selected cases with or without distal esophageal resection. Laparoscopic antireflux surgery was introduced recently [83, 84]. Reports to date suggest that it is safe and effective. Laparoscopic fundoplication is theoretically associated with reduced postoperative morbidity, a decrease in duration of hospital stay, and a shorter downtime before patients can return to work. This new technique may play a significant role in future short-term and long-term strategies for treating patients with GERD.

Empiric treatment of GERD (by physicians)

Empiric treatment by physicians without extensive testing is appropriate and cost-effective for many patients with classic reflux symptoms. Empiric treatment usually consists of lifestyle modifications, nonsystemic antacids (phase I), and systemic treatment either with an HRA in a twice-daily dosage or with cisapride (phase II). In the presence of alarm (trigger) symptoms, such as anorexia, weight loss, dysphagia, odynophagia, vomiting, blood in the stools, and pulmonary symptoms, empiric treatment should not be employed. Additionally, institution of treatment prior to diagnostic testing is unwarranted: (i) when reflux symptoms are very severe; (ii) when symptoms are refractory after 2 weeks of empiric treatment; and (iii) when symptoms recur after discontinuation of empiric treatment. High-risk patients with severe coincident diseases in whom a complication of GERD might be devastating also are not candidates for empiric treatment.

Maintenance therapy for GERD

There is general agreement that GERD is a chronic relapsing disorder. Although recurrent reflux symptoms and mild esophagitis can be controlled in some cases by nonsystemic measures (phase I), many patients with GERD will experience rapid clinical or endoscopic relapse when a successful antireflux treatment program is discontinued. In 1988 Hetzel *et al.* [48] demonstrated 60% and 82% relapse rates of endoscopically confirmed esophagitis within 4 and 6 months, respectively, of discontinuation of treatment in patients originally healed by omeprazole. Subsequent studies have shown the relapse rate for esophagitis to range from 23 to 96% at 12 months when acute treatment is discontinued without maintenance therapy after complete healing has been achieved (Figures 4.2 & 4.3) [38, 48, 85–94].

Data on placebo-controlled maintenance studies after acute healing by an HRA or prokinetic agent are limited. Two recent trials have compared maintenance (long-term) treatment with HRA versus omeprazole in patients healed initially by omeprazole. In a study by Hallerback *et al.* [86], patients receiving maintenance omeprazole, 10 and 20 mg qd, experienced 12-month endoscopic recurrence rates of 42 and 23%, respectively, and 12-month symptomatic recurrence rates of 38 and 28%, respectively. The endoscopic and symptomatic recurrence rates for both omeprazole regimens were significantly lower than the 54–55% rates reported for maintenance ranitidine 150 mg bid. Significantly lower 12-month endoscopic recurrence rates were also reported by Dent *et al.* [87] for omeprazole 20 mg qd versus ranitidine 150 mg bid (11% versus 75%, respectively).

Lieberman [95] suggested that higher LES pressures may play a role in GERD patients who were maintained in remission for more than 2 years than in those who experienced a relapse (13.1 versus 4.9 mmHg, respectively). A potential role for prokinetic agents in the long-term maintenance therapy for GERD has been supported by several recent 6- and 12-month studies [39, 90, 91]. In a European multicenter study involving 443 patients with grade I or II esophagitis healed initially with conventional

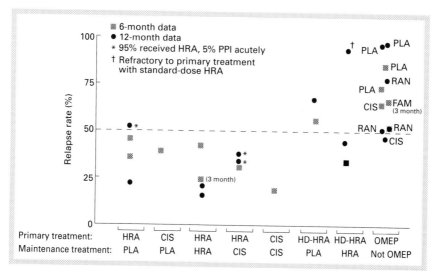

Fig. 4.2 Relapse rates of GERD: effect of HRA, cisapride, and omeprazole as the primary healing agent. Relapse rates are shown on the y-axis. The agent employed for initial (primary) healing of esophagitis is shown on the first horizontal line; the mode of maintenance treatment is shown on the second line. Six-month recurrence rates are designated by squares and 1-year recurrence rates by circles. CIS, cisapride; HD-HRA, high-dose histamine receptor antagonist; HRA, histamine receptor antagonist (standard twice-daily dosing); OMEP, omeprazole; PLA, placebo. References: HRA/PLA [88–91]; CIS/PLA [38]; HRA/HRA [88, 89, 92]; HRA/CIS [90, 91]; CIS/CIS [38]; HD-HRA/PLA (R.M. Murdock, personal communication); HD-HRA/HRA [85] (R.M. Murdock, personal communication); OMEP/Not OMEP [48, 86, 87, 91–94].

regimens of HRA or omeprazole [90], endoscopic recurrence rates at 12 months were significantly lower with cisapride 10 mg bid (34%) and 20 mg hs (32%) than with placebo (51%). Of interest, 94.5% of these patients achieved healing of esophagitis with an acute course of HRA; only 4.5% required omeprazole.

Recently, Italian investigators [93] reported that omeprazole alone at a dosage of 20 mg qd resulted in significantly lower endoscopic recurrences than other single-agent regimens (ranitidine 150 mg three times a day (tid) and cisapride 10 mg tid) after acute healing by omeprazole. Of interest, the combination of omeprazole plus cisapride was more effective than cisapride alone, and the combination of ranitidine and cisapride was more effective than ranitidine alone. Another recent study [94] showed that patients who were treated acutely with omeprazole 20 mg qd plus cisapride 5 mg tid and who subsequently received a maintenance regimen of cisapride 5 mg tid achieved a greater endoscopic remission rate than patients receiving only omeprazole 20 mg qd acutely and no maintenance

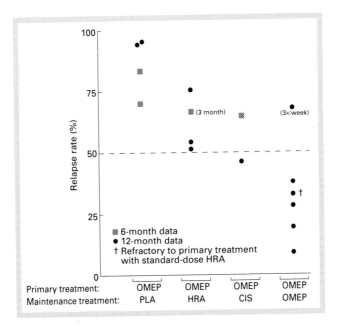

Fig. 4.3 Relapse rates of GERD after acute healing by omeprazole. Relapse rates are shown on the *y*-axis. The use of omeprazole for initial (primary) healing of esophagitis is shown on the first horizontal line; the mode of maintenance treatment is shown on the second line. Six-month recurrence rates are designated by squares and 1-year recurrence rates by circles. CIS, cisapride; HRA, histamine receptor antagonist (standard twice-daily dosing); OMEP, omeprazole; PLA, placebo. References: OMEP/PLA [48, 91, 94]; OMEP/HRA [86, 87, 92, 93]; OMEP/CIS [91, 93]; OMEP/OMEP [85–87, 93].

treatment. Another recent study [96] reported that sucralfate in a 2-g suspension bid significantly reduced endoscopic recurrences at 6 months compared to placebo (31% versus 65%, respectively).

A review of the maintenance literature indicates that GERD patients treated acutely with regular-dose HRA or cisapride experience relapse rates of less than 45% at 6 and 12 months on discontinuation of the acute regimen [39, 88–91]. When maintenance regimens with HRA or cisapride are employed, recurrence rates are below 35% in most cases. In contrast, when omeprazole is used for acute treatment, recurrence rates approximate 70–80% at 6 and 12 months in patients receiving placebo maintenance. These provocative observations suggest that the mode of initial antireflux therapy may affect the agent required to achieve long-term remission: for patients treated previously with omeprazole, only omeprazole will be effective in maintaining remission [85–87, 97]. In contrast, if either an HRA or cisapride is used successfully in acute treatment, one may expect successful maintenance with either agent [39, 89–91]. Further studies will be needed to determine the role of selection bias in the high recurrence rates observed with omeprazole.

Another confounding factor when interpreting maintenance data is the severity of reflux esophagitis at the time of initial treatment. In general, HRAs and prokinetic drugs are more successful in controlling symptoms and healing esophagitis in patients with endoscopy-negative GERD and grades I and II reflux esophagitis. About 70–80% of patients with GERD fit these categories. A prospective long-term study [98] conducted in Barcelona in 107 patients with symptomatic GERD provides further insight on long-term outcomes in this patient group. All study participants were treated for 2 months with lifestyle modifications, high-dose antacid, and domperidone. If no clinical response was observed, an HRA, either cimetidine or ranitidine, was added to the regimen for an additional 6 months. If there was no response to the combination regimen, patients underwent antireflux surgery. A number of interesting observations were reported.

1   Of these patients with symptomatic GERD, 51% had normal endoscopic examinations and 20% had grade I esophagitis.

2   Approximately one-third of patients responded to the initial treatment, while another one-third required the addition of HRA to achieve relief, and the final one-third went on to antireflux surgery.

3   At 3- and 6-year follow-up, more than 80% of patients who responded initially to non-HRA, nonsurgical therapy could be maintained on non-HRA, nonsurgical treatment.

4   Of those patients initially requiring HRA, more than 60% could be 'stepped down' to non-HRA, nonsurgical treatment.

This study suggests that most patients with symptomatic GERD can be maintained over the long term with phase I nonsystemic treatment plus a prokinetic agent.

Thus, several choices for maintaining GERD patients in remission have been evaluated in clinical trials (Table 4.5). In the USA, only ranitidine and omeprazole have received FDA approval for maintenance therapy. On the other hand, the HRAs, the PPIs, and cisapride are used for maintenance therapy in Canada and many European countries.

The long-term safety profiles of PPIs remain unresolved. Long-term use of omeprazole with hypergastrinemia has clearly stimulated enterochromaffin-like (ECL) cell hyperplasia. In rats, this may be associated with the development of carcinoid tumors of the stomach. Development of carcinoid tumors with omeprazole has not been observed in humans,

Table 4.5 Maintenance therapy for GERD.

HRA	
Ranitidine	150 mg bid*
Cimetidine	400 mg bid
Famotidine	20 mg bid
Nizatidine	150 mg bid
Prokinetic agent	
Cisapride	10–20 mg bid†
	20 mg hs†
PPI	
Omeprazole	20 mg od*†
	? 10 mg od
Lansoprazole	30 mg od
Lifestyle modifications	
+	
High-dose antacids (20 mEq ANC 1 and 3 hpc)	
+/−	
Domperidone (10 mg 30 minutes ac)	

* FDA approved.
† Indicated in Canada, UK, and other countries.
bid, two times a day; hs, at bedtime; ANC, acid-neutralizing capacity; hpc, hours after eating; ac, before meals.

however. The potential consequences of long-term potent acid suppression include atrophic gastritis, gastrin levels greater than 500 pg/ml in more than 10% of patients, and perhaps parietal cell hyperplasia [54–56]. The role of *Helicobacter pylori* in some of these phenomena has not yet been clearly defined.

Summary

This chapter discusses a stepped approach to treating patients with symptomatic GERD. Management options begin with empiric treatment using nonsystemic agents, but also utilizing HRA and cisapride when necessary as part of empiric treatment. In refractory patients, once a diagnosis of GERD is established, medical treatment may proceed to HRAs in high-dose regimens, to PPIs in single-agent regimens, or to combination regimens of standard/high-dose HRA or PPI plus a prokinetic agent. Antireflux surgery should be considered in selected patients. Some guidelines for empiric treatment of GERD are suggested. Readers are reminded that many patients with symptomatic GERD will likely require long-term maintenance to minimize symptomatic and endoscopic recurrence. The efficacy of an agent for long-term maintenance may well be affected by the treatment employed initially to achieve clinical remission. PPIs and high-dose HRAs should be reserved for patients who do not respond to either an HRA or cisapride alone and for those who present with complicated GERD, as indicated by grade III or IV endoscopic esophagitis, a benign esophageal stricture, or Barrett's esophagus.

References

1 Nebel OT, Fornes MF, Castell DO. Symptomatic gastroesophageal reflux: incidence and precipitating factors. *Am J Dig Dis* 1976;**21**:953–6.
2 Heartburn across America: a Gallup Organization national survey. Princeton: The Gallup Organization, 1988.
3 Prevalence, behavior and knowledge of gastrointestinal disorders. Princeton: The Gallup Organization, 1995.
4 Jones RH, Lydeard SE, Hobbs FDR *et al.* Dyspepsia in England and Scotland. *Gut* 1990;**31**:401–5.
5 Ahtaridis G, Snape WJ Jr, Cohen S. Lower esophageal sphincter pressure as an index of gastroesophageal acid reflux. *Dig Dis Sci* 1981;**26**:993–8.
6 Holloway RH, Hongo M, Berger K, McCallum RW. Gastric distention: a mechanism for postprandial gastroesophageal reflux. *Gastroenterology* 1985;**89**:799–84.
7 Castell DO. Medical therapy for reflux esophagitis: 1986 and beyond. *Ann Intern Med* 1986;**104**:112–14.
8 Johnson LF, DeMeester TR. Evaluation of elevation of the head of the bed, bethanechol, and antacid foam tablets on gastroesophageal reflux. *Dig Dis Sci* 1981;**26**:673–80.
9 Hamilton JW, Boisen RJ, Yamamoto DT, Wagner JL, Reichelderfer M. Sleeping on a wedge diminishes exposure of the esophagus to refluxed acid. *Dig Dis Sci* 1988;**33**:518–22.
10 Barnardo DE, Lancaster-Smith M, Strickland ID, Wright JT. A double-blind controlled trial of 'Gaviscon' in patients with symptomatic gastro-oesophageal reflux. *Curr Med Res Opin* 1975;**3**:388–91.
11 Castell DO, Boag Dalton C, Becker D, Sinclair J, Castell JA. Alginic acid decreases postprandial upright reflux: comparison with equal-strength antacid. *Dig Dis Sci* 1992;**37**:589–93.
12 Williams RM, Orlando RC, Bozymski EM *et al.* Multicenter trial of sucralfate suspension for the treatment of reflux esophagitis. *Am J Med* 1987;**83**(Suppl.3B):61–6.
13 Simon B, Mueller P. Comparison of the effect of sucralfate and ranitidine in reflux esophagitis. *Am J Med* 1987;**83**(Suppl.3B):43–7.
14 Elsborg L. Oesophageal reflux disease: diagnosis, pathophysiology and treatment with special reference to the role of sucralfate. *Scand J Gastroenterol* 1987;**22**(Suppl.127):101–9.
15 Behar J, Brand DL, Brown FC *et al.* Cimetidine in the treatment of symptomatic gastroesophageal reflux: a double blind controlled trial. *Gastroenterology* 1978;**74**:441–8.
16 Wesdorp E, Bartelsman J, Pape K, Dekker W, Tytgat GN. Oral cimetidine in reflux esophagitis: a double blind controlled trial. *Gastroenterology* 1978;**74**:821–4.

17 Palmer RH, Frank WO, Rockhold FW, Wetherington JD, Young MD. Cimetidine 800 mg twice daily for healing erosions and ulcers in gastroesophageal reflux disease. *J Clin Gastroenterol* 1990;**12**(Suppl.2):S29–34.

18 Sontag S, Robinson M, McCallum RW, Barwick KW, Nardi R. Ranitidine therapy for gastroesophageal reflux disease: results of a large double-blind trial. *Arch Intern Med* 1987;**147**:1485–91.

19 Roufail W, Belsito A, Robinson M, Barish C, Rubin A. Ranitidine for erosive esophagitis: a double-blind, placebo-controlled study. *Aliment Pharmacol Ther* 1992;**6**:597–607.

20 Sabesin SM, Berlin RG, Humphries TJ *et al.* Famotidine relieves symptoms of gastroesophageal reflux disease and heals erosions and ulcerations. *Arch Intern Med* 1991;**151**:2394–400.

21 Quik RPF, Cooper MJ, Gleeson M *et al.* A comparison of two doses of nizatidine versus placebo in the treatment of reflux oesophagitis. *Aliment Pharmacol Ther* 1990;**4**:201–11.

22 Cloud ML, Offen WW, Robinson M. Nizatidine versus placebo in gastroesophageal reflux disease: a 12-week, multicenter, randomized, double-blind study. *Am J Gastroenterol* 1991;**86**:1735–42.

23 Colin-Jones DG. Histamine-2-receptor antagonists in gastro-oesophageal reflux. *Gut* 1989;**30**:1305–8.

24 Pope C E II. Acid-reflux disorders. *N Engl J Med* 1994;**331**:656–60.

25 Klinkenberg-Knol EC, Jansen JMBJ, Festen HPM, Meuwissen SGM, Lamers CBHW. Double-blind multicentre comparison of omeprazole and ranitidine in the treatment of reflux oesophagitis. *Lancet* 1987;**1**:349–51.

26 Havelund T, Laursen LS, Skoubo-Kristensen E *et al.* Omeprazole and ranitidine in treatment of reflux oesophagitis: double blind comparative trial. *B M J* 1988;**296**:89–92.

27 Vantrappen G, Rutgeerts L, Schurmans P, Coenegrachts J-L. Omeprazole (40 mg) is superior to ranitidine in short-term treatment of ulcerative reflux esophagitis. *Dig Dis Sci* 1988;**33**:523–9.

28 Sandmark S, Carlsson R, Fausa O, Lundell L. Omeprazole or ranitidine in the treatment of reflux esophagitis: results of a double-blind, randomized, Scandinavian multicenter study. *Scand J Gastroenterol* 1988;**23**:625–32.

29 Zeitoun P, Rampal P, Barbier P, Isal JP, Eriksson S, Carlsson R. Omeprazole (20 mg o.m.) versus ranitidine (150 mg b.i.d.) in reflux esophagitis: results of a double-blind randomized trial. *Gastroenterol Clin Biol* 1989;**13**:457–62.

30 The Italian Reflux Oesophagitis Study Group. Omeprazole produces significantly greater healing of erosive or ulcerative reflux oesophagitis than ranitidine. *Eur J Gastroenterol Hepatol* 1991;**3**:511–17.

31 Collen MJ, Lewis JH, Benjamin SB. Gastric acid hypersecretion in refractory gastroesophageal reflux disease. *Gastroenterology* 1990;**98**:654–61.

32 Goularte TA, Lichtenberg DA, Craven DE. Gastric colonization in patients receiving antacids and medicinal modalities: a mechanism for pharyngeal colonization. *Am J Infect Control* 1986;**14**:88.

33 Driks MR, Craven DE, Celli BR *et al.* Nosocomial pneumonia in intubated patients given sucralfate as compared with antacids or histamine type 2 blockers: the role of gastric colonization. *N Engl J Med* 1987;**317**:1376–82.

34 Edoga JK *et al.* G E R D surgery revisited. *Laparoscopy in Focus* 1994;**2**:1–4.

35 Pera M, Cameron AJ, Trastek VF, Carpenter HA, Zinsmeister AR. Increasing incidence of adenocarcinoma of the esophagus and esophagogastric junction. *Gastroenterology* 1993;**104**:510–13.

36 Cucchiara S, Staiano A, Capozzi C, Di Lorenzo C, Boccieri A, Auricchio S. Cisapride for gastro-oesophageal reflux and peptic oesophagitis. *Arch Dis Child* 1987;**62**:454–7.

37 McCallum RW, Prakash C, Campoli-Richards DM, Goa KL. Cisapride: a preliminary review of its pharmacodynamic and pharmacokinetic properties, and therapeutic use as a prokinetic agent in gastrointestinal motility disorders. *Drugs* 1988;**36**:652–81.

38 Toussaint J. Gossuin A, Deruyttere M, Huble F, Devis G. Healing and prevention of relapse of reflux esophagitis by cisapride. *Gut* 1991;**32**:1280–5.

39 Van Outryve M, Vanderlinden I, Dedullen G, Rutgeerts L. Dose–response study with cisapride in gastroesophageal reflux disease. *Curr Ther Res* 1988;**43**:408–15.

40 Wiseman LR, Faulds D. Cisapride: an updated review of its pharmacology and therapeutic efficacy as a prokinetic agent in gastrointestinal motility disorders. *Drugs* 1994;**47**:116–52.

41 Dodds W, Champion M, Orr W, Robinson M, Spechler S. Oral cisapride in GERD: a double-blind placebo-controlled multicenter trial. *Gastroenterology* 1989;**96**:A126.

42 Faruqui S, Sigmund C, Smith R *et al.* Cisapride in the treatment of GERD: a double-blind, placebo-controlled multicenter dose–response trial. *Gastroenterology* 1992;**102**:A66.

43 Propulsid. Prescribing information. Titusville, NJ: Janssen Pharmaceutica Inc, Sept 1995.

44 Galmiche JP, Brandstatter G, Evreux M *et al.* Combined therapy with cisapride and cimetidine in severe reflux oesophagitis: a double blind controlled trial. *Gut* 1988;**29**:675–81.

45 Wienbeck M, the Ranpride Study Group. Does a motor stimulating agent improve the therapeutic effect of H_2-blockers in reflux esophagitis? *Gastroenterology* 1986;**90**:A1691.

46 Collen MJ, Johnson DA, Sheridan MJ. Basal acid output and gastric acid hypersecretion in gastroesophageal reflux disease. *Dig Dis Sci* 1994;**39**:410–17.

47 Euler AR, Murdock RH Jr, Wilson TH, Silver MT, Parker SE, Powers L. Ranitidine is effective therapy for erosive esophagitis. *Am J Gastroenterol* 1993;**88**:520–4.

48 Hetzel DJ, Dent J, Reed WD *et al.* Healing and relapse of severe peptic esophagitis after treatment with omeprazole. *Gastroenterology* 1988;**95**:903–12.

49 Barradell LB, Faulds D, McTavish D. Lansoprazole: a review of its pharmacodynamic and pharmacokinetic properties and its therapeutic efficacy in acid-related disorders. *Drugs* 1992;**44**:225–50.

50 Berstad A, Hatlebakk JG. Lansoprazole in the treatment of reflux oesophagitis: a survey of clinical studies. *Aliment Pharmacol Ther* 1993;**7**(Suppl.1):34–6.

51 Brunner G, Creutzfeldt W, Harke U, Lamberts R. Efficacy and safety of long term treatment with omeprazole in patients with acid related diseases resistant to ranitidine. *Can J Gastroenterol* 1989;**3**(Suppl.A):72–6A.

52 Freston JW. Clinical significance of hypergastrinemia: relevance to gastrin monitoring during omeprazole therapy. *Digestion* 1992;**51**(Suppl.1):102–14.

53 Lamberts R, Creutzfeldt W, Struber HG, Brunner G, Solcia E. Long-term omeprazole therapy in peptic ulcer disease: gastrin, endocrine cell growth, and gastritis. *Gastroenterology* 1993;**104**:1356–70.

54 Klinkenberg-Knol EC, Festen HPM, Jansen JBMJ *et al.* Long-term treatment with omeprazole for refractory reflux esophagitis: efficacy and safety. *Ann Intern Med* 1994;**121**:161–7.

55 Weinstein WM, Ang ST, Ippoliti AF, Lieberman DA. Fundic gland polyps in patients on long term omeprazole therapy: a light and electron microscopic study of the gastric mucosa. *Gastroenterology* 1994;**106**:A210.

56 Ang ST, Lieberman DA, Ippoliti AF, Weber L, Weinstein WM. Long-term omeprazole therapy in patients with Barrett's esophagus is associated with parietal cell hyperplasia. *Gastroenterology* 1994;**106**:A1016.

57 Hay AM, Man WK. Effect of metoclopramide on guinea pig stomach: critical dependence on intrinsic stores of acetylcholine. *Gastroenterology* 1979;**76**:492–6.

58 Albibi R, McCallum RW. Metoclopramide: pharmacology and clinical application. *Ann Intern Med* 1983;**98**:86–95.

59 Dilawari JB, Misiewicz JJ. Action of oral metoclopramide on the gastrooesophageal junction in man. *Gut* 1973;**14**:380–2.

60 McCallum RW, Kline MM, Curry N, Sturdevant RAL. Comparative effects of metoclopramide and bethanechol on lower esophageal sphincter pressure in reflux patients. *Gastroenterology* 1975;**68**:1114–18.

61 Cohen S, Morris DW, Schoen HJ, DiMarino AJ. The effect of oral and intravenous metoclopramide on human lower esophageal sphincter pressure. *Gastroenterology* 1976;**70**:484–7.

62 Fink SM, Lange RC, McCallum RW. Effect of metoclopramide on normal and delayed gastric emptying in gastroesophageal reflux patients. *Dig Dis Sci* 1983;**28**:1057–61.

63 McCallum RW, Ippoliti AF, Cooney C, Sturdevant AL. A controlled trial of metoclopramide in symptomatic gastroesophageal reflux. *N Engl J Med* 1977;**296**:354–7.

64 Bright-Asare P, El-Bassoussi M. Cimetidine, metoclopramide, or placebo in the treatment of symptomatic gastroesophageal reflux. *J Clin Gastroenterol* 1980;**2**:149–56.

65 Guslandi M, Testoni PA, Passaretti S *et al.* Ranitidine vs metoclopramide in the medical treatment of reflux esophagitis. *Hepatogastroenterology* 1983;**30**:96–8.

66 Tonnesen H, Andersen JR, Christoffersen P, Kaas-Claesson N. Reflux oesophagitis in heavy drinkers: effect of ranitidine and alginate/metoclopramide. *Digestion* 1987;**38**:69–73.

67 Lieberman DA, Keeffe EB. Treatment of severe reflux esophagitis with cimetidine and metoclopramide. *Ann Intern Med* 1986;**104**:21–6.

68 Ganzini L, Casey DE, Hoffman WF, McCall AL. The prevalence of metoclopramide-induced tardive dyskinesia and acute extrapyramidal movement disorders. *Arch Intern Med* 1993;**153**:1469–75.

69 Farrell RL, Roling GT, Castell DO. Stimulation of the incompetent lower esophageal sphincter: a possible advance in therapy of heartburn. *Am J Dig Dis* 1973;**18**:646–50.

70 Hollis JB, Castell DO. Effects of cholinergic stimulation on human esophageal peristalsis. *J Appl Physiol* 1976;**40**:40–3.

71 Phaosawasdi K, Malmud LS, Tolin RD, Stelzer F, Applegate G, Fisher RS. Cholinergic effects on esophageal transit and clearance. *Gastroenterology* 1981;**81**:915–20.

72 Farrell RL, Roling GT, Castell DO. Cholinergic therapy of chronic heartburn: a controlled trial. *Ann Intern Med* 1974;**80**:573–6.

73 Thanik KD, Chey WY, Shah AN, Gutierrez JG. Reflux esophagitis: effect of oral bethanechol on symptoms and endoscopic findings. *Ann Intern Med* 1980;**93**:805–8.

74 Reynolds JC. Prokinetic agents: a key in the future of gastroenterology. *Gastroenterol Clin North Am* 1989;**18**:437–57.

75 Valenzuela JE, Defilippi C, Gutierrez F. Effect of domperidone on patients with symptomatic gastroesophageal reflux. *Dig Dis Sci* 1980;**25**:716(A-3).

76 Goethals C. Domperidone in the treatment of postprandial symptoms suggestive of gastroesophageal reflux. *Curr Ther Res* 1979;**27**:874–80.

77 Masci E, Testoni PA, Passaretti S, Guslandi M, Tittobello A. Comparison of rani-

tidine, domperidone maleate, and ranitidine + domperidone maleate in the short-term treatment of reflux oesophagitis. *Drugs Exp Clin Res* 1985;**11**:687–92.

78 Guslandi M, Dell'Oca M, Molteni V, Romano R, Passaretti S, Ballarin E. Famotidine vs domperidone versus a combination of both in the treatment of reflux esophagitis: interim report. *Gastroenterology* 1989;**96:191A.**

79 Battle WS, Nyhus LM, Bombeck CT. Nissen fundoplication and esophagitis secondary to gastroesophageal reflux. *Arch Surg* 1973;**106**:588–92.

80 Butterfield WC. Current hiatal hernia repairs: similarities, mechanisms, and extended indications — an autopsy study. *Surgery* 1971;**69**:910–16.

81 DeMeester TR, Johnson LF, Kent AH. Evaluation of current operations for the prevention of gastroesophageal reflux. *Ann Surg* 1974;**180**:511–25.

82 Spechler SJ, Department of Veterans Affairs Gastroesophageal Reflux Disease Study Group. Comparison of medical and surgical therapy for complicated gastroesophageal reflux disease in veterans. *N Engl J Med* 1992;**326**:786–92.

83 Cuschieri A, Hunter J, Wolfe B, Swanstrom LL, Hutson W. Multicenter prospective evaluation of laparoscopic antireflux surgery: preliminary report. *Surg Endosc* 1993;**7**:505–10.

84 Waring JP, Hunter JG, Oddsdottir M, Wo J, Katz E. The preoperative evaluation of patients considered for laparoscopic antireflux surgery. *Am J Gastroenterol* 1995;**90**:35–8.

85 Lundell L, Backman L, Ekstrom P *et al.* Prevention of relapse of reflux esophagitis after endoscopic healing: the efficacy and safety of omeprazole compared with ranitidine. *Scand J Gastroenterol* 1991;**26**:248–56.

86 Hallerback B, Unge P, Carling L *et al.* Omeprazole or ranitidine in long-term treatment of reflux esophagitis. *Gastroenterology* 1994;**107**:1305–11.

87 Dent J, Yeomans ND, Mackinnon M *et al.* Omeprazole v ranitidine for prevention of relapse in reflux esophagitis: a controlled double blind trial of their efficacy and safety. *Gut* 1994;**35**:590–8.

88 Koelz HR, Birchler R, Bretholz A *et al.* Healing and relapse of reflux esophagitis during treatment with ranitidine. *Gastroenterology* 1986;**91**:1198–205.

89 Berlin R, Ebel D, Cook T. Famotidine 20 HS and 40 HS vs placebo in the maintenance therapy of reflux esophagitis: results of a double-blind, multicenter trial. *Gastroenterology* 1989;**96**:A39.

90 Blum AL, Adami B, Bouzo MH *et al.* Effect of cisapride on relapse of esophagitis: a multinational, placebo-controlled trial in patients healed with an antisecretory drug. *Dig Dis Sci* 1993;**38**:551–60.

91 Tytgat GNJ, Anker Hansen OJ, Carling L *et al.* Effect of cisapride on relapse of reflux oesophagitis, healed with an antisecretory drug. *Scand J Gastroenterol* 1992;**27**:175–83.

92 Bianchi-Porro G, Pace F, Sangaletti O *et al.* High-dose famotidine in the maintenance treatment of refractory esophagitis: results of a 'medium-term' open study. *Am J Gastroenterol* 1991;**86**:1585–7.

93 Vigneri S, Termini R, Leandro G *et al.* A comparison of five maintenance therapies for reflux esophagitis. *N Engl J Med* 1995;**333**:1106–10.

94 Kimmig JM. Treatment and prevention of relapse of mild oesophagitis with omeprazole and cisapride: comparison of two strategies. *Aliment Pharmacol Ther* 1995;**9**:281–6.

95 Lieberman DA. Medical therapy for chronic reflux esophagitis: long-term follow-up. *Arch Intern Med* 1987;**147**:1717–20.

96 Tytgat GNJ, Koelz H-R, Vosmaer GDC. Sucralfate maintenance therapy in reflux esophagitis. *Am J Gastroenterol* 1995;**90**:1233–7.

97 Antonson CW, Robinson MG, Hawkins TM, McIntosh DL, Campbell DR. High doses of histamine antagonists do not prevent relapses of peptic esophagitis following therapy with a proton pump inhibitor. *Gastroenterology* 1990;**98**:A16.
98 Kuster E, Ros E, Toledo-Pimentel V *et al*. Predictive factors of the long term outcome in gastro-oesophageal reflux disease: six year follow up of 107 patients. *Gut* 1994;**35**:8–14.

« 5 »
Gastroparesis: Pathogenesis and Evaluation

John G. Moore

Delayed gastric emptying in the absence of mechanical obstruction is known as gastroparesis. It is an uncommon, though well-known, complication of diabetes (gastroparesis diabeticorum) and may contribute to symptoms in subsets of patients with gastroesophageal reflux disease and irritable bowel syndrome, two common disorders in Western societies [1, 2]. Patients with gastroparesis may be asymptomatic, or they may display a gamut of upper gastrointestinal (GI) symptoms, including, alone or in combination, persistent belching, bloating, abdominal pain, anorexia, early satiety, nausea with or without vomiting, and weight loss. In some patients, these symptoms may be life threatening. Indeed, gastric bypass or surgical revisions are sometimes employed as 'last-ditch' treatments, and in up to 20% of patients with chronic gastroparesis, long-term nutritional supplementation may be required [3]. In this chapter, the pathogenesis and both the traditional and newer approaches to the evaluation of this disorder are reviewed.

Pathogenesis

Delayed gastric emptying has a variety of mechanical and nonmechanical causes, as listed in Table 5.1. In the clinical setting, the symptoms of delayed gastric emptying due to mechanical causes cannot be distinguished reliably from those due to nonmechanical causes (i.e. gastroparesis) and, therefore, the more frequent conditions associated with gastric outlet obstruction (e.g. a peptic ulcer or tumor) must first be addressed and ruled out. 'True' gastroparesis, then, is diagnosed by exclusion and is due to primary failure of one or more of the neuro-muscular components essential to the gastric emptying process in health.

Regulation of gastric emptying in health

A review of the traditional concepts of liquid- and solid-meal gastric

87

Table 5.1 Causes of delayed gastric emptying.

Mechanical obstruction
Status post gastric surgery
Duodenal, pyloric, gastric ulcer
Gastric malignancy
Bezoar

Nonmechanical obstruction

Neuromuscular
Gastroparesis diabeticorum
Muscular, myotonic dystrophy
Scleroderma, dermatomyositis, and polymyositis
Amyloidosis
Hollow viscera neuropathy–myopathy ('pseudo-obstruction')

Infiltrative
Malignancy

Infectious
Chronic viral

Gastric surgery
Vagotomy, with or without resection

Psychiatric disorders
Anorexia nervosa
Bulimia

Metabolic
Hyperglycemia
Hyperthyroidism, hypothyroidism

Idiopathic
Gastric arrhythmias (may accompany many of the above disorders)
   Arrhythmia with retrograde propulsion
    Bradygastria
    Tachygastria

Use of medication

---

emptying in health is important here. Figure 5.1 depicts the emptying pattern of a mixed liquid and solid meal, in which the liquid (orange juice) and the solid (beef stew) portions, labeled with different radionuclides, were administered to healthy volunteers [4]. The percent of emptying over time was monitored by externally positioned gamma-detectors placed over the gastric region. As is evident, liquid emptying, depicted by a curvilinear regression line, is more rapid than solid emptying, depicted by a more linear emptying curve. This is a typical emptying pattern for mixed liquid–solid meals. Nonnutrient liquid meals given alone empty

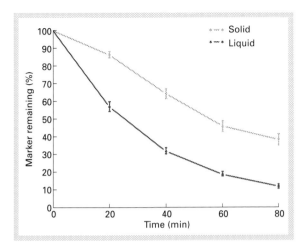

Fig. 5.1 Gastric emptying of liquid and solid foods. Note the near-linear and slower emptying of solids as compared to liquids. Solid-meal emptying is biphasic, with an initial lag period of variable length, depending on meal size and composition, followed by a linear decay. With the 300-g meal employed in this study [44], the mean lag period was approximately 8.6 minutes. The biphasic nature of solid emptying is not depicted in the figure because of the long sampling intervals of 20 minutes. In this study, a 300-g combined solid and liquid meal, labeled with technetium-99m(^{99m}Tc) sulfur colloid (solid phase) and indium-111 (^{111}In) (liquid phase), was ingested at 0 minutes. Percent retention refers to the percentage of the radiolabeled marker remaining in the stomach over time (minutes). Each point represents the mean ± SEM for 32 studies in eight male subjects (four studies each). (From Brophy *et al.* [4].)

exponentially, while nutrient liquids and liquids ingested with nutrient solids assume an increasingly linear pattern (with increasing nutrient meal content), presumably because of feedback inhibition from nutrient-sensitive small bowel receptors [5, 6].

Figure 5.2 is a schematic of the neuromuscular controls and regions integral to the normal gastric emptying process for liquid- and solid-meal components. The proximal stomach receives and stores foodstuffs and acts, therefore, as a reservoir. The neuromuscular properties of the proximal stomach are distinctive: (i) receptive relaxation, the ability to relax in anticipation of swallowed foodstuffs; and (ii) accommodation, the capacity to distend without increasing intragastric pressure. These properties are vagally mediated and due, it has recently been proposed [7], to local release of nitric oxide (NO), a potent smooth-muscle relaxant. The contraction following relaxation of the proximal stomach is slow and sustained, giving rise to a fundal–duodenal pressure gradient that assists in the movement of both liquids and solids from the proximal to the distal

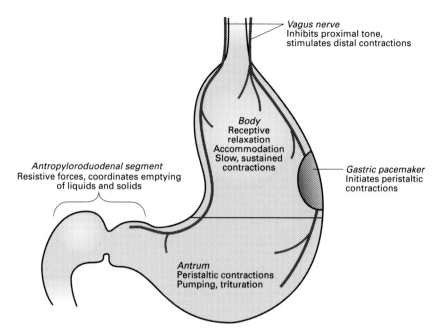

Fig. 5.2 Schema of anatomic and neuromuscular elements important in the normal gastric emptying of liquid and solid foodstuff. Liquid-meal emptying requires a fundal–duodenal pressure gradient to promote distal flow; the antropyloroduodenal segment controls the time and the amount of transpyloric liquid transfer. Solid-meal emptying also requires fundal pressures to promote distal flow but, more importantly, it requires peristaltic antral contractions to grind digestible food particles into sizes that permit transpyloric transfer. The timing and amount of solid-food transpyloric flow are controlled by the antropyloroduodenal segment, which is primarily a resistive/permissive force. Thus, the emptying of both liquids and solids requires a coordinated, sequential participation of both the gastric fundus and the antrum. Vagus nerve stimulation inhibits proximal fundal tone and stimulates antral contractions.

stomach. Until recently, it was believed that the caudally directed pressure gradient thus generated was all that was required for liquid emptying. However, this simplified concept is now untenable: liquid emptying into the duodenum is pulsatile, as is solid emptying, requiring the participation of antral wall propulsive and pyloric–duodenal resistive forces in a coordinated effort [8].

The principal function of the distal stomach is to retain and grind solid foodstuffs until their particle size is small enough (< 1.0 mm) to permit passage into the duodenum. The motor activity of the distal stomach is characterized by peristaltic waves sweeping aborally from the mid-stomach to the duodenum. The pacesetter for this electrically generated activity resides in a pacemaker located in the longitudinal muscle of the greater curvature. In humans, the pacemaker discharges at a frequency of 3/min, spreads circumferentially and distally, and in the presence of food or another distending source (e.g. air) converts to action potentials and muscle contractions. The peristaltic wave thus generated is lumen-obliterating in the distal 2 cm of the antrum; solid food is retained here for further grinding and trituration before emptying occurs.

An additional motor form, termed the *migrating motor complex* (MMC), is responsible for the emptying of indigestible solids — solid food particles, usually in excess of 5 mm, which cannot be emptied with digestible solids. The MMCs are powerful 'housekeeping' waves that are inhibited by feeding, are stimulated by fasting, and occur every 60–120 minutes in the fasted, healthy human. The occurrence of MMCs coincides with rises in the plasma hormone motilin, which presumably acts on gastric smooth muscle to initiate the wave [9, 10]. A circadian rhythm has been described for the MMC, in which the daytime speed of propagation (centimeters per minute) is about twice the nighttime speed (Figure 5.3) [11].

The rate at which the stomach empties its solid and liquid contents is controlled by mucosal receptors in the small intestine that are sensitive to caloric, osmolar, and acid loads. Calorie-containing meals — equicaloric loads of lipid, carbohydrate, and protein are equipotent — are potent inhibitors of gastric emptying through complex vasovagal–myenteric

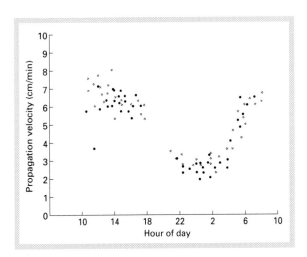

Fig. 5.3 Propagation velocity (centimeters per minute) of MMCs in 10 healthy volunteers (light circles) and 10 patients with irritable bowel syndrome (dark circles) in relation to the 24-hour period. The daytime velocity is more than double the nighttime velocity in both groups. The gap at 1800 hours (6 PM) represents feeding of a 540-kcal meal and its inhibiting influence on the MMC. (From Kumar *et al.* [11]; © 1996 by the American Gastroenterological Association.)

nervous system and humoral feedback arcs. The hormone cholecystokinin (CCK) may be a mediator, and NO liberation may accompany some,
but not all, of the inhibitory responses, depending on the stimulus [12, 13].
Young, premenopausal women empty significantly more slowly than
age-matched men, suggesting that progestational compounds or estradiol
are also inhibitors of gastric emptying [14, 15]. Gastric emptying, however, is unchanged during the menstrual cycle [16]. Assumption of the
upright posture and modest physical activity are physiologic stimulants
of gastric emptying [17, 18]. In addition, a circadian rhythm in gastric
emptying rates has been documented in human volunteers in which
morning-meal emptying rates are about twice as rapid as evening-meal
emptying rates and in accord with the circadian changes observed in
MMC propagation, cited earlier (Figure 5.4) [19]. The mechanisms
explaining these circadian differences in emptying rates are not known.
Finally, day-to-day variability in solid- or liquid-meal emptying rates
within a single subject under identical test conditions may be as great as
100%; the reason for this variability is not known [4].

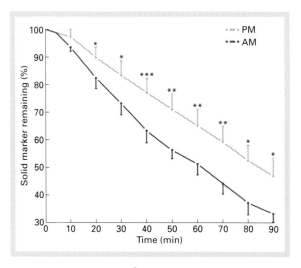

Fig. 5.4 Solid-phase morning (AM) and evening (PM) gastric emptying curves in 16
healthy male volunteers ingesting identical 547-kcal meals at either 8 AM or 8 PM.
Significant differences in mean percentage retention values were noted at all timing
intervals after 10 minutes. Two-tailed paired t-test values: $*0.02 < P > 0.01$;
$**0.01 > P > 0.001$; $***P < 0.001$. (From Goo *et al.* [19]; © 1996 by the American
Gastroenterological Association.)

Gastroparesis

Neuromuscular defects in diabetic patients

Gastroparesis is the end result of neuromuscular failure or excessive inhibitory influence, or both, at one or more key junctures of the gastric emptying process, as shown in Figure 5.5.

1   Fundal hypomotility delays passage of liquid and solid foodstuffs into the distal stomach.

2   Antral hypomotility compromises trituration and delays transpyloric flow of gastric content.

3   Gastric arrhythmias — in the form of bradygastria, tachygastria, or displacement of pacemaker activity to more distal regions with or without retrograde conduction — disrupt peristaltic coordination.

4   Uncoordinated antropyloroduodenal activity, including pyloric 'spasm', prevents gastric chyme from entering the duodenum.

5   Excessive inhibitory feedback at any or all of these junctures could theoretically delay gastric emptying even in an otherwise healthy stomach [20, 21].

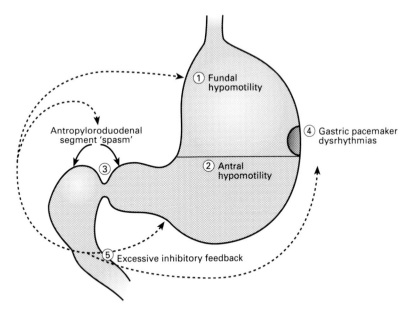

Fig. 5.5 Schema for documented (1–4) and putative (5) mechanisms underlying neuromuscular failure in gastroparesis. Patients with gastroparesis usually have combined defects, if measured, and no single defect has been documented to be specific for any underlying disease. Excessive small bowel inhibitory influence (5) could delay gastric emptying at any or all locations (1, 2, 3, or 4).

However, this last possibility has not been fully documented in any gastroparetic state, nor has any one of these five defects been identified as pathognomonic of any specific disorder, and in most patients with gastroparesis, more than one abnormality is found when gastric emptying is measured. In diabetes mellitus, for example, several manometric and electrographic abnormalities have been described: diminished antral and fundal motility, absent or reduced MMCs, arrhythmias in pacemaker function, and pyloric sphincter dysmotility (spasm) [20–25]. Figure 5.6 depicts the manometric documentation of antral hypomotility and pylorospasm in a diabetic patient [23]. The abnormalities in diabetic gastroparesis have been attributed to a decrease in vagal tone ('autovagotomy'). Indeed, basal gastric acid secretion, primarily vagus mediated, is decreased in diabetic gastroparesis, and other autonomic dysfunctions are also found in diabetic patients with delayed emptying [24, 25]. On the other hand, surgical truncal vagotomy is often accompanied by rapid liquid emptying, not the delayed emptying pattern found in diabetic individuals [26]. In addition, postmortem examination of diabetic stomachs has failed to demonstrate neural damage consistent with autovagotomy [27].

The delay in gastric emptying observed in many diabetic patients may

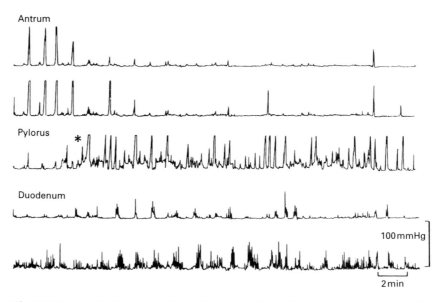

Fig. 5.6 Manometrically recorded antral hypomotility and episode of pylorospasm (*) in a diabetic patient following a meal. Note that antral and duodenal phasic activity is mixed with tonic activity. (From Mearin *et al.* [23]; © 1996 by the American Gastroenterological Association.)

be attributable, at least in part, to poor diabetic control and hyperglycemia. In a group of patients with types I and II diabetes, Horowitz *et al.* [28, 29] observed a strong correlation between delays in gastric emptying and plasma glucose levels above 270 mg/dl. In healthy volunteers, delays in emptying of a meal from the stomach have been induced by acute hyper-glycemia [30, 31]. Other studies of induced hyperglycemia in healthy volunteers have shown loss of fasting MMC activity at plasma glucose levels exceeding 140 mg/dl, reduced antral motility patterns following oral feeding at plasma glucose levels exceeding 175 mg/dl, and induction of gastric electrical arrhythmias at plasma glucose levels exceeding 230 mg/dl [32, 33]. These effects were not mediated by secondary supraphysiologic insulin release with glucose administration. Furthermore, the induction of gastric arrhythmias with elevated plasma glucose levels, but not of antral hypomotility, was reversed with indomethacin pretreatment.

Other causes of gastroparesis

Few of the other causes of gastroparesis, listed in Table 5.1, have been studied as systematically as diabetes. Scleroderma and other collagen–vascular disorders, amyloidosis, and malignant infiltration (e.g. gastric lymphoma) produce features of both nerve and muscle damage in the gastric wall [34]. Involvement of other organs dominates the clinical presentation in these disorders, and symptomatic gastroparesis is unusual. The role of gastric arrhythmias as a causal factor in delayed gastric emptying is uncertain. Gastric arrhythmias are often an associated finding, among other abnormal findings, in studies of gastroparetic patients. They may also occur spontaneously in volunteers without associated symptoms [35]. However, in isolated cases, as illustrated in the patient study represented in Figure 5.7, removal of the arrhythmogenic focus contributed to clinical improvement [36].

It should be emphasized that mechanical and nonmechanical causes of delayed gastric emptying may coexist in the same patient. This is best illustrated by the patient with pyloric channel obstruction due to either ulcer or tumor and secondary antral 'pump' failure. It is also noteworthy that in the hospitalized patient, a variety of drugs may contribute to delayed gastric emptying, and it will be necessary to discontinue these agents before any diagnostic testing is performed. The anticholinergics and opiates are commonly implicated in this regard, but many other drugs administered to the hospitalized patient may contribute (Table 5.2). Immobility and the recumbent posture, the norm for many hospitalized

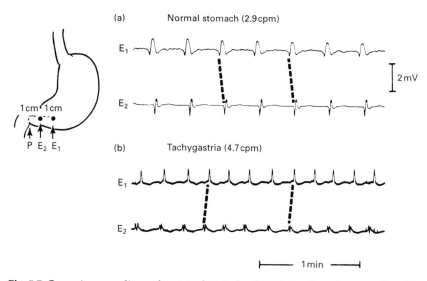

Fig. 5.7 Operative recordings of gastric electrical activity taken from the serosal surface of the antrum in (a) a healthy human stomach and (b) a 5-month-old patient with gastric retention. Dotted lines indicate that propagation is in the orad direction in the patient, in contrast to the usual aborad direction. In addition, the patient recording exhibits more rapid electrical activity (tachygastria). E, electrode; P, pylorus. (From Telander *et al.* [36]; © 1996 by the American Gastroenterological Association.)

Table 5.2 Medications that can cause delay in gastric emptying.

Use may lead to clinically evident gastroparesis
Anticholinergics
Opiates
L-dopa
Tricyclic antidepressants
Phenothiazines
Somatostatin

Use rarely leads to clinically evident gastroparesis
Calcium channel blockers
Sympathomimetics (beta-agonists)
Progesterone
Aluminum antacids
Sucralfate
Potassium salts
Alcohol (in high concentrations)
Cannabis
Gamma-aminobutyric acid (GABA)
Cholera toxin
Nicotine

patients, are known to influence gastric emptying and contribute to the relatively high frequency of delayed emptying in the hospitalized compared with the ambulant patient [17, 18].

Evaluation of gastric emptying

Traditional methods

Figure 5.8 outlines an algorithmic approach to patients with delayed gastric emptying. Early satiety, weight loss, excessive abdominal bloating and pain, anorexia, nausea with food ingestion with or without vomiting,

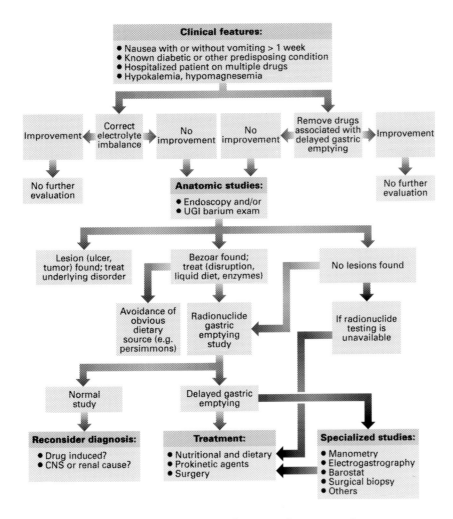

Fig. 5.8 Approach to evaluating patients with suspected gastroparesis.

and vomiting of food items ingested more than 8 hours earlier all suggest delayed gastric emptying irrespective of cause. Unfortunately, there is a poor correlation between clinical symptoms and objective evidence of delayed gastric emptying [34]. Patients with persistent symptoms may demonstrate normal meal emptying rates; conversely, asymptomatic patients may demonstrate marked gastric retention when tested by sensitive radioisotopic techniques.

In the clinical setting, conditions causing mechanical obstruction (e.g. peptic ulcer with pyloric stenosis or tumors) must be addressed first and ruled out. Although these diagnoses can be secured by either endoscopy or radiography, endoscopy is preferred because of its superior diagnostic yield and the capability of offering specific therapy (e.g. bezoar dissolution). Conventional barium studies of the upper GI tract reliably detect organic lesions. However, if lesions are not present, these studies will demonstrate delayed emptying only in severe cases. Barium radiography is insensitive, nonphysiologic (in that barium sulfate meals are not representative of normal meal components), and nonquantitative. Gastric aspiration tests, with or without dye recovery methods, are quantitative, inexpensive, and safe. However, they are invasive, requiring nasogastric intubation, and measure only liquid-meal emptying rates. Solids and liquids empty at different rates (see Figure 5.1) and are not always in agreement. For example, normal liquid and delayed solid gastric emptying may be observed in many diabetic patients [37, 38].

Scintigraphy

The most accurate and sensitive measure of gastric emptying employs radionuclide markers incorporated into either the liquid or the solid phase (or both with simultaneous studies) of the meal [39]. Liquid- and solid-marker emptying is tracked independently and simultaneously by externally positioned gamma-scintillation cameras. The test is physiologic (ordinary meals are employed), noninvasive, and quantitative. However, the study is expensive, is not widely available, and must be standardized within each nuclear medicine laboratory. Test results vary from laboratory to laboratory because of the lack of uniformity in size, composition, and caloric content of the test meal administered. Each of these factors influences meal emptying rates, as do the physiologic factors of gender, body posture, physical activity, and time of day [14, 17–19, 40]. In addition, a host of technical factors (including radiomarker species and collimation) influence test results [41, 42]. For example, anterior imaging alone artificially exaggerates the early 'lag' phase of solid-meal emptying due to shifting of the labeled food mass to a more anterior position in the antrum and toward the anterior detector during meal digestion.

Geometric-mean corrected data, requiring anterior and posterior gastric imaging projections, considerably reduce but do not eliminate the early delay in emptying, as illustrated in Figure 5.9. This figure depicts the emptying curves of radionuclide-labeled solid-phase meals administered to 16 healthy subjects, with data acquired in either the anterior projection alone or the combined anterior and posterior projection with geometric-mean calculations [43]. Data acquired solely in the anterior projection overestimated both the time to half-emptying ($T_{\frac{1}{2}}$) (73.0 versus 63.8 minutes) and the lag phase (19.0 versus 7.0 minutes), when compared with the geometric-mean calculated data. In another scintigraphy-based solid-meal gastric emptying study [42], involving 32 healthy subjects ingesting 300-g meals, an average percent difference of 38.1 was found in $T_{\frac{1}{2}}$ between geometric-mean and anterior-projection-alone methods (60.3 versus 83.4 minutes, respectively) [42]. The lag phase for this meal size was calculated at 8.6 minutes [44]. These observations are pertinent to the

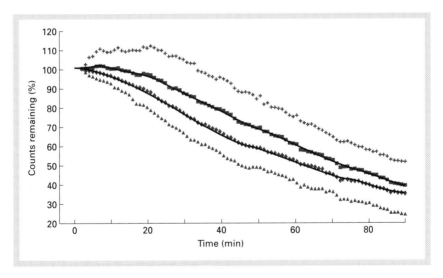

Fig. 5.9 Scintigraphy-based gastric emptying curves outlined in 16 healthy subjects. From top to bottom, the curves represent: standard error of measurement of the anterior alone-acquired data (+); anterior-alone mean value data (■); geometric-mean acquired data (◆); and standard error of measurement of the geometric-mean corrected data (▲). Note the shortening of the time to half-emptying ($T_{\frac{1}{2}}$) and the 'lag' period of the geometric-mean data, when compared with the anterior-only acquired data. (From Katz *et al.* [43].)

application of curve-fitting formulas to grouped data. Recommendations for complex curve-fitting formulas have been made by at least three groups of investigators [45–47], who did not employ geometric-mean correction. These nonlinear, curve-fitting formulas were based, in part, on the recognition of a consistently observed and prolonged early delay in solid-phase emptying. With geometric-mean corrected data, in contrast, the emptying curves most closely conform to a linear fit, even taking into account an early short lag period. If data are acquired discontinuously (e.g. every 20 minutes; see Figure 5.1), the lag phase may be missed; if data are acquired continuously (e.g. every minute), the lag phase will be detected. In diabetic patients with gastroparesis, the lag phase (early delay in emptying) is about twice the duration in diabetic patients without gastroparesis and normal controls [48]. The delay is attributed to prolonged retention of food in the proximal stomach and reduced antral motility.

Thus, the proper interpretation of scintigraphic measurements of gastric emptying can be obtained only in laboratories with standardized techniques for measuring gastric emptying rates with appropriate correction techniques and established control population values. It should be understood that even the best scintigraphic studies provide only gross measurements of meal emptying rates and limited information concerning the dynamics of the emptying process itself. This is because of the lack of resolution with the technique and the inability to define wall motion in relation to moment-to-moment transpyloric chyme transfer.

For clinical purposes, gastric emptying data have been expressed in a variety of ways, including $T_{\frac{1}{2}}$, slope, percentage retention at a specific time, lag time to emptying, mean transit time, and power function analysis [41, 42, 44]. No one expression has been found to be superior in distinguishing normal from abnormal patient studies. For most clinical studies, calculations of $T_{\frac{1}{2}}$ and the slope of the regression line have been the most commonly and easily understood expressions.

Newer techniques

More recent technical innovations, employing ultrasound or magnetic resonance imaging (MRI), electrogastrography (EGG), barostat measurements of fundal tone, and intragastric axial force measurements — in addition to conventional manometric studies — provide much more detail on the dynamics of the emptying process. Gastric manometry identifies antral hypomotility, pyloric spasm, antropyloroduodenal incoordination, and absence of MMCs [22]. Mucosal and cutaneous EGG studies have helped to define the role of the gastric pacemaker in generating peristaltic contractions and to identify abnormalities in gastroparesis [49].

It is believed that the pacesetter potentials identified by the cutaneous EGG phase trigger the onset of action potentials that, in turn, trigger muscle contractions. The pacesetter potential, therefore, sets the frequency, velocity, and direction of peristaltic wave spread, while the amplitude of the action potential determines the strength of contraction [50, 51]. Delayed gastric emptying occurs when few or no contractions are present or when ectopic pacemakers, usually antral in location, 'pace' the frequency either too rapidly (tachygastria) or too slowly (bradygastria), and/or in the reverse, orad direction (reverse peristalsis). These abnormalities have been detected in the postoperative stomach and, in isolated examples, have been corrected by externally applied pacing techniques [52]. Refinements in cutaneous EGG techniques and data analysis have established this methodology as a practical tool for exploring a variety of problems in gastric pathophysiology. The number and positioning of cutaneous electrodes in relation to the stomach are critical because of the low signal-to-noise ratio. In addition, specialized computer-assisted statistical programs are required to transform the raw slow-wave gastric pacemaker signal for study interpretation.

Figure 5.10 displays the raw signal and power spectral analyses of control and induced-hyperglycemia studies in a single healthy volunteer from the research of Hasler *et al.* [33] cited earlier. The induction of hyperglycemia produced a significant increase in signal activity in the tachygastric range (4.5–9.0 cycles per minute (cpm), normal range, 2.0–4.5 cpm), with concurrent reduction in antral motor activity. Because EGG is a noninvasive technique, measurements may be obtained simultaneously and in combination with more invasive modalities (e.g. manometric tubes) that measure gastric motor contractile events and gastric emptying rates. In this regard, a recent study by Chen *et al.* [53], in which simultaneous surface EGG and scintigraphy measurements were performed in 43 patients with symptoms of delayed gastric emptying, showed that an abnormal EGG pattern predicted delayed gastric emptying with an accuracy of 90%. It is thus possible that the surface EGG will be useful in the screening and identification of patients with gastroparesis.

The gastric barostat, a device that measures pressure and isobaric volume changes in a fundal balloon, has been used to identify fundal hypomotility in postgastrectomy patients [54]. Figure 5.11 compares the

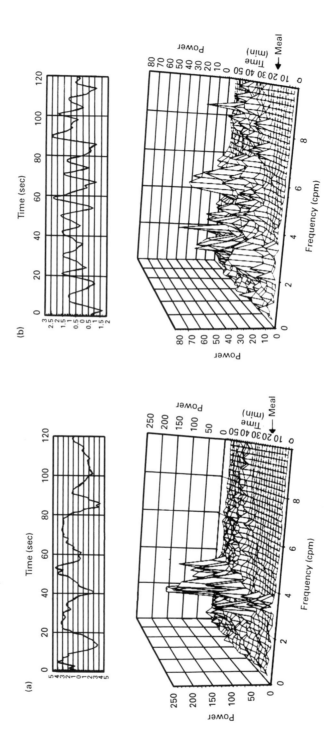

Fig. 5.10 Sample EGG results from (a) a healthy volunteer and (b) a healthy volunteer undergoing hyperglycemic clamping to plasma glucose levels of 230 mg/dl. The top panels represent the raw slow-wave records; the bottom panels, the respective power spectral analysis conversion records. Note that the hyperglycemia induced a significant increase in signal activity in the tachygastric range (4.5–9.0 cpm). (From Hasler *et al.* [33].)

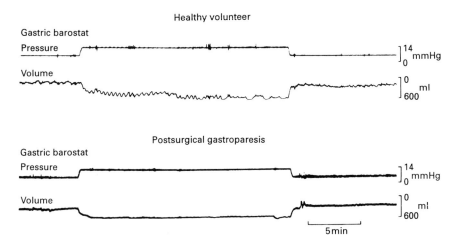

Healthy volunteer

Fig. 5.11 Dynamic response of the stomach to distention by air in a fundally placed barostat bag. Note the intense phasic activity in measurements obtained from the healthy volunteer and the lack of phasic activity in the patient with postsurgical gastroparesis. Not depicted in this patient is the lower-than-normal resting gastric tone typical in patients with postsurgical gastroparesis. (From Aspiroz & Malagelada [54]; © 1996 by the American Gastroenterological Association.)

responses of a healthy stomach and a postsurgical gastroparetic stomach to distention of the barostat bag by air. In this study, gastroparetic stomachs had significantly larger barostat bag volumes at lower intra-gastric pressures, as well as impaired tone, when compared with the normal stomach.

Ultrasonography has demonstrated that the transpyloric flow of chyme is pulsatile and occurs with coordinated progression of antral contractions and pyloric and proximal duodenal relaxation [55]. However, antral flow measures are indirectly determined (by changes in antral volumes) and the technique is not adaptable to solid-meal measurements.

MRI-based gastric imaging studies are capable of providing real-time information on transpyloric flow and volume emptying in relation to gastric contractile events in the human subject [56]. Further improvements in MRI would include the development of a solid-meal emptying marker and the ability to scan in the erect position.

A new approach to intraluminal manometry has been the development of an axial force transducer [57]. This pressure transducer, attached to a 1.5 ml inflatable balloon and placed intragastrically, measures longitudinally directed axial, or 'push', forces rather than circumferentially directed forces, which are measured by standard manometry. Simultaneous measurement of axial forces, scintigraphy to measure gastric emptying rates, and antroduodenal manometry in healthy subjects have shown excellent correlation of axial forces with emptying rates for both solids and liquids. Approximately 20% of the axial forces were unassociated with manometrically recorded pressure waves, suggesting that the transpyloric flow of gastric chyme may not necessarily require gastric contractile activity, much less lumen-occluding contraction [58].

Finally, it is well known that the small bowel exerts an inhibitory influence on gastric emptying through food-induced release of enterogastrones (e.g. CCK and somatostatin). Nutrients delivered anywhere along the small bowel retard gastric emptying, and several disorders of small bowel motility are associated with delayed emptying [6, 34]. Lin [21] has proposed that gastric emptying can be delayed by inappropriately intense inhibitory small bowel feedback from ordinary meals in intact subjects or by exposure of nutrients to excessively long segments of small bowel in patients following gastric surgery. Delayed gastric emptying could then result from excessive inhibitory feedback in an otherwise healthy or partially intact stomach.

Summary

It is no longer tenable to view gastric motor function as a two-compartment model in which the fundus simply serves as a reservoir and regulator of liquid emptying and the antrum is responsible for the preparation and delivery of solid foodstuffs into the small bowel. It is a much more complex, interactive system in which the propulsive forces generated by fundal tone and antral contracting waves act in balance with the resistive forces of the pylorus and duodenum to regulate transpyloric flow of both liquids and solids. In the gastroparetic stomach, a combination of contractile and coordination defects exists in which the space-and-time sequencing of motor events may be more important than whether and where the contraction occurs or its absolute strength.

Gastric scintigraphy provides the most sensitive clinical measure of gastric emptying available. However, a lack of resolution limits its usefulness in elucidating the neuromuscular defects underlying gastroparesis. A greater understanding of these defects will likely emerge from studies employing different techniques simultaneously. Practical considerations will inhibit this approach in humans, but it is now feasible to simultaneously measure transpyloric flow rates and wall motion with MRI or ultrasound in combination with standard manometric or axial force pressure measurements. Other combinations of technologies are possible, however, and will be necessary to enlarge our understanding of gastroparetic disorders.

Acknowledgment

This work was supported by DVA Medical Research Funds.

References

1 McCallum RW, Berkowitz DM, Lerner E. Gastric emptying in patients with gastroesophageal reflux. *Gastroenterology* 1981;**80**:285–91.

2 Urbain JLC, Siegel JA, Debie NC, Pauwels SP. Effects of cisapride on gastric emptying in dyspeptic patients. *Dig Dis Sci* 1988;**33**:779–83.

3 Kendall BJ, McCallum RW. Gastroparesis and the current use of prokinetic drugs. *Gastroenterologist* 1993;**1**:107–14.

4 Brophy CM, Moore JG, Christian PE, Egger MJ, Taylor AT. Variability of gastric emptying measurements in man employing standardized radiolabeled meals. *Dig Dis Sci* 1986;**31**:799–806.

5 Hunt JN, Spurrell WR. The pattern of emptying of the human stomach. *J Physiol (Lond)* 1951;**113**:157–68.

6 Meyer JH. The physiology of gastric motility and gastric emptying. In: Yamada T, ed. *Textbook of Gastroenterology.* Philadelphia: JB Lippincott Co, 1991:137–57.

7 Desai KM, Sessa WC, Vane JR. Involvement of nitric oxide in the reflex relaxation of the stomach to accommodate food or fluid. *Nature* 1991;**351**:477–9.

8 Horowitz M, Dent J, Fraser R, Sun W, Hebbard G. Role and integration of mechanisms controlling gastric emptying. *Dig Dis Sci* 1994;**39**(12):7–13S.

9 Itoh Z, Nakaya M, Suzuki T, Arai H, Wakabayashi K. Erythromycin mimics exogenous motilin in gastrointestinal contractile activity in the dog. *Am J Physiol* 1984;**247**:G688–94.

10 Peeters T, Matthijs G, Depoortere I, Cachet T, Hoogmartens J, Vantrappen G. Erythromycin is a motilin receptor agonist. *Am J Physiol* 1989;**257**:G470–4.

11 Kumar D, Wingate D, Ruckebusch Y. Circadian variation in the propagation velocity of the migrating motor complex. *Gastroenterology* 1986;**91**:926–30.

12 Burks TF. Muscle receptors, neurotransmitters, and drugs. *Dig Dis Sci* 1994;**39**(12):S6–8.

13 Allesher HD, Daniel EE. Role of NO in pyloric, antral, and duodenal motility and its interaction with other inhibitory mediators. *Dig Dis Sci* 1994;**39**(12):73–5S.

14 Datz FL, Christian PE, Moore J. Gender-related differences in gastric emptying. *J Nucl Med* 1987;**28**:1204–7.

15 Hutson WR, Roehrkasse RL, Wald A. Influence of gender and menopause on gastric emptying and motility. *Gastroenterology* 1989;**96**:11–17.

16 Horowitz M, Maddern GJ, Chatterton BE *et al.* The normal menstrual cycle has no effect on gastric emptying. *Br J Obstet Gynaecol* 1985;**92**:743–6.

17 Moore JG, Datz FL, Christian PE, Greenberg E, Alazraki N. Effect of body posture on radionuclide measurements of gastric emptying. *Dig Dis Sci* 1988;**33**:1592–5.

18 Moore JG, Datz FL, Christian PE. Exercise increases solid meal gastric emptying rates in men. *Dig Dis Sci* 1990;**35**:428–32.

19 Goo RH, Moore JG, Greenberg E, Alazraki NP. Circadian variation in gastric

emptying of meals in humans. *Gastroenterology* 1987;**93**:515–18.

20 Malagelada J-R, Azpiroz F, Mearin F. Gastroduodenal motor function in health and disease. In: Sleisenger MH, Fordtran JS, eds. *Gastrointestinal Disease: Pathophysiology/ Diagnosis/Management*, 5th edn. Philadelphia: WB Saunders Co, 1993:486–508.

21 Lin HC. Abnormal intestinal feedback in disorders of gastric emptying. *Dig Dis Sci* 1994;**39**(12):54–6S.

22 Camilleri M, Malagelada J-R. Abnormal intestinal motility in diabetics with gastroparesis syndrome. *Eur J Clin Invest* 1984;**14**:420–7.

23 Mearin F, Camilleri M, Malagelada J-R. Pyloric dysfunction in diabetics with recurrent nausea and vomiting. *Gastroenterology* 1986;**90**:1919–25.

24 Feldman M, Corbett DB, Ramsey EJ, Walsh JR, Richardson CT. Abnormal gastric function in longstanding insulin-dependent diabetic patients. *Gastroenterology* 1979;**77**12–17.

25 Keshavarzian A, Iber FL, Vaeth J. Gastric emptying in patients with insulin-requiring diabetes mellitus. *Am J Gastroenterol* 1987;**82**:29–35.

26 Clarke RJ, Alexander-Williams J. The effect of preserving antral innervation and of a pyloroplasty on gastric emptying after vagotomy in man. *Gut* 1973;**14**:300–7.

27 Yoshida MM, Schuffler MD, Sumi SM. There are no morphologic abnormalities of the gastric wall or abdominal vagus in patients with diabetic gastroparesis. *Gastroenterology* 1988;**94**:907–14.

28 Horowitz M, Harding PE, Maddox AF *et al.* Gastric and oesophageal emptying in patients with type 2 (non-insulin-dependent) diabetes mellitus. *Diabetologia* 1989;**32**:151–9.

29 Fraser RJ, Horowitz M, Maddox AF, Harding PE, Chatterton BE, Dent J. Hyperglycaemia slows gastric emptying in type 1 (insulin-dependent) diabetes mellitus. *Diabetologia* 1990;**33**:675–80.

30 Aylett P. Gastric emptying and change of blood glucose, as affected by glucagon and insulin. *Clin Sci* 1962;**22**:171–8.

31 MacGregor IL, Gueller R, Watts HD, Meyer JH. The effect of acute hyperglycemia on gastric emptying in man. *Gastroenterology* 1976;**70**:190–6.

32 Barnett JL, Owyang C. Serum glucose concentration as a modulator of interdigestive gastric motility. *Gastroenterology* 1988;**94**:739–44.

33 Hasler WL, Soudah HC, Dulai G, Owyang C. Mediation of hyperglycemia-evoked gastric slow-wave dysrhythmias by endogenous prostaglandins. *Gastroenterology* 1955;**108**:727–36.

34 Lin HC, Meyer JH. Disorders of gastric emptying. In: Yamada T, ed. *Textbook of Gastroenterology*. Philadelphia: JB Lippincott Co, 1991:1213–40.

35 Stoddard CJ, Smallwood RH, Duthie HL. Electrical arrhythmias in the human stomach. *Gut* 1981;**22**:705–12.

36 Telander RL, Morgan KG, Kreulen DL, Schmalz PF, Kelly KA, Szurszewski JH. Human gastric atony with tachygastria and gastric retention. *Gastroenterology* 1978;**75**:497–501.

37 Loo FD, Palmer DW, Soergel KH, Kalbfleisch JH, Wood CM. Gastric emptying in patients with diabetes mellitus. *Gastroenterology* 1984;**86**:485–94.

38 Havelund T, Oster-Jorgensen E, Eshoj O, Larsen ML, Lauritsen K. Effects of cisapride on gastroparesis in patients with insulin-dependent diabetes mellitus. *Acta Med Scand* 1987;**222**:339–43.

39 Heading RC, Tothill P, McLoughlin GP, Shearman DJC. Gastric emptying rate measurement in man: a double isotope scanning technique for simultaneous study of liquid and solid components of a meal. *Gastroenterology* 1976;**71**:45–50.

40 Moore JG, Christian PE, Coleman RE. Gastric emptying of varying meal weight and composition in man. *Dig Dis Sci* 1981;**26**:16–22.

41 Christian PE, Datz FL, Moore JG. Technical considerations in radionuclide gastric emptying studies. *J Nucl Med Tech* 1987;**15**(4):200–7.

42 Moore JG, Christian PE, Taylor AT, Alazraki N. Gastric emptying measurements: delayed and complex emptying patterns without appropriate correction. *J Nucl Med* 1985;**26**:1206–10.

43 Katz N, Toney MO, Heironimus JD II, Smith TE. Gastric emptying: comparison of anterior only and geometric mean correction methods employing static and dynamic imaging. *Clin Nucl Med* 1994;**19**:396–400.

44 Christian PE, Datz FL, Moore JG. Confirmation of short solid-food lag phase by continuous monitoring of gastric emptying. *J Nucl Med* 1991;**32**:1349–52.

45 Barber DC, Duthie HL, Howlett PJ *et al.* Principal components: a new approach to the analysis of gastric emptying. In: *Dynamic Studies With Radioisotopes in Medicine.* Vienna: IAEA, 1975:185–96.

46 Elashoff JD, Reedy TJ, Meyer JH. Analysis of gastric emptying data. *Gastroenterology* 1982;**83**:1306–12.

47 Dugas MC, Schade RR, Lhotsky D, Van Thiel D. Comparison of methods for analyzing gastric isotope emptying. *Am J Physiol* 1982;**243**:G237–42.

48 Urbain JLC, Vekemans MC, Bouillon R *et al.* Characterization of gastric antral motility disturbances in diabetics using a scintigraphic technique. *J Nucl Med* 1993;**34**:576–81.

49 Chen JDZ, McCallum RW. Clinical applications of electrogastrography. *Am J Gastroenterol* 1993;**88**:1324–36.

50 Cullen JJ, Kelly KA. The future of intestinal pacing. *Gastroenterol Clin North Am* 1994;**23**:391–402.

51 Kelly KA. Pacing the gut. *Gastroenterology* 1992;**103**:1967–9.

52 Hocking MP, Vogel SB, Sninsky CA. Human gastric myoelectric activity and gastric emptying following gastric surgery and with pacing. *Gastroenterology* 1992;**103**:1811–16.

53 Chen JDZ, Lin ZY, Yi XB, McCallum RW. Diagnostics of delayed gastric emptying using surface electrogastrography. *Gastroenterology* 1995;**108**:A639.

54 Azpiroz F, Malagelada J-R. Gastric tone measured by an electronic barostat in health and postsurgical gastroparesis. *Gastroenterology* 1987;**92**:934–43.

55 King PM, Adam RD, Pryde A, McDicken WN, Heading RC. Relationship of human antroduodenal motility and transpyloric fluid movement: non-invasive observations with real-time ultrasound. *Gut* 1984;**25**:1384–91.

56 Fraser R, Schwizer W, Borovicka J, Asal K, Fried M. Gastric motility measurement by MRI. *Dig Dis Sci* 1994;**39**(12):20–3S.

57 Vassallo MJ, Camilleri M, Prather CM, Hanson RB, Thomforde GM. Measurement of axial forces during emptying from the human stomach. *Am J Physiol* 1992;**263**:G230–9.

58 Camilleri M, Prather CM. Axial forces during gastric emptying in health and models of disease. *Dig Dis Sci* 1994;**39**(12):14–7S.

« 6 »

Treatment of Gastroparesis

Malcolm C. Champion

The physiology of delayed as well as normal gastric emptying, together with the causes of gastroparesis, has already been reviewed in Chapter 5. This chapter reviews the therapy for gastroparesis, with particular emphasis on gastric prokinetic agents.

Symptoms

The symptoms of gastroparesis include anorexia, postprandial epigastric fullness and bloating, nausea, and epigastric pain. In addition, patients may complain of early satiety and may vomit undigested food often eaten several hours earlier. Symptoms initially can be intermittent and may or may not become continuous, depending on the underlying condition and its severity. Conversely, patients with gastroparesis may have few or no symptoms; yet, at the time of endoscopy, there will be retained food in the stomach (bezoar). Diabetic patients also may be asymptomatic and present with either labile or difficult-to-control diabetes.

Treatment of underlying condition

Gastroparesis generally is associated with diabetes mellitus, is idiopathic, or follows gastric surgery. Delayed gastric emptying also can play a role in functional dyspepsia, gastroesophageal reflux disease (GERD), progressive systemic sclerosis and chronic intestinal pseudo-obstruction. Figure 6.1 reviews the relative incidence of common gastroparetic conditions, based on gastric emptying studies at one clinical center [1].

Many potentially correctable conditions can give rise to gastroparesis. Delayed emptying due to peptic ulcer disease or inflammatory conditions in the stomach often improves with appropriate treatment. Treatment of metabolic and endocrine abnormalities usually leads to amelioration of symptoms and enhanced gastric motility. A surgical approach may be necessary to resolve some causes of delayed gastric emptying, for

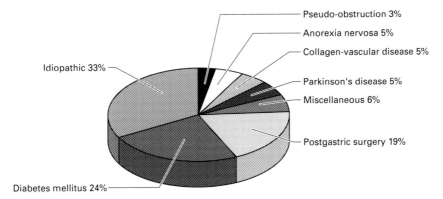

Fig. 6.1 Relative incidence of common gastroparetic conditions. (From Kendall & McCallum [1]. Reprinted from *Gastroenterologist* VI, **1**, 107–14, 1993 by permission of Little, Brown and Company (Inc.).)

example, pyloric stenosis caused by previous peptic ulcer disease. Finally, several drugs have been implicated in delaying gastric emptying (Table 6.1). All patients with symptoms of gastroparesis should have their medications reviewed.

Diet

Patients with gastroparesis experience difficulty in eating regular-sized meals and will benefit from having small frequent meals throughout the day. Patients with gastroparesis also are prone to bezoar formation. This appears to be due to a decrease or absence in the stomach of phase III of the migrating motor complex (MMC), which is responsible for clearing

Table 6.1 Drugs that cause gastroparesis.

May cause gastroparesis	Rarely cause gastroparesis
• Anticholinergic	• Calcium channel blockers
• Opiates	• Sympathomimetic (beta-agonists)
• L-Dihydroxyphenylalanine (L-DOPA)	• Progesterone
• Tricyclic antidepressants	• Aluminum antacids
• Phenothiazines	• Sucralfate
• Somatostatin	• Potassium salts
	• Alcohol (high concentrations)
	• Cannabis
	• Gamma-aminobutyric acid (GABA)
	• Cholera toxin
	• Nicotine

undigested material from the stomach in the fasting state [2, 3]. It is therefore appropriate to advise patients to follow a diet avoiding the leguminous vegetables.

A low-residue diet also may be beneficial but may exacerbate the constipation that accompanies gastroparesis, for example, in patients with diabetic autonomic neuropathy. Patients often find that restricting the fat content of meals will reduce their gastroparetic symptoms. Fat stimulates the release of cholecystokinin, which is a potent inhibitor of gastric emptying.

Drug therapy

Numerous studies have demonstrated a poor correlation between symptoms and the gastric emptying rate on radionuclide studies. Preliminary evidence [4, 5] suggests that findings on electrogastrography (EGG) may show a better correlation with symptoms. There is also a poor correlation between individual symptomatic improvement after prokinetic treatment and improvement in gastric emptying. This raises the question of the usefulness of gastric emptying and EGG studies in the evaluation of patients with presumed gastroparesis. Symptomatic patients need to be treated regardless of whether such studies reveal an abnormality. Asymptomatic patients with evidence of delayed emptying, particularly those with diabetes, also will benefit from treatment. Treatment for gastroparesis will result in better glycemic control and improved nutrition.

Treatment can either take the form of short-term pulse therapy, for at least 4–8 weeks, when the patient is symptomatic, or be continuous depending on the underlying condition and the severity of symptoms. Certainly in diabetic patients, long-term therapy is indicated. Several days or weeks may elapse between the initiation of treatment and clinical improvement, owing to delayed drug absorption in some patients with gastroparesis.

Clinical experience has shown that prokinetic agents can take at least 2–4 weeks to exert their maximal effect. Ideally, a therapeutic trial should last at least 4–8 weeks before considering an increase in dose or an alternative therapy. In certain conditions, such as diabetes and progressive systemic sclerosis, the dose of medication may need to be increased with time as the disease process becomes more severe.

Administration of a gastric prokinetic agent should be timed so that peak plasma levels and therapeutic activity coincide with eating. This is normally achieved by taking the medication at least 30 minutes before meals. If the patient misses a meal, the medication should still be taken to maintain steady-state plasma levels. In addition to mealtime dosing, the evening, or hs, dose is important. Gastric prokinetic agents improve gastroduodenal coordination and appear to restore a more normal inter-digestive MMC [2, 3, 6, 7]. This is particularly important in the overnight fasting state, when the stomach clears undigested material in the third phase of the MMC. Although unproven, an evening dose of medication seems a logical approach to minimize bezoar formation.

Prokinetic drugs

The gastric prokinetic drugs to be discussed in detail are metoclopramide, domperidone, cisapride, and erythromycin. Their pharmacology is reviewed, followed by their efficacy in common gastroparetic conditions. The pharmacokinetics of these agents are summarized in Table 6.2 [8–11].

Metoclopramide

Metoclopramide is a procainamide derivative with both gastric prokinetic and antiemetic properties. The gastric prokinetic properties result from antagonism of gastric dopamine receptors and augmented release of acetylcholine from the myenteric plexus [12]. Metoclopramide exerts its antiemetic action on the chemoreceptor trigger zone on the floor of the fourth ventricle and crosses the blood–brain barrier to affect the inter-cerebral vomiting center [8]. Metoclopramide is not a pure cholinomimetic because it does not influence gastric, pancreatic, or biliary secretions [12].

Metoclopramide increases gastric emptying by increasing the tone and amplitude of gastric contraction, relaxing the pyloric sphincter, and increasing antral peristalsis [13]. These actions also result in improved antroduodenal coordination [12, 13]. In diabetics, metoclopramide has been shown [2] to increase peristaltic activity similar to phase III of the MMC.

Side effects

The major limiting factor in the use of metoclopramide is the side-effects profile. Side effects are usually dose related and have been reported in at least 20–40% of patients [12–15]. Neurologic side effects due to intra-

Table 6.2 Pharmacokinetic properties of metoclopramide, domperidone, cisapride, and erythromycin in normal volunteers.

Drug	Absorption t_{max} (minutes)	Bioavailability (%)	Elimination half-life (hours)	Metabolism (liver and/or gut wall)	Excretion
Metoclopramide [8]	60–180	32–97	2.6–5.0	Partial	Urine 80%
Domperidone [9]	15–75	13–17	6.5–16.0	Extensive	Urine 31% Feces 60%
Cisapride [10]	60–120	40–50	7–10	Extensive	Urine 50% Feces 50%
Erythromycin* [11]	30–240*	30–60*	1.4–2.0*	Concentrated in liver	Principally in bile

* Depends on formulation.
t_{max}, Mean time for maximum plasma concentration.

cerebral dopamine antagonism have been reported [14] in up to 10% of patients at the recommended dose of 10 mg four times a day (qid), with the most common problems being drowsiness and lassitude. In a recent review [15], the relative risk for tardive dyskinesia was 1.67 and for drug-induced parkinsonism 4.0. Metoclopramide-treated patients had a significantly greater severity of tardive dyskinesia, drug-induced parkinsonism, and subjective akathisia than controls. Metoclopramide-treated patients with diabetes also had a significantly greater severity of tardive dyskinesia than metoclopramide-treated patients who were not diabetic. Hyperprolactinemia is another common problem, which can result in mastalgia, gynecomastia, galactorrhea, and amenorrhea.

Dose

In acute gastroparesis, metoclopramide may be administered parenterally by either the intravenous (IV), intramuscular, or subcutaneous route. The subcutaneous route may be useful for self-administration when the patient is unable to tolerate oral metoclopramide. The parenteral dose is 10 mg every 6 hours, but may vary depending on the indication. Parenteral administration may be augmented by oral intake, with tapering of the parenteral dose as symptoms improve. The usual dose of oral metoclopramide in adults is 10 mg at least 30 minutes before the three main meals and at bedtime. An increase in dose to 20 mg is generally not well tolerated due to side effects. A suppository form of metoclopramide is available in Europe but not in North America.

Domperidone

More recently, a dopamine antagonist has been developed that does not readily cross the blood–brain barrier. Like metoclopramide, domperidone, a benzimidazole derivative, exerts its gastric prokinetic action by dopamine receptor blockade in the stomach and duodenum. Its antiemetic action occurs only in the chemoreceptor trigger zone.

Domperidone improves antral peristalsis, duodenal contractility, and antroduodenal coordination [9]. The compound does not affect gastric acid secretion, secretory volume, pH, or serum gastrin levels [16].

Side effects

Domperidone is associated with fewer side effects than metoclopramide, with an overall incidence of 2–7% [9, 17, 18]. The main side effects are dry mouth, headache, and endocrinologic problems related to hyperpro-lactinemia. Like other dopamine antagonists, domperidone stimulates prolactin release from the pituitary. This can result in mastalgia, gyne-comastia, galactorrhea, or menstrual irregularities. There is no direct correlation between dose and prolactin response, although the increase in prolactin secretion rises with increasing doses of both domperidone and metoclopramide [12, 18]. Somnolence and extrapyramidal side effects occur in less than 0.01% of domperidone-treated patients, compared with an incidence of up to 10% in patients treated with metoclopramide. There is no parenteral formulation of domperidone, as large IV doses have been associated with cardiac arrhythmias [19].

Dose

The recommended initial dosage for oral domperidone is 10 mg before meals and at bedtime. Domperidone 20 mg qid is well tolerated and appears to be a more effective dosage for the treatment of gastroparesis. Some investigators have found that 30 mg qid is well tolerated in severe gastroparesis. A suppository form of domperidone is available in Europe but not in North America.

Cisapride

Cisapride, a benzamide derivative, appears to exert its effect throughout the entire gastrointestinal (GI) tract by enhancement of the physiologic release of acetylcholine at the postganglionic nerve endings of the myenteric plexus [20]. Studies [20] indicate that this intestinal effect is most likely due to an agonist effect of 5-hydroxytryptamine (5-HT) at the 5-HT$_4$ receptor. Cisapride also is an antagonist at the 5-HT$_3$ receptor and other, as yet unidentified, 5-HT receptors may be involved.

Cisapride increases lower esophageal sphincter (LES) pressure and strengthens peristalsis in the distal esophagus, thereby decreasing esophageal acid contact time. The compound stimulates gastric emptying independent of the plasma motilin concentration [21]. Cisapride has been shown to stimulate antral and pyloric motility as well as improve antroduodenal coordination. In the small bowel and colon it increases peristalsis and decreases transit time [10, 22]. It has not been shown [10] to affect gastric or pancreatic secretion.

Side effects

Cisapride appears to be well tolerated and is associated with fewer side effects than the dopamine antagonists. The overall incidence of side effects in placebo-controlled studies was approximately 3% above the incidence with placebo. The most frequent side effects were transient loosening of stools, transient abdominal cramping, and borborygmi [22]. Cisapride is metabolized mainly via the cytochrome P450 (CYP) 3A4 isoenzyme. Coadministration of cisapride with certain antifungal agents or macrolide antibiotics that inhibit this enzyme may result in high plasma levels of cisapride and produce prolongation of the QT interval on electrocardiography; isolated cases of cardiac arrhythmias have been reported. As a result, cisapride is contraindicated for concomitant use with ketoconazole, itraconazole, fluconazole, miconazole, troleandomycin, erythromycin, and clarithromycin [23]. This contraindication applies to oral and IV, but not topical, administration.

Dose

The recommended dose of cisapride for the treatment of gastroparesis is 10 mg half an hour before meals and at bedtime. In severe gastroparesis, a 20-mg dose is well tolerated and is often an effective initial regimen. The author has long-term experience treating diabetic patients with severe gastroparesis with cisapride doses of 30–40 mg qid with no apparent increase in side effects. Cisapride is available as tablets and in a liquid suspension. No parenteral formulation is available. A suppository form of cisapride is available in Europe but not in North America.

Erythromycin

Erythromycin [11] and related 16-membered macrolides have been shown [24–26] to bind to motilin receptors on GI smooth-muscle membrane, thereby acting as a motilin agonist. It is interesting to note that this prokinetic compound appears to be more effective via an IV route than orally [24]. There also appears to be decreased efficacy with long-term use. Whether this is due to poor drug absorption, tachyphylaxis, or another mechanism remains to be defined. In the rabbit [27], the motilin receptor appears to be downregulated with continued erythromycin dosing. The clinical importance of these observations needs further evaluation. However, if symptoms return after initial improvement, the decreased efficacy of oral erythromycin has to be considered.

Erythromycin accelerates gastric emptying by increasing the amplitude of antral contractions and improving antroduodenal coordination [28]. In the fasting state, erythromycin 1–3 mg/kg has been shown [29] to induce contractions identical to interdigestive MMC phase III activity. In healthy volunteers and diabetic patients with gastroparesis, larger doses of erythromycin (250–500 mg orally) produced a brief increase in gastric antral velocity, without a change in small bowel motility [30]. With erythromycin the emptying rates of solids and liquids become similar, suggesting a loss of gastric discrimination between the two forms [31]. This effect appears to be due to stimulation of phase III MMC activity postprandially, contrary to the normal physiologic interdigestive MMC, which occurs after 2–3 hours of fasting. These strong postprandial antral contractions against an open pylorus have raised concerns that the treatment of gastroparesis with erythromycin may impair the orderly digestion and absorption of nutrients because of the rapid delivery of large food particles to the small bowel [32].

Side effects

Not surprisingly, the most frequent side effects are gastrointestinal, including abdominal pain, diarrhea, nausea, and vomiting. Mildly elevated transaminases (alanine aminotransferase (ALT), aspartate aminotransferase (AST)), cholestatic jaundice, and cholestatic hepatitis are other important side effects. The risk of hepatotoxicity appears to be greater with the estolate and succinate salts than with the erythromycin base preparation. Hepatotoxicity also appears to be related to the dose used and the duration of therapy. This may be important in the long-term treatment of gastroparesis.

Dose

The effective IV dose of erythromycin for gastric prokinetic action appears to be 3–6 mg/kg three times a day (tid). In clinical studies, oral doses have ranged from 250 mg tid to 500 mg qid.

Comparative studies

Five studies have compared the efficacy of these prokinetic agents in gastroparetic conditions (Table 6.3) [33–37].

Table 6.3 Comparison of prokinetic agents.

Study	Number of patients	Route	Duration	Diagnosis	Regimen	Study design	Parameter studied	Results
McHugh et al. [33]	8	IV	Acute	DG	Cisapride 2.5, 5, 10 mg vs metoclopramide 10 mg vs placebo	SBR	GE solid	C>P M>P C 10 mg > M 10 mg
Feldman and Smith [34]	9	IV	Acute	DG	Cisapride 5 mg vs metoclopramide 10 mg vs placebo	DBC	GE Radio-opaque markers	C>P M=P
De Caestecker et al. [35]	19	Oral	8 weeks	DG	Cisapride 10 mg tid vs metoclopramide 10 mg tid vs placebo	DBC	Symptoms Esoph. emptying GE liquid Whole-gut transit	M=C C=P M=P M=C C=P M=P M=C C=P M=P M=C C=P M=P
Erbas et al. [36]	13	Oral	3 weeks	DG	Metoclopramide 10 mg tid vs erythromycin 250 mg tid	DBC	Symptoms GE solid	M=E M=E
Champion et al. [37]	10	Oral	4 weeks	9 DG 11 I	Domperidone 20 mg qid vs cisapride 10 mg qid	Open	Symptoms Total Individual GE solid	D=C D<C D=C

C, Cisapride; D, domperidone; DBC, double-blind crossover; DG, diabetic gastroparesis; E, erythromycin; Esoph., esophageal; GE, gastric emptying; I, idiopathic gastroparesis; M, metoclopramide; P, placebo; SBR, single-blind randomized.

Metoclopramide has been compared with cisapride in two placebo-controlled IV studies [33, 34]. In eight patients with diabetic gastroparesis, metoclopramide and cisapride significantly improved solid-phase gastric emptying, but cisapride 10 mg IV was significantly more effective than metoclopramide 10 mg IV [33]. In nine diabetic patients, cisapride 5 mg IV significantly improved the gastric emptying of indigestible radio-opaque markers, relative to placebo, while metoclopramide 10 mg IV did not [34]. This finding suggests an improvement in phase III of the MMC, with enhanced removal of indigestible solids from the stomach.

A randomized crossover study [35] compared oral metoclopramide 10 mg tid, cisapride 10 mg tid, and placebo in 19 patients with diabetic mellitus. The sole criterion for inclusion into the study was evidence of autonomic neuropathy, with most patients having no evidence of delayed liquid- or solid-phase gastric emptying. At 8 weeks there was no significant difference in symptom improvement or in liquid- or solid-phase gastric emptying between the three treatment groups.

Metoclopramide 10 mg tid was compared with erythromycin 250 mg tid in a 3-week crossover trial of 13 patients with diabetic gastroparesis [36]. At the end of the study, gastric emptying improved significantly from baseline with both metoclopramide and erythromycin, but there was no significant difference in gastric emptying when metoclopramide was compared with erythromycin. The total symptom score improved significantly in both treatment groups, with a more pronounced improvement with erythromycin.

Domperidone was compared with cisapride in a nonrandomized crossover study [37] in nine patients with diabetic gastroparesis and one with idiopathic gastroparesis. At the end of the 4-week treatment period, domperidone 20 mg qid and cisapride 10 mg qid showed a significant improvement from baseline in solid-phase gastric emptying and total symptom score. Domperidone significantly improved the symptoms of early satiety and anorexia, while cisapride improved epigastric fullness and pain, nausea, and bloating. There was no significant difference when domperidone was compared to cisapride in gastric emptying or symptoms at the end of the 4 week period.

Other drugs

Several other therapeutic agents have prokinetic properties with potential clinical use in gastroparesis.

Bethanechol

Bethanechol, a cholinomimetic agent that stimulates the parasympathetic nervous system, appears to stimulate gastric motility by increasing gastric tone and restoring a more normal MMC [2, 3]. In patients with reflux esophagitis and gastroparesis, it was not effective in improving gastric emptying whereas metoclopramide was [38]. In the past, bethanechol has often been used adjunctively with a dopamine antagonist. With the availability of cisapride, cotherapy with bethanechol and a dopamine antagonist is unlikely to be common practice, particularly because of the safety profile and questionable efficacy.

Side effects associated with bethanechol result from overstimulation of the parasympathetic nervous system. These include abdominal discomfort, excessive salivation, flushing of the skin, and excessive sweating.

Naloxone

Opiate peptides appear to act as neurotransmitters for both gastric motility and secretion. Naloxone, a parenteral opiate antagonist, appears to have an inhibitory effect on gastric emptying when used in a dose of 2 mg IV [39], while 5 mg IV accelerates gastric emptying [40]. Further studies are needed to define the role of naloxone and its oral equivalent, naltrexone, in the therapy for gastroparesis. To date, the potential gastric motility effects of naltrexone have not been studied.

Fedotozine

Fedotozine, a peripheral opioid agonist that acts on kappa-receptors in the gut wall, has been shown to modify visceral sensitivity [41] and enhance GI motility [42] in animals. In patients with functional dyspepsia, fedotozine has improved symptoms of gastroparesis [43]. Its role in gastroparesis remains to be defined. However, the main clinical area of interest with fedotozine is in the treatment of functional dyspepsia and irritable bowel syndrome.

Clebopride

Clebopride, a benzamide derivative, is a more selective blocker of the dopamine-2 receptors. It appears to have antiemetic [44] and gastric prokinetic [45] properties, and has been shown [46] to increase LES pressure. Clebopride has been used for reflux esophagitis and gastro-paresis, and as an antiemetic. Despite its dopamine receptor selectivity, extrapyramidal side effects remain a problem.

Zacopride

Zacopride, which appears to have gastric prokinetic and antiemetic properties, is undergoing preliminary evaluation. It seems to act as a serotonin antagonist, along with some dopamine antagonism and choli-nergic activity [47].

Renzapride

Renzapride, a substituted benzamide similar to metoclopramide, appears to exert its prokinetic effect not by dopamine antagonism but by agonist activity at the 5-HT$_4$ receptors [48]. In nine diabetic patients with gas-troparesis, renzapride 2 mg significantly improved solid/liquid gastric emptying compared to its effect in controls [49].

Clonidine

Clonidine, a specific alpha-2-adrenergic receptor agonist, has shown efficacy in diarrhea associated with diabetic autonomic neuropathy [50]. In an open study [51] involving diabetic patients with evidence of autonomic neuropathy, clonidine 0.3 mg/day improved upper GI symptoms in 6/6 patients and liquid-phase gastric emptying in 3/4 patients with abnormal gastric emptying. These findings suggest that adrenergic modulation may play a role in the pathophysiology of diabetic gastroparesis.

New prokinetic agents

The future development of new prokinetic agents appears to be focused on the motilin and 5-HT receptors. These are reviewed in Chapter 14.

Treatment of gastroparetic condition

In single oral-dose and IV studies, metoclopramide [8, 12], domperidone [9, 52], cisapride [10, 22], and erythromycin [53, 54] have shown efficacy in a variety of gastroparetic conditions (Table 6.4). The reader is referred to the above-mentioned review articles, which summarize these studies.

Table 6.4 Treatment of gastroparesis using parenterally or orally administered prokinetic agents: acute studies.

Condition underlying gastroparesis	Metoclopramide	Domperidone	Cisapride	Erythromycin
Diabetes	+	+	+	+
Dyspepsia	+	+	+	
Postsurgery	+	+	(+)	+
Idiopathic	+	(+)	+	+
PAN	(+)	(+)	+	+
GERD	(+)	(+)	+	
PSS	(+)	(+)	+	+
Myotonic dystrophy	+		+	
Intestinal pseudo-obstruction			+	+

+, Beneficial effect; ( ), small numbers in trial; PAN, primary anorexia nervosa; PSS, progressive systemic sclerosis.

This chapter focuses on double-blind, placebo and other controlled studies. Many studies evaluated a patient population with gastroparesis of diverse etiology. When relevant, this chapter discusses findings in the context of specific gastroparetic conditions. This approach results in some overlap, with the same studies being reviewed under more than one gastroparetic condition. Gastroparesis associated with functional dyspepsia or chronic intestinal pseudo-obstruction is discussed in Chapters 7 and 8.

Diabetes mellitus

The reported prevalence of gastroparesis associated with type I diabetes mellitus has varied from 9.9% to as high as 76% [55, 56]. Incidence rates of 32% and 50% also have been reported [57, 58]. This variability depends on the type of patients studied and the criteria used to make the diagnosis of gastroparesis. Diabetic gastroparesis is certainly more common in type I diabetes but can also occur in type II diabetes. In one study [59] in patients with type II diabetes receiving oral hypoglycemics, 30% had delayed solid-phase gastric emptying and 25% had delayed liquid-phase gastric emptying. Gastroparesis can present in diabetic patients with and without diabetic neuropathy [60, 61], but clinically may be more common when there is evidence of peripheral neuropathy. In diabetic gastroparesis, solid- but not liquid-phase gastric emptying appears to be consistently delayed [58, 62–64].

Treatment

Hyperglycemia has been shown [65, 66] to delay gastric emptying in diabetic individuals, and improving glycemic control alone can often improve gastric emptying as well as the symptoms of gastroparesis. In healthy volunteers, hyperglycemia, but not hyperinsulinemia, inhibited postprandial antral motility and induced gastric dysrhythmias on EGG. The induction of dysrhythmias appears to be prostaglandin mediated, as it is inhibited by oral indomethacin [67]. This observation may partially explain the antral hypomotility and gastric dysrhythmias found in diabetic gastroparesis. Treatment of the hyperglycemia and gastroparesis is important in both types of diabetes. In type I, improved gastric emptying will mean that the postprandial glucose increase will correspond with the rise in insulin levels, resulting in better glycemic control with less hyperglycemia and hypoglycemia. In type II, hyperglycemia has been shown [68] to delay the absorption of the oral hyperglycemic agent glipizide.

Short-term studies in diabetic gastroparesis are summarized in Table 6.5 [35, 69–78] and long-term studies in Table 6.6 [79–83]. Studies in patients with idiopathic or diabetic gastroparesis are summarized in Table 6.7 [84–91].

Metoclopramide

In studies [69, 70] in which metoclopramide 10 mg tid or qid was compared with placebo for 3 weeks, both treatment groups demonstrated a significant improvement in symptoms and one [69] showed improvement in liquid-phase gastric emptying. In an open study [71], metoclopramide 10 mg tid for 4 weeks produced improvement in symptoms but not gastric emptying of liquids when 12 diabetic patients were compared with a control group.

In a previously described randomized crossover study [35] of 19 diabetic patients with evidence of autonomic neuropathy, there was no significant difference in symptoms or in solid- or liquid-phase gastric emptying after 8 weeks of treatment with metoclopramide 10 mg tid, cisapride 10 mg tid, or placebo. In 40 diabetic patients, metoclopramide 10 mg qid for 3 weeks produced significant improvements in nausea and postprandial fullness and reductions in nausea, vomiting, fullness, and early satiety, compared with placebo [72]. In the metoclopramide-treated group, gastric emptying of a liquid/solid test meal improved from baseline but not compared with placebo.

The true efficacy of metoclopramide as a prokinetic agent in these studies remains questionable. Long-term symptom improvement may be due more to the antiemetic action of metoclopramide on the chemo-receptor trigger zone and the vomiting center rather than to the gastric prokinetic action.

Domperidone

Horowitz *et al.* [73] studied the effects of acute and chronic administration of domperidone in 12 diabetic patients. In the acute study using dom-peridone 40 mg orally, solid and liquid emptying rates were increased significantly compared with placebo. After chronic administration (35–51 days), domperidone 20 mg after meals had no significant effect on solid emptying but was still effective in increasing liquid emptying when compared with 22 controls. Symptoms of gastroparesis also improved after chronic administration. In another study [74], involving 19 diabetic patients, domperidone 20 mg qid for 4 weeks significantly improved total symptom scores and solid-phase gastric emptying compared with placebo. There was also improvement in the symptoms of nausea and early satiety.

In a multicenter study [75] involving 89 patients with type I diabetes (47 with gastroparesis and 42 with symptoms but normal gastric emp-tying), administration of domperidone 20 mg qid for 4 weeks during an initial single-blind phase produced improvement from baseline in all symptoms of gastroparesis. In the subsequent double-blind phase, 64 patients were randomized to receive domperidone 20 mg qid or placebo for another 4 weeks. Those receiving placebo experienced a significant worsening of symptoms compared to the domperidone-treated group. Patients with delayed gastric emptying responded better to domperidone than those with normal gastric emptying in the single-blind phase and deteriorated more rapidly on placebo in the double-blind phase.

Cisapride

In placebo-controlled studies of cisapride 10 mg qid for 4–8 weeks, symptoms and solid-phase gastric emptying improved significantly in two studies [76, 77] and neither improved in two other studies [35, 78]. In a placebo-controlled study evaluating cisapride 10 mg qid, there were no significant differences in symptom score [78], but there was a significant improvement in gastric emptying at 6 weeks in patients with severe gastroparesis [84].

Table 6.5 Short-term randomized studies in diabetic gastroparesis.

Study	Number of patients	Duration (weeks)	Regimen	Study design	Parameters studied	Results
METOCLOPRAMIDE						
Snape et al. [69]	10	3	Metoclopramide 10 mg qid vs placebo	DB	Symptoms GE liquid	M > P M > P
Ricci et al. [70]	13	3	Metoclopramide 10 mg qid vs placebo	DBC	Symptoms	M > P
Schade et al. [71]	12	4	Metoclopramide 10 mg tid	CO	Symptoms GE liquid	M > B M = B
De Caestecker et al. [35]	19	8	Metoclopramide 10 mg tid vs cisapride 10 mg qid vs placebo	DBC	Symptoms Esoph. emptying GE liquid GE solid Whole-gut transit	M = P M = P M = P M = P M = P
McCallum et al. [72]	40	3	Metoclopramide 10 mg qid vs placebo	DB	Symptoms GE liquid* GE solid*	M > P M > B M = P
DOMPERIDONE						
Horowitz et al. [73]	12	*	Domperidone 20 mg tid	CO	Symptoms GE liquid GE solid	D > N D > N D = N

Study	N	Wks	Treatment	Design	Evaluation	Result
Champion et al. [74]	19	4	Domperidone 20 mg qid vs placebo	DB	Symptoms	D > P
					GE solid	D > P
Patterson et al. [75]	89	4	Domperidone 20 mg qid	SB	Symptoms	D > B
Patterson et al. [75]	64	4	Domperidone 20 mg qid vs placebo	DB	Symptoms	D > P

CISAPRIDE

Study	N	Wks	Treatment	Design	Evaluation	Result
Horowitz et al. [76]	20	4	Cisapride 10 mg qid vs placebo	DB	Symptoms	C > P
					Esoph. emptying	C = P
					GE liquid	C > P
					GE solid	C > P
Champion et al. [77]	18	4	Cisapride 10 mg qid vs placebo	DB	Symptoms	C > P
					GE solid	C > P
De Caestecker et al. [35]	19	8	Cisapride 10 mg qid vs metoclopramide 10 mg tid vs placebo	DBC	Symptoms	C = P
					Esoph. emptying	C = P
					GE liquid	C = P
					GE solid	C = P
					Whole-gut transit	C = P
Havelund et al. [78]	15	4	Cisapride 10 mg qid vs placebo	DBC	Symptoms	C = P
					GE solid	C = P

ERYTHROMYCIN (no controlled studies*)

*See text.
B, Baseline evaluation; C, cisapride; CO, comparison; D, domperidone; DB, double-blind controlled; DBC, double-blind crossover; Esoph, esophageal; GE, gastric emptying; M, metoclopramide; N, normal range; P, placebo; SB, single-blind.

Table 6.6 Treatment of diabetes mellitus: long-term open studies.

Study	Number of patients	Duration (months)	Regimen	Study design	Parameter studied	Results
DOMPERIDONE						
Koch et al. [79]	6	6	Domperidone 20 mg qid	Open	Symptoms	Significant
					GE solid	NS
					EGG	Significant
CISAPRIDE						
Champion et al. [80]	12	12	Cisapride 10 mg qid (n = 10)	Open	Symptoms	Significant
			Cisapride 20 mg qid (n = 2)		GE solid	Significant
					HbAlc	NS
Wolfsen and Patterson [81]	12	13	Cisapride 10–20 mg tid	Open	Symptoms	Improved in seven patients (58%)
						Improved and d/c in two patients (17%)
						No improvement in three patients (25%)
Patterson et al. [82]	7	24	Cisapride 20 mg tid	Open	Symptoms	Significant
					GE solid	Significant
Horowitz and Roberts [83]	1	12	Cisapride 10 mg tid	DBC	Symptoms	Significant
					GE liquid	Significant
					GE solid	Significant
					HbA1c	NS

C, cisapride; DBC, double-blind crossover; d/c, discontinued medication; GE, gastric emptying; HbAlc, glycosylated hemoglobin; NS, not significant compared with baseline values; Significant, significant compared with baseline values.

Table 6.7 Short-term and long-term studies in diabetic and idiopathic gastroparesis.

Study	Number of patients	Duration	Regimen	Study design	Parameter studied	Results
SHORT-TERM RANDOMIZED STUDIES						
Richards et al. [84]	D 7 I 29 S 2	6 weeks	Cisapride 20 mg tid vs placebo	DB	Symptoms GE solid	C = P = B C > P
LONG-TERM OPEN STUDIES						
Rothstein et al. [85]	D 7 I 7	6 months	Cisapride 10 mg tid	Open	Symptoms GE solid EGG	Significant Significant Improved*
Valenzuela et al. [86]	D 3 I 9	≥ 6 months*	Cisapride 20 mg tid	Open	Symptoms GE solid	40% improvement Significant
Abell et al. [87]	D 7 I 12	12 months	Cisapride 10 mg tid	Open	Symptoms GE liquid GE solid	Significant Significant Significant
Cooper et al. [88]	D 5 I 5	24 months	Cisapride 20 mg tid	Open	Symptoms GE solid	Significant Significant
Kendall et al. [89]	D 5 I 27	24 months	Cisapride 20 mg tid	Open	Symptoms GE solid	NS Significant
McCallum et al. [90]	D 1 I 5	9 months (3–13)	Cisapride 20 mg tid	Open	Symptoms GE solid	52% improvement Significant
Valenzuela et al. [91]	9*	15 ± 4 months	Cisapride 20 mg tid	Open	Symptoms Nausea Early satiety GE solid	Significant Significant Significant

* See text.

B, Baseline; C, cisapride; D, diabetic gastroparesis; DB, double-blind; GE, gastric emptying; I, idiopathic gastroparesis; NS, not significant compared with baseline values; P, placebo; S, progressive systemic sclerosis; Significant, significant compared with baseline values.

Erythromycin

There have been no placebo-controlled studies with erythromycin in patients with diabetic gastroparesis. In the initial article on the gastric prokinetic effect of erythromycin, Janssens *et al.* [24] followed 10 patients with type I diabetes and gastroparesis. IV erythromycin shortened the prolonged gastric emptying time for both liquids and solids to normal when compared with 10 healthy subjects. Gastric emptying also improved, but to a lesser degree, in the 10 patients after 4 weeks of treatment with oral erythromycin 250 mg tid. In another study [92], two patients with type I diabetes were among 10 patients who received erythromycin 500 mg qid for 4 weeks. For the study population as a whole, solid-phase gastric emptying and symptoms improved significantly from baseline. Five patients were followed for a total of 8.4 months, with the erythromycin dosage being adjusted to minimize symptoms.

In 20 type II diabetic patients with symptoms of gastroparesis and delayed solid-phase gastric emptying, erythromycin 250 mg tid for 2 weeks significantly improved from baseline that component of gastric emptying and the fasting blood sugar [93]. Symptoms were not evaluated in this study.

Erythromycin has been studied [94] in 12 patients with diabetes and 19 without who received chronic ambulatory peritoneal dialysis (CAPD). In four patients, the gastroparesis had been unresponsive to cisapride and metoclopramide. Intraperitoneal erythromycin, 100 mg for each 21 of dialysate, improved symptoms in all 31 patients. The authors thought that this was an effective means of administering a prokinetic agent to patients undergoing CAPD.

Long-term studies in diabetes mellitus

There are only limited data on the long-term efficacy of prokinetic agents in patients with diabetic gastroparesis. As it is not possible to conduct long-term placebo-controlled studies in gastroparesis, we must rely on results from open studies. Long-term trials in diabetic gastroparesis are summarized in Table 6.6; studies in patients with diabetic or idiopathic gastroparesis are reviewed in Table 6.7.

Long-term data have been reported with domperidone and cisapride. Six patients with type I diabetes and gastroparesis who were administered domperidone 20 mg qid were followed for 6 months [79]. Total symptom scores improved significantly; gastric emptying improved but not significantly. A normal 3-cpm EGG pattern, absent at the initial evaluation, was evident in all patients at the end of the study.

There have been four long-term studies [80–83] with cisapride in patients with diabetic gastroparesis. The first study [80] was an extension of a placebo-controlled study in 18 diabetics [77]. Twelve patients completing the placebo-controlled study were followed for 12 months. At the end of the 12 months there was a significant improvement in total symptom scores as well as epigastric pain, bloating, and constipation. In addition, solid-phase gastric emptying improved significantly in the first month and further improved at 12 months. All patients initially received cisapride 10 mg qid, and in two patients the dosage was increased to 20 mg qid during the study period.

In 9/12 patients with type I diabetes who were resistant to metoclopramide, cisapride 10–20 mg tid produced symptom improvement at 13 months (with two also discontinuing cisapride) [81]. In another study [82], cisapride 20 mg tid improved symptoms and solid-phase gastric emptying at 24 months. Finally in one patient, there was a significant 12-month improvement in total symptom scores as well as solid- and liquid-phase gastric emptying with cisapride 10 mg tid [83]. Glycosylated hemoglobin (HbA1c), an index of glycemic control, was measured in two studies [80, 83] and did not improve.

Cisapride also has been evaluated in study populations with diabetic *and* idiopathic gastroparesis. Rothstein *et al.* [85] reported normalization of EGG electroactivity in 4/12 patients and improvement in 6/12. Patients in whom the EGG normalized had a greater gastric emptying rate than those with continued dysrhythmias. In a total of 78 patients with diabetic or idiopathic gastroparesis [86–91] followed for 6–24 months, cisapride produced consistent significant improvements in solid-phase gastric emptying; significant symptom improvement was reported in 3/6 studies [87, 88, 91].

Idiopathic gastroparesis

Studies in idiopathic gastroparesis are summarized in Table 6.8 [95–100]. Studies evaluating patients with idiopathic or diabetic gastroparesis were summarized in Table 6.7. Two studies of gastroparesis of different causes including idiopathic gastroparesis are reviewed in Table 6.10.

Table 6.8 Short-term and long-term studies in idiopathic gastroparesis.

Study	Number of patients	Duration	Regimen	Study design	Parameter studied	Results
SHORT-TERM RANDOMIZED STUDIES						
Domperidone						
McCallum *et al.* [95]	5	3 weeks	Domperidone 20–30 mg qid vs placebo	DBC	Symptoms	D > P
Cisapride						
Corinaldesi *et al.* [96]	12	2 weeks	Cisapride 10 mg tid vs placebo	DBC	Symptoms GE solid	C = P C > P
Jian *et al.* [97]	28	6 weeks	Cisapride 10 mg tid vs placebo	DB	Symptoms GE liquid GE solid (59%)*	C = P C > P C > P
LONG-TERM OPEN STUDIES						
Cisapride						
Dworkin *et al.* [98]	10	13.5 months*	Cisapride 10–20 mg tid	Open	Symptoms GE solid	Significant Significant
Fette *et al.* [99]	15	6 months	Cisapride 10–20 mg tid	Open	GE solid	Significant
Stagias *et al.* [100]	21	18 months	Cisapride 10–20 mg tid	Open	Symptoms GE solid	Improved Improved

* See text.

C, Cisapride; D, domperidone; DB, double-blind; DBC, double-blind controlled; DBC, double-blind crossover; GE, gastric emptying; P, placebo; Significant, significant improvement compared with baseline.

Metoclopramide

Fifty-five patients with symptoms of gastroparesis and evidence of delayed emptying with an abnormal barium burger radiologic study were randomized to metoclopramide 10 mg qid or placebo for 3 weeks [101] (see Table 6.10). In the 29 patients with idiopathic gastroparesis, metoclopramide significantly decreased symptom scores.

Domperidone

In a double-blind crossover study [95] in five patients with idiopathic gastroparesis, domperidone 20–30 mg qid for 3 weeks significantly improved symptoms compared with placebo. Gastric emptying was not evaluated in this study.

Cisapride

Three double-blind studies [84, 96, 97] evaluating cisapride 10 or 20 mg tid for 2–6 weeks in patients with idiopathic gastroparesis did not show symptom improvement compared with placebo but did show enhanced gastric emptying. In contrast, in yet another crossover study [114] (see Table 6.10), cisapride 10 mg tid for 3 weeks did improve symptoms compared with placebo as well as improved gastric emptying of solids.

Erythromycin

There have been no controlled studies with erythromycin. In 10 patients with idiopathic gastroparesis (along with four with diabetic gastroparesis), there were significant improvements in solid-phase gastric emptying and symptoms after erythromycin 500 mg qid for 4 weeks [92]. These findings were similar to results of another open study [102] of two patients with idiopathic gastroparesis taking erythromycin 100 mg tid or 300 mg qid who had not responded to domperidone or metoclopramide.

Long-term studies

Long-term studies in patients with diabetic or idiopathic gastroparesis have already been summarized in the discussion on diabetic gastroparesis. A total of 46 patients with idiopathic gastroparesis have been followed for 6–18 months [98–100]. The dose of cisapride varied from 10 to

20 mg tid. The three studies demonstrated significant improvements from baseline in solid-phase gastric emptying and symptoms.

Postsurgical gastroparesis

Upper GI symptoms in patients following gastric surgery are usually multifactorial in etiology. Gastric surgery, particularly truncal vagotomy, produces abnormalities in gastric motor activity, resulting in more rapid emptying of liquids but slower emptying of solids. Other factors include the dumping syndrome, size of the gastric remnant, bile gastritis, and small bowel bacterial overgrowth. Studies of prokinetic agents in patients with postsurgical gastroparesis are summarized in Table 6.9 [103–108]. Three studies of gastroparesis of different causes are reviewed in Table 6.10 [101, 109–114].

Metoclopramide

Several studies have demonstrated the efficacy of metoclopramide in acute and chronic postsurgical gastroparesis. Most were performed in the 1970s, were of short duration, and relied on symptom improvement or a worsening of symptoms on discontinuation of metoclopramide [12]. There have been two small controlled studies in a total of 27 patients with metoclopramide 10 mg tid or qid with symptoms of gastroparesis after vagotomy and gastric surgery [104, 105]. Metoclopramide significantly improved symptoms compared with placebo and in one study was superior to carbachol 1 mg tid (a parasympathomimetic) [104]. In another study by Davidson, of 20 patients with postsurgical gastroparesis taking metoclopramide 10 mg qid for 2–4 weeks, there was excellent or good relief of symptoms in 45% of patients, fair improvement in 25%, and no change in symptoms in 35% [105]. In a double-blind study in gastroparesis associated with diabetes ($n = 13$) and duodenal surgery ($n = 10$), Saltzman et al. [113] showed that IV and oral metoclopramide significantly improved the gastric emptying of a semisolid meal; metoclopramide 10 mg qid for 3 weeks significantly improved the symptoms of gastroparesis compared with placebo. In 55 patients with symptoms of gastroparesis and evidence of delayed gastric emptying, metoclopramide 10 mg qid for 3 weeks significantly improved symptoms in 21 patients who had had a vagotomy and drainage procedure [101].

Table 6.9 Short-term studies in postsurgical gastroparesis.

Study	Number of patients	Duration (weeks)	Regimen	Study design	Parameter studied	Results
METOCLOPRAMIDE						
Stadaas and Aune [103]	10	2	Metoclopramide 10 mg tid vs carbachol 1 mg tid vs placebo	DBC	Symptoms	M > C M > P C = P
McClelland and Horton [104]	17	4	Metoclopramide 10 mg qid vs placebo	DB	Symptoms	M > P
Davidson et al. [105]	20	2–4	Metoclopramide 10 mg tid	Open	Symptoms	Excellent 4 Good 5 Fair 5 Poor 6
DOMPERIDONE						
Molino et al. [106]	12	4	Domperidone 10 mg tid	Open	Symptoms	D > B
CISAPRIDE						
van der Mijle et al. [107]	24	3	Cisapride 10 mg qid	Open	Symptoms GE solid RS	Improved* in 11/24 Improved* in 7/13 Improved* in 3/13
ERYTHROMYCIN						
Ramirez et al. [108]	9	2	Erythromycin 125–250 mg tid	Open	Symptoms	E = B*

*See text.
B, Baseline; C, carbachol; DB, double-blind controlled; DBC, double-blind crossover; E, erythromycin; GE, gastric emptying; M, metoclopramide; P, placebo; RS, Roux limb stasis.

Table 6.10 Studies in primary anorexia nervosa, progressive systemic sclerosis, myotonic dystrophy, and miscellaneous gastroparesis.

Study	Number of patients	Duration (weeks)	Regimen	Study design	Parameter studied	Results
PRIMARY ANOREXIA NERVOSA						
Stacher et al. [109]	12	6	Cisapride 10 mg tid vs placebo	DB	GE semisolid	C > P
Young et al. [110]	34	8	Cisapride 10 mg tid vs placebo	DB	Symptoms	C > P*
					GE solid (n = 9)*	C = P
PROGRESSIVE SYSTEMIC SCLEROSIS						
Horowitz et al. [111]	8	4	Cisapride 10 mg qid	Open	Symptoms	Significant
MYOTONIC DYSTROPHY						
Horowitz et al. [112]	10	4	Cisapride 10 mg qid	Open	Symptoms	Significant
					Esoph. emptying	NS
					GE liquid	NS
					GE solid	Significant
MISCELLANEOUS						
Perkel et al. [101]		3	Metoclopramide 10 mg qid vs placebo	DB	Symptoms	NS
Diabetes	5				D	
Idiopathic	29				I + S	M > P
Postsurgery	21				All patients	M > P
Saltzman et al. [113]		3	Metoclopramide 10 mg qid vs placebo	DBC	Symptoms	M > P
Diabetes	13				GE semisolid	M > P
Postsurgery	10					
McCallum et al. [114]		3	Cisapride 10 mg tid vs placebo	DBC	Symptoms	C > P
Diabetes	8				GE solid	Significant
Idiopathic	7					
Postsurgery	7					

*See text.

C, cisapride; D, diabetic; DB, double-blind controlled; DBC, double-blind crossover; Esoph, esophageal; GE, gastric emptying; I, idiopathic; M, metoclopramide; NS, not significant compared with baseline values; P, placebo; S, postgastric surgery; Significant, significant compared with baseline values.

Domperidone

Domperidone 10 mg tid for 4 weeks improved the symptoms of post-vagotomy gastric stasis in 10/12 patients compared with baseline [106].

Cisapride

In a 3-week crossover study, McCallum *et al.* [114] evaluated cisapride 10 mg tid and placebo in 22 patients, of whom seven had postsurgical gastroparesis. The other 15 patients in the study had diabetic ($n = 8$) or idiopathic ($n = 7$) gastroparesis. There were significant improvements in gastric emptying and symptoms in the cisapride group compared with placebo. In another study [107], cisapride 10 mg qid for 3 weeks produced symptom relief in 11/24 patients with gastric stasis following Roux-en-Y surgery. Seven patients with gastroparesis and three with Roux-en-Y stasis had symptomatic improvement and accelerated emptying. This improvement was sustained in all but one patient after 6 more months of therapy. In the 13 patients whose symptoms did not improve, there was no improvement in gastric emptying.

Erythromycin

Recent studies have demonstrated the efficacy of IV erythromycin in improving gastroparesis associated with esophagectomy [115], Whipple resection [116], and gastric surgery for peptic ulcer disease [117, 118]. Oral erythromycin was evaluated in an open study [108] of nine patients with gastroparesis following vagotomy and antrectomy. After erythromycin 150 mg (range, 125–250 mg) tid orally for 2 weeks, symptoms improved in only 3/9 patients. This was not significant when all nine patients were compared to their baseline symptom scores.

Primary anorexia nervosa (PAN)

Delayed gastric emptying has been reported to be common in patients with PAN. Even without documented gastroparesis, many symptoms encountered in these patients suggest gastric dysmotility or a delay in gastric emptying. Acute IV use of metoclopramide, domperidone, cisapride, and erythromycin has been shown to be effective in PAN; the long-term efficacy of prokinetic agents remains unclear.

There have been two short-term placebo-controlled studies with cisapride (Table 6.10). Stacher *et al.* [109] evaluated cisapride 10 mg tid versus placebo for 6 weeks in 12 patients with PAN. Cisapride accelerated gastric emptying in 6/6 patients, five patients gained weight, and four patients had symptom improvement. In the placebo group, gastric emptying improved in 3/6 patients, four gained weight, and one had symptom improvement. At the end of 6 weeks, all patients received cisapride for a further 6 weeks. There was further improvement in 5/6 patients who initially received cisapride. In the patients who were previously randomized to placebo, 4/6 had improvement in gastric emptying, five gained weight, and four had symptom improvement. In the other study [110], 34 patients with PAN were treated with cisapride 10 mg tid or placebo for 8 weeks. There was no significant improvement in gastric emptying in the nine patients with gastroparesis treated with cisapride. However, postprandial abdominal discomfort associated with PAN did improve significantly compared with placebo. It was thought that cisapride may aid psychiatric therapy in patients with PAN.

Progressive systemic sclerosis (PSS)

Patients with PSS have frequent GI involvement, presenting with esophageal and gastric emptying abnormalities that may be associated with small bowel dysfunction. In IV studies, metoclopramide, domperidone, cisapride, and erythromycin have shown efficacy in improving esophageal or gastric dysmotility, or both. There are no placebo-controlled studies with prokinetic agents in patients with PSS; an open study has been reported (Table 6.10).

Horowitz *et al.* [111] studied the acute and chronic effects of cisapride on gastric emptying in eight patients with PSS. There was a significant improvement in both solid and liquid emptying after administration of cisapride 10 mg IV. After 4 weeks of cisapride 10 mg qid orally, there was a significant improvement in symptoms compared to baseline. In a patient with scleroderma, erythromycin 200 mg tid for 9 months effectively resolved the symptoms of gastroparesis and led to a 4-kg weight gain [119].

Recently, octreotide, a long-acting somatostatin analog, has been shown to restore the MMC to normal, decrease rectal and bowel distention, and improve bacterial overgrowth in patients with PSS [120]. Plasma motilin levels, which are normally high in patients with scleroderma, were inhibited by octreotide injection, suggesting that the intestinal motility evoked was independent of motilin. Symptom improvement has been reported [120–122] in a total of 11 patients with PSS receiving octreotide 50 µg daily for 3 weeks.

Myotonic dystrophy

Patients with myotonic dystrophy may have symptoms of gastroparesis and delayed gastric emptying, presumably due to gastric smooth-muscle involvement. In 10 patients with this disease, Horowitz *et al.* [112] found that cisapride 10 mg qid for 4 weeks significantly improved the gastric emptying of solids and associated symptoms (Table 6.10). Cisapride appears to be a drug to consider in patients with myotonic dystrophy and symptoms of gastroparesis.

Summary

The efficacy of four gastric prokinetic agents — metoclopramide, domperidone (not yet available in the USA), cisapride, and erythromycin — have been reviewed.

Metoclopramide is an effective parenterally administered prokinetic agent. The long-term efficacy of the gastric prokinetic action of metoclopramide has been questioned. Long-term symptom improvement may be due more to the antiemetic action on the chemoreceptor trigger zone and the vomiting center than to the drug's prokinetic action. The use of metoclopramide is limited by the high incidence of side effects.

Domperidone is an effective gastric prokinetic agent in diabetic gastroparesis. Studies in other gastroparetic conditions demonstrate a less clear-cut efficacy. Domperidone is associated with fewer side effects than metoclopramide. For physicians who wish to use a dopamine antagonist, domperidone, with its better side-effects profile, is the drug of choice. The antiemetic action of the dopamine antagonists makes these agents particularly effective in gastroparetic patients with significant nausea.

Cisapride is an effective prokinetic in many gastroparetic conditions. It is the only prokinetic agent with proven efficacy in long-term studies. With fewer side effects than the dopamine antagonists, it is the prokinetic agent of choice in gastroparesis. This recommendation is made with the recognition that cisapride is not approved in the USA for the treatment of gastroparesis. The potential for drug–drug interactions with certain antifungal agents and macrolide antimicrobials has led to two important considerations.

1   There is no recommendation for how long to discontinue cisapride

before using one of these agents or for how long to discontinue an interacting agent before restarting cisapride. The prescribing physician should review the half-lives of the drugs in question and make a decision on the basis of the estimated time to eliminate the drug from the body.

2   The combination of cisapride and erythromycin in severe gastroparesis should no longer be considered.

Erythromycin has proven to be an effective gastric prokinetic agent in many acute oral and IV studies. The clinical efficacy of erythromycin for long-term (more than 2 weeks) use is not well established. Currently, erythromycin seems to be used in the short-term or acute management of gastroparesis, particularly as erythromycin is one of the two available parenteral prokinetic agents. A new generation of macrolide prokinetic drugs is undergoing preclinical testing and should be available for clinical studies in the near future.

Approach to the patient with gastroparesis (Figure 6.2)

The diagnosis of gastric dysmotility or gastroparesis can be made by history alone. Patients with symptoms of anorexia, early satiety, nausea, vomiting, and postprandial epigastric pain or fullness should be considered for a trial of a prokinetic agent. An upper GI series or, ideally, an endoscopy should be performed to rule out a mechanical obstruction or acid-mediated disease. These investigations may demonstrate retained food in the stomach. There also may be associated GERD secondary to gastric stasis. Given the poor correlation between symptoms and findings on gastric motility testing, it is reasonable to recommend that these investigations be reserved for the atypical patient or the patient with a typical presentation who does not improve with an adequate trial of therapy. Because prokinetic agents take time to exert their maximal effect, therapy should be continued for at least 4–8 weeks before considering alternative therapy or an increase in dose. Patients with severe gastroparesis may also have delayed delivery of the drug to the small bowel, which further delays the onset of the drug's therapeutic action.

Gastroparesis, like many other motility disorders, is often cyclic or intermittent in its severity. In patients with intermittent symptoms, pulse therapy for 4–8 weeks with a prokinetic agent is often effective. Treatment can be administered on return of symptoms, with the patient taking no medication between symptom episodes. In diabetic gastroparesis, PSS and other gastroparetic conditions associated with more severe symptoms, continuous therapy is necessary. In diabetic gastroparesis, the

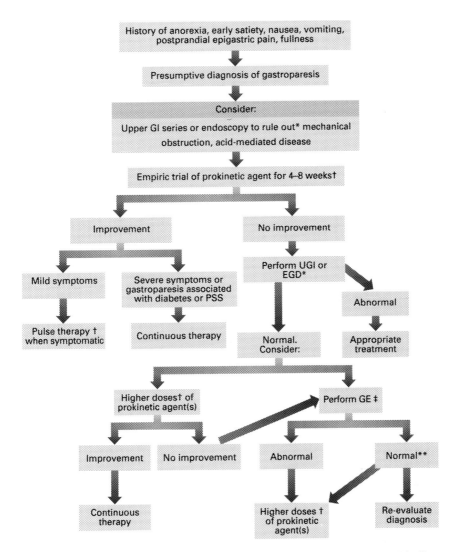

Fig. 6.2 Algorithm for the treatment of gastroparesis in the 'typical' patient. *Ideally esophagogastroduodenoscopy. †See text. ‡Gastric emptying study should ideally be performed after discontinuation of prokinetic treatment for at least 2 weeks. Alternatively, perform gastric emptying study while the patient is on prokinetics. If abnormal, continue prokinetics. If normal, discontinue prokinetics for 2 weeks and repeat gastric emptying study. **Gastric emptying study may be normal in patients with symptoms of gastroparesis. These patients often improve with continued use of prokinetic agent (3–6 months). EGD, esophagogastroduodenoscopy; GE, gastric emptying study; UGI, upper GI barium series.

prokinetic agent should be continued whether or not the patient is symptomatic, as improved gastric emptying results in better glycemic control.

Initially, IV administration may have to be considered in some gastroparetic conditions. The drug of choice is metoclopramide 10 mg every 6 hours. Erythromycin 250–500 mg every 8 hours should be reserved for patients who do not improve with or who cannot tolerate metoclopramide. Patients administered metoclopramide can be given oral therapy at the same time.

The drug of choice for oral therapy is cisapride 10–20 mg half an hour before meals and at bedtime. In single-agent or combination therapy, the effective dose of domperidone is 20 mg qid and of metoclopramide, 10 mg qid. With its better side-effects profile, domperidone is the dopamine antagonist of choice for the treatment of gastroparesis. However, in the USA, metoclopramide is an alternative, because domperidone is not available. Dopamine antagonists are particularly effective in patients with significant nausea and may be considered as primary or combination therapy in these patients. When severe symptoms of gastroparesis are present, combination therapy with a dopamine antagonist and cisapride may be considered. The rationale for combining two prokinetic agents is their different modes of action on improving gastric motility. Cisapride increases acetylcholine release at the myenteric plexus, thereby accelerating gastric emptying. Antagonism of the dopamine receptor improves gastric motility by releasing the 'breaking' action of dopamine. Effective dosing for combination therapy is domperidone 20 mg qid plus cisapride 20 mg qid.

In severe gastroparesis, cisapride is well tolerated in larger doses. The author has treated at least 40 patients with diabetic gastroparesis with a combination of domperidone 20 mg qid plus cisapride 20–40 mg qid. Large doses of prokinetic agents should be used only when clinically necessary and when the benefits outweigh the risks. The dosage should be increased slowly, with small increments every 4–8 weeks. Candidates for high-dose prokinetic therapy include diabetics with severe gastroparesis who have difficulty maintaining an adequate caloric intake due to the gastroparesis.

Acknowledgment

Dr Champion would like to thank Anna Micucci for her secretarial assistance in preparing this manuscript.

References

1 Kendall BJ, McCallum RW. Gastroparesis and the current use of prokinetic drugs. *Gastroenterologist* 1993;**1**:107–14.

2 Malagelada J-R, Rees WDW, Mazzotta LJ, Go VLW. Gastric motor abnormalities in diabetic and postvagotomy gastroparesis: effect of metoclopramide and bethanechol. *Gastroenterology* 1980;**78**:286–93.

3 Fox S, Behar J. Pathogenesis of diabetic gastroparesis: a pharmacologic study. *Gastroenterology* 1980;**78**:757–63.

4 Lin ZY, Pan J, McCallum RW, Chen JDZ. Do gastric myoelectrical abnormalities predict delayed gastric emptying? *Gastroenterology* 1995;**108**:A639.

5 Koch KL, Stern RM, Stewart WR, Vasey MW. Gastric emptying and gastric myoelectrical activity in patients with diabetic gastroparesis: effect of long-term domperidone treatment. *Am J Gastroenterol* 1989;**84**:1069–73.

6 Schuurkes JAJ, Helsen LFM, Van Nueten JM. Improved gastroduodenal coordination by the peripheral dopamine-antagonist domperidone. In: Wienbeck M, ed. *Motility of the Digestive Tract*. New York: Raven Press, 1982:565–72.

7 Stacher G, Gaupmann G, Mittelbach G, Schneider C, Steinringer H, Langer B. Effects of oral cisapride on interdigestive jejunal motor activity, psychomotor function, and side-effect profile in healthy man. *Dig Dis Sci* 1987;**32**:1223–30.

8 McCallum RW. Review of the current status of prokinetic agents in gastroenterology. *Am J Gastroenterol* 1985;**80**:1008–16.

9 Champion MC. Minireview: domperidone. *Gen Pharmacol* 1988;**19**:499–505.

10 McCallum RW. Cisapride: a new class of prokinetic agent. *Am J Gastroenterol* 1991;**86**:135–49.

11 United States Pharmacopeial Convention Inc. Erythromycin. In: *USP Drug Information for the Health Care Professional*. Taunton, MA: Rand McNally, 1995;**I**:1244–5.

12 Albibi R, McCallum RW. Metoclopramide: pharmacology and clinical application. *Ann Intern Med* 1983;**98**:86–95.

13 Pinder RM, Brogden RN, Sawyer PR, Speight TM, Avery GS. Metoclopramide: a review of its pharmacological properties and clinical use. *Drugs* 1976;**12**:81–131.

14 Bateman DN, Rawlins MD, Simpson JM. Extrapyramidal reactions with metoclopramide. *BMJ* 1985;**291**:930–2.

15 Ganzini L, Casey DE, Hoffman WF, McCall AL. The prevalence of metoclopramide-induced tardive dyskinesia and acute extrapyramidal movement disorders. *Arch Intern Med* 1993;**153**:1469–75.

16 Weihrauch TR, Forster CFR, Krieglstein J. Evaluation of the effect of domperidone on human oesophageal and gastroduodenal motility by intraluminal manometry. *Postgrad Med J* 1979;**55**(Suppl.1):7–10.

17 Miederer SE. A German multicentre trial with domperidone in dyspeptic disorders. *Therapeut Today* 1987;**6**:43–8.

18 Brogden RN, Carmine AA, Heel RC, Speight TM, Avery GS. Domperidone: a review of its pharmacological activity, pharmacokinetics and therapeutic efficacy in the symptomatic treatment of chronic dyspepsia and as an antiemetic. *Drugs* 1982;**24**:360–400.

19 Roussak JB, Carey P, Parry H. Cardiac arrest after treatment with intravenous domperidone. *BMJ* 1984;**289**:1579.

20 Reyntjens A, Verlinden M, Aerts T. Development and clinical use of the new gastrointestinal prokinetic drug cisapride 15 (R51 619). *Drug Dev Res* 1986;**8**:251–65.

21 Kawagishi T, Nishizawa Y, Okuno Y, Sekiya K, Morii H. Effect of cisapride on gastric emptying of indigestible solids and plasma motilin concentration in diabetic autonomic neuropathy. *Am J Gastroenterol* 1993;**88**:933–8.

22 Wiseman LR, Faulds D. Cisapride: an updated review of its pharmacology and therapeutic efficacy as a prokinetic agent in gastrointestinal motility disorders. *Drugs* 1994;**47**:116–52.

23 Propulsid. Prescribing information. Titusville, NJ: Janssen Pharmaceutica Inc, September, 1995.

24 Janssens J, Peeters TL, Vantrappen G et al. Improvement of gastric emptying in diabetic gastroparesis by erythromycin: preliminary studies. *N Engl J Med* 1990;**322**:1028–31.

25 Itoh Z, Nakaya M, Suzuki T, Arai H, Wakabayashi K. Erythromycin mimics exogenous motilin in gastrointestinal contractile activity in the dog. *Am J Physiol* 1984;**247**:G688–94.

26 Kondo Y, Torii K, Omura S, Itoh Z. Erythromycin and its derivatives with motilin-like biological activities inhibit the specific binding of ^{125}I-motilin to duodenal muscle. *Biochem Biophys Res Commun* 1988;**150**:877–82.

27 Depoortere I, Peeters TL, Vantrappen G. Erythromycin modulates motilin receptor density in rabbit. *Gastroenterology* 1989;**96**:A119.

28 Annese V, Janssens J, Vantrappen G et al. Erythromycin accelerates gastric emptying by inducing antral contractions and improved gastroduodenal coordination. *Gastroenterology* 1992;**102**:823–8.

29 Tomomasa T, Kuroume T, Arai H, Wakabayashi K, Itoh Z. Erythromycin induces migrating motor complex in human gastrointestinal tract. *Dig Dis Sci* 1986;**31**:157–61.

30 Sarna SK, Soergel KH, Koch TR et al. Effects of erythromycin on human gastrointestinal motor activity in the fasted and fed states. *Gastroenterology* 1989;**96**:A440.

31 Janssens J, Vantrappen G, Urbain JL et al. The motilin agonist erythromycin normalises impaired gastric emptying in diabetic gastroparesis. *Gastroenterology* 1989;**96**:A237.

32 Lin HC, Sanders SL, Gu Y-G, Doty JE. Erythromycin accelerates solid emptying at the expense of gastric sieving. *Dig Dis Sci* 1994;**39**:124–8.

33 McHugh S, Lico S, Meindok H, Diamant NE. Intravenous cisapride in diabetic gastroparesis. *Gastroenterology* 1986;**90**:A1545.

34 Feldman M, Smith HJ. Effect of cisapride on gastric emptying of indigestible solids in patients with gastroparesis diabeticorum: a comparison with metoclopramide and placebo. *Gastroenterology* 1987;**92**:171–4.

35 De Caestecker JS, Ewing DJ, Tothill P, Clarke BF, Heading RC. Evaluation of oral cisapride and metoclopramide in diabetic autonomic neuropathy: an eight-week double-blind crossover study. *Aliment Pharmacol Ther* 1989;**3**:69–81.

36 Erbas T, Varoglu E, Erbas B, Tastekin G, Akalin S. Comparison of metoclopramide and erythromycin in the treatment of diabetic gastroparesis. *Diabetes Care* 1993;**16**:1511–14.

37 Champion MC, Braaten J, Gulenchyn K. Domperidone (Motilium) compared to cisapride (Prepulsid) in the management of gastroparesis. *Am J Gastroenterol* 1991;**86**:1309.

38 Fink SM, Lange RC, McCallum RW. Effect of metoclopramide on normal and delayed gastric emptying in gastroesophageal reflux patients. *Dig Dis Sci* 1983;**28**:1057–61.

39 Champion MC, Sullivan SN, Chamberlain M, Vezina W. Naloxone and morphine inhibit gastric emptying of solids. *Can J Physiol Pharmacol* 1982;**60**:732–4.

40 Mittal RK, Frank EB, Lange RC, McCallum RW. Effects of morphine and naloxone on esophageal motility and gastric emptying in man. *Dig Dis Sci* 1986;**31**:936–42.

41 Coffin B, Jian R, Lemann M *et al*. Fedotozine increases threshold of discomfort to gastric distension in healthy subjects. *Gastroenterology* 1992;**102**:A437.

42 Pascaud X, Honde C, Le Gallou B *et al*. Effects of fedotozine on gastrointestinal motility in dogs: mechanism of action and related pharmacokinetics. *J Pharm Pharmacol* 1990;**42**:546–52.

43 Fraitag B, Homerin M, Hecketsweiler P. Double-blind dose-response multicenter comparison of fedotozine and placebo in treatment of nonulcer dyspepsia. *Dig Dis Sci* 1994;**39**:1072–7.

44 Lenz HJ, Schuler U, Hicking W, Ehninger G. Phase I-trial of clebopride, a new antiemetic, in chemotherapy-induced nausea and vomiting. *Eur J Clin Pharmacol* 1990;**38**:525.

45 Bavestrello L, Caimi L, Barbera A. A double-blind comparison of clebopride and placebo in dyspepsia secondary to delayed gastric emptying. *Clin Ther* 1985;**7**:468–73.

46 Bovero E, Poletti M, Vigneri S. The effects of clebopride on esophageal motility: a double-blind randomized manometric study. *Curr Ther Res* 1989;**46**:895–902.

47 Smith WL, Alphin RS, Jackson CB, Sancilio LF. The antiemetic profile of zacopride. *J Pharm Pharmacol* 1989;**41**:101–5.

48 Craig DA, Clarke DE. Peristalsis evoked by 5-HT and renzapride: evidence for putative 5-HT$_4$ receptor activation. *Br J Pharmacol* 1991;**102**:563–4.

49 Mackie ADR, Ferrington C, Cowan S, Merrick MV, Baird JD, Palmer KR. The effects of renzapride, a novel prokinetic agent, in diabetic gastroparesis. *Aliment Pharmacol Ther* 1991;**5**:135–42.

50 Fedorak RN, Field M, Chang EB. Treatment of diabetic diarrhea and clonidine. *Ann Intern Med* 1985;**102**:197–9.

51 Rosa-E-Silva L, Troncon LEA, Oliveira RB, Iazigi N, Gallo L Jr, Foss MC. Treatment of diabetic gastroparesis with oral clonidine. *Aliment Pharmacol Ther* 1995;**9**:179–83.

52 Champion MC, Hartnett M, Yen M. Domperidone, a new dopamine antagonist. *Can Med Assoc J* 1986;**135**:457–61.

53 Peeters TL. Erythromycin and other macrolides as prokinetic agents. *Gastroenterology* 1993;**105**:1886–99.

54 Weber FH Jr, Richards RD, McCallum RW. Erythromycin: a motilin agonist and gastrointestinal prokinetic agent. *Am J Gastroenterol* 1993;**88**:485–90.

55 Feldman M, Schiller LR. Disorders of gastrointestinal motility associated with diabetes mellitus. *Ann Intern Med* 1983;**98**:378–84.

56 van Dijl PW, Hofma SJ, van Doormaal JJ, Piers DA, Beekhuis H, Kleibeuker JH. Low prevalence of symptomatic gastric and esophageal motor dysfunction in diabetes mellitus. *Gastroenterology* 1989;**96**:A524.

57 Keshavarzian A, Iber FL, Vaeth J. Gastric emptying in patients with insulin-requiring diabetes mellitus. *Am J Gastroenterol* 1987;**82**:29–35.

58 Horowitz M, Harding PE, Maddox A *et al*. Gastric and oesophageal emptying in insulin-dependent diabetes mellitus. *J Gastroenterol Hepatol* 1986;**1**:97–113.

59 Horowitz M, Maddox AF, Wishart JM, Harding PE, Chatterton BE, Shearman DJC. Relationships between oesophageal transit and solid and liquid gastric emptying in diabetes mellitus. *Eur J Nucl Med* 1991;**18**:229–34.

60 Clouse RE, Lustman PJ. Gastrointestinal symptoms in diabetic patients: lack of association with neuropathy. *Am J Gastroenterol* 1989;**84**:868–72.

61 Campbell IW, Heading RC, Tothill P, Buist TAS, Ewing DJ, Clarke BF. Gastric emptying in diabetic autonomic neuropathy. *Gut* 1977;**18**:462–7.

62 Loo FD, Palmer DW, Soergel KH, Kalbfleisch JH, Wood CM. Gastric emptying in patients with diabetes mellitus. *Gastroenterology* 1984;**86**:485–94.

63 Wegener M, Borsch G, Schaffstein J, Luerweg F, Leverkus F. Gastrointestinal transit disorders in patients with insulin-treated diabetes mellitus. *Dig Dis* 1990;**8**:23–36.

64 Wright RA, Clemente R, Wathen R. Diabetic gastroparesis: an abnormality of gastric emptying of solids. *Am J Med Sci* 1985;**289**:240–2.

65 Fraser RJ, Horowitz M, Maddox AF, Harding PE, Chatterton BE, Dent J. Hyperglycaemia slows gastric emptying in type 1 (insulin-dependent) diabetes mellitus. *Diabetologia* 1990;**33**:675–80.

66 Horowitz M, Harding PE, Maddox AF *et al.* Gastric and oesophageal emptying in patients with type 2 (non-insulin-dependent) diabetes mellitus. *Diabetologia* 1989;**32**:151–9.

67 Hasler WL, Soudah HC, Dulai G, Owyang C. Mediation of hyperglycemia-evoked gastric slow-wave dysrhythmias by endogenous prostaglandins. *Gastroenterology* 1995;**108**:727–36.

68 Groop LC, DeFronzo RA, Luzi L, Melander A. Hyperglycaemia and absorption of sulphonylurea drugs. *Lancet* 1989;**2**:129–30.

69 Snape WJ Jr, Battle WM, Schwartz SS, Braunstein SN, Goldstein HA, Alavi A. Metoclopramide to treat gastroparesis due to diabetes mellitus: a double-blind, controlled trial. *Ann Intern Med* 1982;**96**:444–6.

70 Ricci DA, Saltzman MB, Meyer C, Callachan C, McCallum RW. Effect of metoclopramide in diabetic gastroparesis. *J Clin Gastroenterol* 1985;**7**:25–32.

71 Schade RR, Dugas MC, Lhotsky DM, Gavaler JS, Van Thiel DH. Effect of metoclopramide on gastric liquid emptying in patients with diabetic gastroparesis. *Dig Dis Sci* 1985;**30**:10–15.

72 McCallum RW, Ricci DA, Rakatansky H *et al.* A multicenter placebo-controlled clinical trial of oral metoclopramide in diabetic gastroparesis. *Diabetes Care* 1983;**6**:463–7.

73 Horowitz M, Harding PE, Chatterton BE, Collins PJ, Shearman DJC. Acute and chronic effects of domperidone on gastric emptying in diabetic autonomic neuropathy. *Dig Dis Sci* 1985;**30**:1–9.

74 Champion MC, Gulenchyn K, O'Leary T, Irving P, Edwards A, Braaten J. Domperidone (Motilium) improves symptoms and solid phase gastric emptying in diabetic gastroparesis. *Am J Gastroenterol* 1987;**82**:975.

75 Patterson D, Koch K, Abell T, Wald A, Falk GW, Long J. A multi-center placebo-controlled study of domperidone in diabetic gastroparesis. *Gastroenterology* 1993;**104**:A564.

76 Horowitz M, Maddox A, Harding PE *et al.* Effect of cisapride on gastric and esophageal emptying in insulin-dependent diabetes mellitus. *Gastroenterology* 1987;**92**:1899–907.

77 Champion MC, Gulenchyn K, Braaten J, Irvine P, O'Leary T, Edwards A, Gay J. Cisapride improves symptoms and solid phase gastric emptying in diabetic gastroparesis (DGP). *Diabetes* 1988;**37**(Suppl.1):84A.

78 Havelund T, Oster-Jorgensen E, Eshoj O, Lytken Larsen M, Lauritsen K. Effects of cisapride on gastroparesis in patients with insulin-dependent diabetes mellitus: a double-blind controlled trial. *Acta Med Scand* 1987;**222**:339–43.

79 Koch KL, Stern RM, Stewart WR, Vasey MW. Gastric emptying and gastric

myoelectrical activity in patients with diabetic gastroparesis: effect of long-term domperidone treatment. *Am J Gastroenterol* 1989;**84**:1069–75.

80 Champion MC, Gulenchyn K, Braaten J, Irvine P, O'Leary T, Gay J. Long term (1 year) efficacy of cisapride (Prepulsid) in diabetic gastroparesis (DGP). *Diabetes* 1989;**38**(Suppl.2):26A.

81 Wolfsen HC, Patterson DJ. Long term cisapride treatment in patients with refractory diabetic gastropathy (DG). *Am J Gastroenterol* 1989;**89**:1172.

82 Patterson DJ, Eisenberg B, Skinner SF. Cisapride is effective long-term therapy for diabetic gastroparesis. *Gastroenterology* 1993;**104**:A564.

83 Horowitz M, Roberts AP. Long-term efficacy of cisapride in diabetic gastroparesis. *Am J Med* 1990;**88**:195–6.

84 Richards RD, Valenzuela GA, Davenport KG, Fisher KLK, McCallum RW. Objective and subjective results of a randomized, double-blind, placebo-controlled trial using cisapride to treat gastroparesis. *Dig Dis Sci* 1993;**38**:811–16.

85 Rothstein RD, Alavi A, Reynolds JC. Electrogastrography in patients with gastroparesis and effect of long-term cisapride. *Dig Dis Sci* 1993;**38**:1518–24.

86 Valenzuela G, Fisher K, Davenport K, Plankey M, McCallum RW. Long term subjective and objective effects of cisapride in the treatment of gastroparesis. *Gastroenterology* 1990;**98**:A399.

87 Abell TL, Camilleri M, DiMagno EP, Hench VS, Zinsmeister AR, Malagelada J-R. Long-term efficacy of oral cisapride in symptomatic upper gut dysmotility. *Dig Dis Sci* 1991;**36**:616–20.

88 Cooper T, Cutts T, Abell TL, West L, Cardoso S. Long-term cisapride therapy improves quality of life measures in patients with symptoms of gastroparesis. *Gastroenterology* 1991;**100**:A432.

89 Kendall BJ, Kendall ET, McCallum RW. Cisapride in the long term treatment of chronic gastroparesis: a two year open label study. *Gastroenterology* 1993;**104**:A14.

90 McCallum RW, Plankey MW, Fisher KL. Chronic oral cisapride therapy increases solid meal gastric emptying and improves symptoms in patients with gastric stasis. *Gastroenterology* 1987;**92**:A1525.

91 Valenzuela G, Plankey M, Fisher K, McCallum R. The safety and efficacy of long term cisapride in the treatment of gastroparesis. *Gastroenterology* 1989;**96**:A521.

92 Richards RD, Davenport K, McCallum RW. The treatment of idiopathic and diabetic gastroparesis with acute intravenous and chronic oral erythromycin. *Am J Gastroenterol* 1993;**88**:203–7.

93 Pan D-Y, Chen G-H, Chang C-S *et al.* Effect of oral erythromycin on patients with diabetic gastroparesis. *Chin Med J (Taipei)* 1995;**55**:447–51.

94 Gallar P, Oliet A, Vigil A, Ortega O, Guijo G. Gastroparesis: an important cause of hospitalization in continuous ambulatory peritoneal dialysis patients and the role of erythromycin. *Perit Dial Int* 1993;**12**(Suppl.2):S183–6.

95 McCallum RW, Ricci D, DuBovik S. Effect of domperidone on gastric emptying and symptoms of patients with idiopathic gastric stasis. *Gastroenterology* 1984;**86**:1179.

96 Corinaldesi R, Stanghellini V, Raiti C, Rea E, Salgemini R, Barbara L. Effect of chronic administration of cisapride on gastric emptying of a solid meal and on dyspeptic symptoms in patients with idiopathic gastroparesis. *Gut* 1987;**28**:300–5.

97 Jian R, Ducrot F, Ruskone A *et al.* Symptomatic, radionuclide and therapeutic assessment of chronic idiopathic dyspepsia: a double-blind placebo-controlled evaluation of cisapride. *Dig Dis Sci* 1989;**34**:657–64.

98 Dworkin BM, Rosenthal WS, Casellas AR *et al.* Open label study of long-term

effectiveness of cisapride in patients with idiopathic gastroparesis. *Dig Dis Sci* 1994;**39**:1395–8.

99 Fette C, Nagrani M, Traube M. Effect of long-term oral cisapride on gastric emptying in patients with symptoms suggestive of gastroparesis. *Gastroenterology* 1989;**96**:A149.

100 Stagias JG, Zubal G, Traube M. Effects of long-term oral cisapride treatment in idiopathic gastric stasis syndrome. *Gastroenterology* 1993;**104**:A586.

101 Perkel MS, Hersh T, Moore C, Davidson ED. Metoclopramide therapy in fifty-five patients with delayed gastric emptying. *Am J Gastroenterol* 1980;**74**:231–6.

102 Klutman NE, Eisenach JB. Erythromycin therapy for gastroparesis. *South Med J* 1992;**85**:524–7.

103 Stadaas JO, Aune S. Clinical trial of metoclopramide on postvagotomy gastric stasis. *Arch Surg* 1972;**104**:684–6.

104 McClelland RN, Horton JW. Relief of acute, persistent postvagotomy atony by metoclopramide. *Ann Surg* 1978;**188**:439–47.

105 Davidson ED, Hersh T, Haun C, Brooks WS. Use of metoclopramide in patients with delayed gastric emptying following gastric surgery. *Am Surg* 1977;**43**:40–4.

106 Molino D, Mosca S, Angrisani G, Magliacano V. Symptomatic effects of domperidone in postvagotomy gastric stasis. *Curr Ther Res* 1987;**41**:13–16.

107 van der Mijle HCJ, Beekhuis H, Bleichrodt RP, Kleibeuker JH. Cisapride in treatment of Roux-en-Y syndrome. *Dig Dis Sci* 1991;**36**:1691–6.

108 Ramirez B, Eaker EY, Drane WE, Hocking MP, Sninsky CA. Erythromycin enhances gastric emptying in patients with gastroparesis after vagotomy and antrectomy *Dig Dis Sci* 1994;**39**:2295–300.

109 Stacher G, Abatzi-Wenzel T-A, Wiesnagrotzki S, Bergmann H, Schneider C, Gaupmann G. Gastric emptying, body weight and symptoms in primary anorexia nervosa: long-term effects of cisapride. *Br J Psychiatry* 1993;**162**:398–402.

110 Young GP, Miller G, Szmukler G. Gastric symptoms and gastric emptying in anorexia nervosa: effect of cisapride. *Gastroenterology* 1992;**102**:A537.

111 Horowitz M, Maddern GJ, Maddox A, Wishart J, Chatterton BE, Shearman DJC. Effects of cisapride on gastric and esophageal emptying in progressive systemic sclerosis. *Gastroenterology* 1987;**93**:311–15.

112 Horowitz M, Maddox A, Wishart J, Collins PJ, Shearman DJC. The effects of cisapride on gastric and oesophageal emptying in dystrophia myotonica. *J Gastroenterol Hepatol* 1987;**2**:285–93.

113 Saltzman M, Meyer C, Callachan C, McCallum RW. Effect of metoclopramide on chronic gastric stasis in diabetic and post-gastric surgery patients. *Gastroenterology* 1981;**80**:A1268.

114 McCallum RW, Petersen J, Dubovic S. Effect of cisapride on gastric emptying and symptoms associated with gastroparesis. *Gastroenterology* 1986;**90**:A1541.

115 Hill AD, Walsh TN, Hamilton D *et al.* Erythromycin improves emptying of the denervated stomach after oesophagectomy. *Br J Surg* 1993;**80**:879–81.

116 Yeo CJ, Barry MK, Sauter PK *et al.* Erythromycin accelerates gastric emptying after pancreaticoduodenectomy: a prospective, randomized, placebo-controlled trial. *Ann Surg* 1993;**218**:229–38.

117 Hocking MP. Postoperative gastroparesis and tachygastria — response to electric stimulation and erythromycin. *Surgery* 1993;**114**:538–42.

118 Xynos E, Mantides A, Papageorgiou A, Fountos A, Pechlivanides G, Vassilakis JS. Erythromycin accelerates delayed gastric emptying of solids in patients after truncal vagotomy and pyloroplasty. *Eur J Surg* 1992;**158**:407–11.

119 Dull JS, Raufman J-P, Zakai MD, Strashun A, Straus EW. Successful treatment of gastroparesis with erythromycin in a patient with progressive systemic sclerosis. *Am J Med* 1990;**89**:528–30.

120 Soudah NC, Hasler WL, Owyang C. Effect of octreotide on intestinal motility and bacterial overgrowth in scleroderma. *N Engl J Med* 1991;**325**:1461–7.

121 Owyang   C.   Octreotide   in   gastrointestinal   motility   disorders.   *Gut* 1994(Suppl.3):S11–14.

122 Kobayashi T, Kobayashi M, Naka M, Nakajima K, Momose A, Toi M. Response to octreotide of intestinal pseudoobstruction and pneumatosis cystoides intestinalis associated with progressive systemic sclerosis. *Intern Med* 1993;**32**:607–9.

« 7 »

Functional Dyspepsia

Robert C. Heading

The investigation and management of dyspepsia continue to stimulate interest among gastroenterologists. Reasons for this high level of interest are easy to identify: dyspepsia is a common problem, and patients with dyspeptic symptoms represent a substantial part of every gastro-enterologist's clinical practice. Clinical judgments about the diagnosis, appropriate investigation, and management are often far from easy. Even when all accessible diagnostic resources have been utilized, many dyspeptic patients appear to have no disease process or pathology to which their symptoms can be attributed. Many physicians are just a little uncomfortable when the time comes to explain to these patients the results of their investigations, the diagnosis being made, and the therapy proposed.

This clinical entity — functional dyspepsia — presents a considerable challenge at both the intellectual and scientific levels, and in the context of everyday clinical practice. This review attempts to address both.

Terminology

Agreement about terminology is an important prerequisite to the useful discussion of dyspepsia. Many definitions of dyspepsia have been offered in recent years, and published reviews frequently draw attention to this as evidence of confusion or at least lack of agreement. In fact, real differences between recently published definitions are small (Table 7.1) [1–9]. The essential feature common to all these definitions of dyspepsia seems to be the occurrence of chronic or recurrent upper abdominal pain or discomfort.

The term *functional dyspepsia* now seems to have replaced *nonulcer dyspepsia* to denote dyspepsia for which conventional gastrointestinal (GI) investigation has failed to identify a cause. It is certainly a useful label to attach to a patient in this clinical status, but it is not satisfactory as a diagnosis. If observations on functional dyspepsia are to be systematized, it is necessary first to ask what investigations must return negative results

148

Table 7.1 Some definitions of dyspepsia published in the past 10 years.

Definition	Source
Pain, discomfort, or nausea referable to the upper alimentary tract which may be intermittent or continuous, has been present for a month or more, is not precipitated by exertion nor relieved within 5 minutes by rest.	Talley & Piper, 1986 [1]
Chronic or recurrent ($\geqslant$ 3 months) upper abdominal pain or nausea which may or may not be related to meals.	Talley & Phillips, 1988 [2]
Upper abdominal or retrosternal pain, discomfort, heartburn, nausea, vomiting, or other symptoms considered to be referable to the proximal alimentary tract.	Colin-Jones et al., 1988 [3]
Episodic or persistent abdominal symptoms, often related to feeding, which patients or physicians believe to be due to disorders of the proximal portion of the digestive tract.	Barbara et al., 1989 [4]
Indigestion of more than a few days.	Jones et al., 1990 [5]
Episodic or persistent abdominal symptoms that include abdominal pain or discomfort. The term *dyspepsia* is not applied to patients whose symptoms are thought to be arising from outside the proximal gastrointestinal tract.	Heading, 1991 [6]
Persistent or recurrent abdominal pain or abdominal discomfort centered in the upper abdomen.	Talley et al., 1991 [7]
Upper abdominal pain and/or a combination of at least three other symptoms attributable to the upper alimentary tract during the previous 3 months.	Schlemper et al., 1993 [8]
Episodic, recurrent or persistent abdominal pain or discomfort or any other symptoms referable to the upper alimentary tract, excluding bleeding or jaundice, of duration 4 weeks or longer.	Crean et al., 1994 [9]

before this diagnosis can be properly applied. One definition of functional dyspepsia [7] required that there be no clinical, biochemical, endoscopic, or ultrasonographic evidence of any known organic disease likely to explain the symptoms (e.g. acid-peptic or neoplastic disease of the stomach, esophagus, or duodenum, or disease of the pancreas or hepatobiliary system). However, these authors conceded that it is not always necessary to investigate all these possibilities before making a diagnosis of functional dyspepsia. Nyren et al. [10] presented evidence that upper GI endoscopy alone is probably sufficient to exclude most organic disease in most dyspeptic patients, and Drossman et al. [11] likewise appeared to accept that endoscopy is probably the only obligatory investigation. In fact, the extent of appropriate investigation is a pragmatic clinical judgment rather than something that can be specified in fundamentalist terms. It is evident that upper GI endoscopy will not identify pancreatic or biliary disease, but it is so rare for dyspepsia to be caused by unsuspected disease in the pancreas or the biliary tract that their specific investigation in every dyspeptic patient is not warranted.

Thus, despite numerous publications that might initially seem to suggest controversy and confusion about definitions of dyspepsia and functional dyspepsia, there is, in reality, a very substantial agreement about the symptom complexes with which patients commonly present, and about the fact that in many patients no disease or disorder can be identified to which the symptoms can confidently be attributed.

Epidemiologic observations

The results of epidemiologic studies of dyspepsia are necessarily influenced by the selected definition of the condition and the choice of population being surveyed. Considering the potential differences in both these variables, the agreement in the published literature is remarkable. Reviewing a number of reports from western Europe, Knill-Jones [12] reported period prevalence values ranging from 19% to 41%, with a mean of 32%. Figures of 26% and 29% have recently been reported for adult populations under the age of 65 [13, 14]. Thus, it seems that, overall, recently reported figures are remarkably similar to the 13% prevalence of major dyspepsia and 17% prevalence of minor dyspepsia reported by Doll *et al.* [15] more than 40 years ago.

Epidemiologic data about functional dyspepsia are less easy to come by, if only because the criteria for exclusion of organic disease are variably selected and applied by investigators. For obvious reasons, it is much more difficult to investigate a community-based sample than it is to obtain results from patients seeking medical care for their symptoms. Published prevalence figures for functional dyspepsia vary from 19% to 76%, undoubtedly reflecting methodologic differences between investigators [12]. Conflicting data also exist concerning geographic differences. For example, one study [8] in Japan suggested dyspepsia with a verified peptic ulcer history to be more common than functional dyspepsia, whereas the findings in another study [16] suggested a spectrum of upper GI disease, including functional dyspepsia, much the same as encountered in the West.

One important aspect of the epidemiologic data on dyspepsia is the relatively small proportion of symptomatic individuals who seek medical attention. In studies reported by Jones *et al.* [5, 17–19], only about 35% of individuals with dyspeptic symptoms consulted a physician. Consultation rates were positively associated with age, with low socioeconomic status, and most particularly with anxiety about the possibility that the symptoms were caused by 'serious illness,' with cancer or heart disease typically being identified.

These findings are powerful evidence that for an individual with dyspeptic symptoms the basis of a decision to see a physician is complex. Symptom severity has an influence [14] but is by no means the principal explanation. Anxiety about the significance of the symptoms is likely to be much more important.

It is self-evident that this information has important implications for studies of dyspepsia, especially for investigations of pathogenesis. If only 25% of afflicted individuals ever consult a physician (and perhaps a much smaller proportion ever see a gastroenterologist), those coming to gastroenterology units and participating in clinical research may be unrepresentative of dyspepsia sufferers generally. The results of such clinical research must therefore be interpreted with due caution.

Clinical presentation

A powerful tradition of inherited clinical wisdom is associated with the interpretation of upper GI symptoms. Aphorisms and clinical impressions are handed down from teacher to student and from textbook to textbook: when evidence is obtained showing the perceived wisdom to be mistaken, correction enters the system only very slowly. The work of Edwards and Coghill [20], Horrocks and De Dombal [21], and Talley *et al.* [1, 22] has been exemplary in clarifying some of the basic clinical information that should be at every gastroenterologist's metaphorical fingertips, yet is actually familiar to very few.

For example, the relationship of pain to meals — an element of the folklore of gastroenterologic diagnosis — is of little diagnostic value in distinguishing functional dyspepsia from peptic ulcer disease (Figure 7.1). However, patients with gallbladder disease seldom suffer pain when the stomach is empty. Statistically, the occurrence of pain at night, vomiting, and the relief of pain by milk or food are encountered more often in peptic ulcer disease than in functional dyspepsia [1]. Nevertheless, the occurrence of pain during the night has a lesser predictive

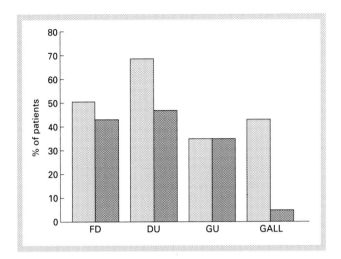

Fig. 7.1 Relationship of pain to meals. FD, functional dyspepsia; DU, duodenal ulcer; GU, gastric ulcer; GALL, gallstones. Pain 0.5 to 3 hours after meals (darker shade); pain before meals or when hungry (lighter shade). (From Talley & Piper [1].)

value for peptic ulcer disease than many would suspect (Figure 7.2), and the relief of pain by food, milk, or antacids is perhaps more complex than might be imagined (Figure 7.3). Antacids are almost equally effective in duodenal ulcer disease and in functional dyspepsia, but milk is much more effective in duodenal ulcer.

Figure 7.4 shows that weight loss is a commonly encountered feature among patients presenting with gastric carcinoma — 85% in one study —

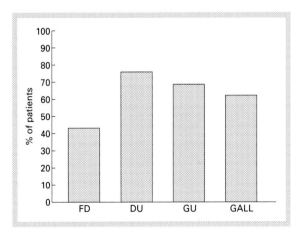

Fig. 7.2 Night pain (i.e., pain severe enough to wake the patient from sleep). FD, functional dyspepsia; DU, duodenal ulcer; GU, gastric ulcer; GALL, gallstones. (From Talley & Piper [1].)

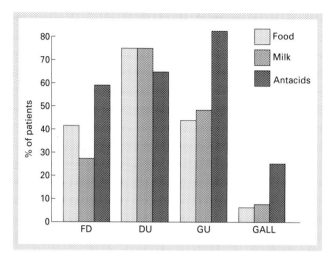

Fig. 7.3 Relief of pain by food, milk, and antacids. FD, functional dyspepsia; DU, duodenal ulcer; GU, gastric ulcer; GALL, gallstones. (From Talley & Piper [1].)

but is also reported by 32% of those with functional dyspepsia [21]. This, too, is perhaps not as well known as it should be, given that the information was published in 1978. Exactly the same point has been made much more recently by Crean *et al.* [9], who reported weight loss in 73% of their patients with gastric carcinoma and in 23% of their patients with functional dyspepsia. Crean *et al.* have also challenged other elements of traditional wisdom in clinical diagnosis. For example, they found that the precise localization of epigastric pain with the 'pointing sign' was not of

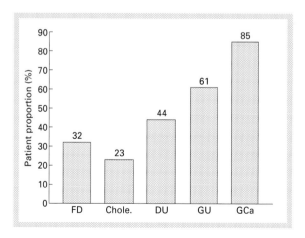

Fig. 7.4 History of weight loss exceeding 3 kg. FD, functional dyspepsia; Chole., cholecystitis; DU, duodenal ulcer; GU, gastric ulcer; GCa, gastric carcinoma. (From Horrocks & De Dombal [21].)

much diagnostic value relative to more diffusely localized upper abdominal pain.

Because the information available from studies such as these is complex and requires that distinctions be drawn between the frequency with which particular features occur in a given condition and their discriminatory value as an aid to diagnosis, it is perhaps rather too tempting to opt out of the rigor of this analysis and retreat in the hope that traditional simplistic diagnostic assumptions will somehow still be adequate. This is regrettable, given the substantial agreement about the interpretation of simple clinical observations that is apparent in the relevant published literature.

In 1988, Colin-Jones *et al.* [3] suggested that a more systematic approach to the analysis of upper GI symptoms in patients with functional dyspepsia might assist in improving characterization of the clinical entity and the further investigation of the underlying pathophysiology. They proposed that symptom clustering often enabled patients to be identified as having reflux-like dyspepsia, dysmotility-like dyspepsia, or ulcer-like dyspepsia. Much interest has been stimulated in the validity and value of this proposed classification. Most evidence to date suggests that the underlying hypothesis may be flawed because most patients with functional dyspepsia do not present with symptom clusters that allow unequivocal allocation to one or another category [23–28]. In a recent population-based study, 83% of the patients studied presented with symptoms which could be associated with more than one symptom category. The current view would seem to be that symptom subgrouping along these lines is not feasible, simply because the majority of dyspeptic patients have features of more than one subgroup. For those with symptoms that do correspond to a single variant of dyspepsia, no evidence yet exists to show that such information permits any useful or practical inference to be drawn.

Pathophysiology and the possible causes of functional dyspepsia

Understandably, the possible causes of functional dyspepsia are of great interest. Substantial reviews of the subject have been published [2, 29, 30]; consequently, only a synopsis of key points is included here.

Acid secretion

There is no persuasive evidence that gastric acid secretion is a significant causal factor in functional dyspepsia. Secretory studies [31] have not shown meaningful abnormalities: provocation tests have failed to relate any aspect of upper GI secretory function to the occurrence of symptoms [32, 33].

Gastroesophageal reflux disease

Good reason exists now to consider unrecognized gastroesophageal reflux disease (GERD) to be responsible for at least some cases of functional dyspepsia. It is now accepted that a significant minority of patients with GERD do not have esophagitis, and it is also evident that many patients with GERD present with a complex dyspeptic history rather than with pure symptoms of heartburn and acid regurgitation [34]. Recent studies [25, 35, 36] using esophageal pH monitoring suggest that previously unrecognized reflux disease may be responsible for about 20% of cases of functional dyspepsia.

Helicobacter pylori infection

For obvious reasons, there has been enormous interest in the possibility that functional dyspepsia may be linked to gastritis caused by *Helicobacter pylori* infection. However, the literature is large and confusing and is therefore most usually interpreted as showing that links between *H. pylori* infection and functional dyspepsia are 'unclear' and that, on a practical basis, there is at present no place for systematic treatment directed to *H. pylori* eradication of functional dyspepsia, except in the context of formal clinical trials [37, 38]. It is then often suggested that occasional treatment of the individual patient may be justified! Critical review of studies investigating the possible association of *H. pylori* infection and functional dyspepsia reveals design weaknesses in many. Consequently, it is fair to conclude that these studies do not justify firm conclusions. Nevertheless, it does appear that the strictly controlled studies have failed to identify any real relationship [39, 40], and this includes studies evaluating the response to eradication therapy in functional dyspepsia patients with *Helicobacter* infection. A recent suggestion [41] that eradication therapy may be symptomatically beneficial in the long term, though not immediately, awaits confirmation.

Gastrointestinal motility disorders

There is overwhelming evidence that delayed postprandial gastric emptying is demonstrable in many patients with functional dyspepsia [42]. Likewise, impaired antral motility has been demonstrated by manometric techniques and is sometimes accompanied by disordered intestinal motility [43, 44]. However, all scintigraphic studies of gastric emptying and manometric studies of contractile activity have identified abnormality in only a proportion of functional dyspepsia subjects: statistically significant differences from controls are certain, but with sufficient overlap of patients and controls to cause difficulty in establishing exactly what the observations mean in biological or clinical terms.

Attempts to correlate symptoms and delayed gastric emptying have shown how difficult it is to establish direct relationships [45, 46]. It remains possible, however, that the standard experimental techniques available hitherto have simply been insufficiently sensitive to recognize the most relevant abnormalities. Much attention is now being paid to increase in antral capacity (and thus altered intragastric distribution of postprandial content), which is now known to be a feature of functional dyspepsia [47–50]. Some data suggest that antral abnormality shows a closer correlation with symptoms than can be obtained with a global gastric emptying measurement. Prolonged antroduodenal manometry appears to be more interpretable than short-term studies and offers a new prospect for relating the abnormalities to symptoms [51]. Prolonged small bowel motility studies in patients with irritable bowel syndrome (IBS) were successful in relating motor abnormalities to pain [52].

A comprehensive study [53] of upper GI function in patients with functional dyspepsia suggested that delayed gastric emptying was associated with a low frequency of *H. pylori* infection, female gender, and young age. Comparison of patients with and without delayed emptying revealed some differences in symptom pattern, and likewise there were some symptom differences when comparison was made between patients with and without *H. pylori* infection. These data are obviously of great interest, although others have failed to confirm the findings [54]. Resolution of this uncertainty awaits further work.

The principal difficulty with all these observations lies in the fact that no very obvious mechanism exists by which most of the observed abnormalities of gastric motor function could be responsible for symptoms. In some circumstances, motor abnormalities are demonstrable when the patient is symptom free, whereas other patients are symptomatic with normal motor function. This remains a major challenge to the clinical investigator interested in GI motility because the existence of a statistically significant association between functional dyspepsia and upper GI motor abnormality is beyond question.

Visceral sensation

Recent interest in the possibility that altered visceral sensation may play a role in the genesis of functional dyspepsia was triggered by an experimental demonstration [55] that inflation of a noncompliant bag positioned in the stomach of patients with functional dyspepsia provoked discomfort at lower inflation pressures than was seen in the healthy controls (Figure 7.5). Of course, the study of pain provocation in the human GI tract by inflating balloons or by direct electrical stimulation has a very long tradition [56–58], and abnormalities of rectal and colonic sensory threshold are well recognized in the IBS [59, 60]. In functional dyspepsia, however, the work of Mearin *et al.* [55] extended previous thinking, first, by showing altered sensation in patients relative to controls despite normal gastric wall compliance (contrasting with the post-vagotomy stomach); secondly, by showing a normal gastric reflex relaxation to cold stress; and thirdly by showing normal somatic (hand) perception of cold. Thus, an abnormality tolerably specific to the mechanisms of gastric perception appeared to be present in the patients.

Further work from the same laboratory and from elsewhere [61–63] has confirmed and extended these observations about the stomach. When

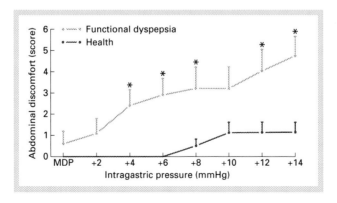

Fig. 7.5 Abdominal discomfort elicited by gastric distention in patients with functional dyspepsia and healthy controls. MDP, minimal distending pressure. *$P < 0.05$ versus controls. (From Mearin *et al.* [55]; © 1996 by the American Gastroenterological Association.)

reviewed in the wider context of visceral sensory function, hyperexcitability of the dorsal horn neuron can be proposed as the key abnormality, potentially being produced either by peripheral tissue irritation or as a response to descending input from the brainstem [64, 65].

Experimental studies of visceral sensation are not easy to conduct, and at present there is considerable confusion concerning the 'effects' of sensory stimulation that are most usefully observed to obtain interpretable information. In human subjects, the perception of pain or discomfort can be recorded, but it is not easily quantified and is susceptible to influence by many other factors. Consequently, other responses to sensory stimulation have been explored, including the RIII biceps femoris reflex [66] and neurohormonal responses [67], as well as the more familiar approach of observing evoked potentials on the electroencephalogram (EEG) [68].

The study of visceral sensation is a rapidly developing field of research interest, and in consequence it is still somewhat confusing. Nevertheless, its importance lies in the fact that sensory abnormalities may explain some of the paradoxes identified from previous GI motility research. The intimate interaction of sensory and motor function in the upper GI tract may explain why altered motility is so frequent in functional dyspepsia yet by itself cannot fully explain the occurrence of symptoms.

Psychosocial factors

Many physicians are convinced by their own experience that functional dyspepsia is associated with psychological abnormalities, such as anxiety or depression, or with stress and coping difficulty in the patient's life. Recent studies that seemed to challenge some of the more simplistic concepts have to be seen in the context of the close relationships that undoubtedly exist between the psyche and GI function. It is still difficult to characterize and define these relationships, however.

Most of the studies [69–73] of functional dyspepsia undertaken in the past 10 years have concluded that both anxiety and depression are more marked in patients than in healthy controls but are probably no different from the anxiety and depression encountered in patients with organic GI disease. Nevertheless, some data [74] suggest that anxiety is greater in functional dyspepsia than in peptic ulcer disease. It seems, however, that contrary to the view of some physicians, there is no particular personality profile associated with patients who have functional dyspepsia [75].

Other researchers have examined stressful life events in the context of dyspepsia, with less consistent findings. Talley and Piper [76] did not identify any relationship between life events and functional dyspepsia, although the design of their study has been criticized [77]. More recently, one study [78] found that stressful life events were more frequent in functional dyspepsia patients than in controls, whereas another [79] failed to find any differences between dyspeptics and controls in the occurrence of positive or negative life events but noted that negative life events were perceived by the patients as having a greater influence on their lives.

Prompted by findings in patients with functional disorders of the lower bowel, one recent study [80] suggested that a history of abuse in childhood (sexual, physical, or emotional) is positively associated with dyspepsia and heartburn. Interestingly, the probability of seeking health care for GI symptoms was highest in individuals reporting abuse in childhood or adult life.

It seems entirely plausible that social influences and psychological status may influence the perception of visceral sensation, and some direct evidence of this exists from studies of gastroesophageal reflux [81]. In this respect, reflux disease may have more in common with functional dyspepsia than is initially apparent.

Therapy

Because many patients seek medical attention for their dyspepsia on account of anxiety about possible 'serious' disease, one of the first obligations for the physician finding normal appearances at upper GI endoscopy is to explain these 'negative' findings and their significance to the patient. Hopefully, some anxieties will thereby be allayed, and if the physician believes that a diagnosis of functional dyspepsia is legitimate, it will be appropriate to consider what further treatment, if any, is required.

Not all patients require pharmacologic therapy. Some who have been reassured by the physician's clinical opinion and by normal results on investigation may express a preference for making some sort of lifestyle change or for following a particular dietary regime. Measures of this sort are not amenable to evaluation by formal clinical trial, and thus their efficacy is unproven. However, provided the proposed lifestyle change or dietary pattern is not too bizarre, few physicians would discourage patients who wished to approach their problem in this fashion.

Drug therapy in functional dyspepsia

Many patients seek drug therapy for their dyspepsia, and pharmacologic intervention certainly has a place. It is highly desirable, however, that physicians be aware of what may reasonably be expected of the drugs that may be prescribed.

Antacids

Antacids are still the most widely used medication in dyspepsia, most being over-the-counter (OTC) purchases for self-medication. Because so many individuals taking antacids in this way have not sought medical attention, there is no information about whether their dyspepsia is organic or functional, and no clear evidence about the efficacy of the medication taken. In functional dyspepsia, three placebo-controlled trials [82–84] of antacid therapy have shown no advantage over placebo. This result may come as no surprise to gastroenterologists but nevertheless deserves to be interpreted with some caution. If patients with functional dyspepsia responding to antacid self-medication are less likely to seek medical attention than those whose symptoms do not respond, the patients seen by doctors and available for recruitment in clinical trials will show a selection bias likely to underestimate the responsiveness to antacids.

Histamine-2 receptor antagonists

In a review of the double-blind placebo-controlled trials of H_2-receptor antagonists published prior to 1990, Talley [85] concluded that approximately half the studies, including those with the largest patient numbers, showed a statistically significant advantage for the active drug over placebo, suggesting that there is a subgroup of functional dyspepsia patients who gain genuine benefit from antisecretory therapy. More recently, a comparison of ranitidine and antacid therapy [86] has shown better symptom relief with ranitidine. In contrast, a comparison of ranitidine and sucralfate [87] suggested better symptom relief with sucralfate. A substantial $n=1$ trial of cimetidine and placebo [88] suggested that approximately half of a group of patients with functional dyspepsia showed a symptomatic response to cimetidine that was comparable to the response seen in patients with esophagitis or peptic ulcer.

The suggestion that a subgroup of patients with functional dyspepsia truly respond to antisecretory therapy thus appears to be correct. Some of these patients are presumably individuals with previously unrecognized GERD, as explained above.

Prokinetic drugs

The efficacy of metoclopramide, domperidone, and cisapride in relieving the symptoms of functional dyspepsia is now well established on the basis of controlled clinical trials. Reviews of the individual studies [85, 89, 90] have been published elsewhere and are not repeated here. Available data suggest that the efficacy of all three drugs is broadly similar, although cisapride has the advantage of causing fewer adverse reactions. It is also the most comprehensively studied of the three prokinetics.

Two recent studies that have compared the effects of cisapride and an H_2-receptor antagonist are of particular interest. In a comparison with cimetidine [91], cisapride was found more effective overall, although the data suggested that the difference was perhaps due to an inferior response to cimetidine by patients with dysmotility-like dyspeptic symptoms. There was no evidence of superior outcomes with the H_2 blocker in other patient subgroups. In a comparison of cisapride and ranitidine in the treatment of functional dyspepsia, Carvalhinhos *et al.* [92] concluded that the response to cisapride was superior with respect to overall symptom evaluation and, more specifically, to epigastric distention. Again, no symptom pattern showing a better response to the H_2 blocker was identified.

These studies are important in challenging the proposition that antisecretory therapy may appropriately be given to patients with some symptom patterns, whereas prokinetic drug therapy may be more appropriate for others. Despite a lack of evidence, the advocacy of antisecretory therapy for ulcer-like or reflux-like dyspepsia and prokinetic therapy for dysmotility-like dyspepsia has seemed to be logical. Unfortunately, the logic is false: dysmotility-like dyspepsia is not specifically associated with objectively demonstrable GI dysmotility, and reflux-like dyspepsia is very poorly correlated with gastroesophageal reflux. Other evidence [28] that the outcome of cisapride therapy is much the same in all symptom subgroups indicates that there is no particular symptom pattern for which cisapride therapy is either especially advantageous or especially disadvantageous. In contrast, a poorer response to H_2 blockade seems possible for some patients, on the basis of the above studies with cimetidine and ranitidine.

Carvalhinhos *et al.* [92] rightly urged caution in the interpretation of their data, simply because the differences between the two treatment groups were small. Nevertheless, the degree of accord with the findings of Halter *et al.* [91] is reassuring.

5-Hydroxytryptamine (5-HT) agonists and antagonists

It is now evident that a number of drugs have overlapping agonist or antagonist action on $5-HT_3$ and $5-HT_4$ receptors [93]. Although the substituted benzamide prokinetics are thought to act primarily as $5-HT_4$ agonists, they are also effective $5-HT_3$ antagonists at high concentrations. Conversely, some drugs such as renzapride and zacopride, primarily identified as $5-HT_3$ antagonists, also have some $5-HT_4$ agonist action. Consequently, there is interest in the $5-HT_3$ antagonists as possible therapeutic agents in functional dyspepsia. This interest has been enhanced by the demonstration that granisetron decreases rectal sensation [94], and although ondansetron apparently does not [95], its administration to patients with IBS diminished postprandial discomfort and flatulence in one study [96].

Studies [97, 98] using the barostat technique have shown that neither ondansetron nor alosetron modifies the perception of gastric distention. Consequently, this class of drugs seems unlikely to have potential for modifying this aspect of functional dyspepsia.

Kappa opioid agonists

Fedotozine is a specific agonist of the kappa opioid receptor with the ability to reduce nociceptive responses to balloon distention of the GI tract [99]. Preliminary data [100] show heightened sensory thresholds to experimental gastric distention in healthy volunteers given fedotozine. In a controlled clinical trial [101], more effective symptom relief was obtained in functional dyspepsia treated with fedotozine than with placebo. Further studies of drugs in this class are awaited with interest.

The practical approach to dyspepsia management

With the plethora of editorials, review articles, and consensus statements on dyspepsia published in medical journals during the past 10 years [3, 4, 6, 102–105], a consistent theme has been endorsement or positive recommendation to try empirical treatment rather than to undertake investigation in younger dyspeptic patients, provided no 'alarm features' are present. Indeed, even in the early 1980s, policies that might reduce 'inappropriate' investigation were being advocated, invariably on the basis that clinical judgment was reasonably reliable in distinguishing high-risk from low-risk dyspepsia, and that provided a failure of empirical therapy led to further investigation, there was economic advantage but no clinical disadvantage in adopting this empirical treatment policy [106, 107]. One consequence of this thinking has been the generation of investigation and treatment algorithms such as the example shown in Figure 7.6 [89]. Minor differences are apparent when algorithms

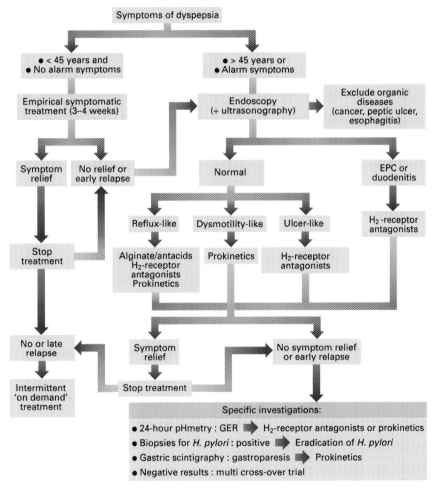

Fig. 7.6 Flow chart for the management of dyspeptic patients. EPC, erosive prepyloric changes at endoscopy; GER, gastroesophageal reflux. (From Galmiche & Vallot [89].)

of different authors are compared, and only the more recent proposals have incorporated assessment of *H. pylori* status, but agreement on the basic pattern of these algorithms has been apparent.

It is arguable that the evidence now available justifies reconsideration of this investigation and therapeutic policy in a more fundamental way. The work of Bytzer *et al.* [108] comparing prompt diagnostic endoscopy with empirical H_2 blockade treatment (and subsequent endoscopy, if required) in the management of dyspepsia established that 1 year after presentation, there were no differences between the two study groups with respect to symptoms or quality-of-life measures. Nevertheless, patients in the group first given empirical H_2 blockade were less satisfied with their medical care, incurred higher drug costs, and took more sick leave than the group managed by prompt endoscopy. These findings thus give compelling support to a strategy of prompt investigation, both from a health economics perspective and from the perspective of the patient, who would like to feel satisfied by his clinical care.

If empirical therapy with an H_2 antagonist can no longer be recommended in preference to prompt endoscopy, it is evident that the distinction between organic and functional dyspepsia should be made earlier in the evolution of the patient's clinical care than has been customary in recent years. When organic disease is identified (in approximately 30% of patients in Bytzer's series [108]), appropriate therapy will be instituted. When a diagnosis of functional dyspepsia is made, the evidence detailed above suggests that prokinetic therapy with cisapride is more likely than any other drug therapy to produce symptom improvement. Logic thus leads to the algorithm shown in Figure 7.7. It is perhaps a slight oversimplification, but it is consistent with the evidence now available on appropriate investigation and therapy.

Persistent and refractory functional dyspepsia

A very small minority of patients continue to seek medical attention for persistent or variable symptoms for which investigation reveals no explanation and all therapy fails. Little useful generalization is possible about the appropriate further assessment of such individuals, and few specific recommendations about treatment can be offered. The identification of any objective abnormality must always invite consideration of previously unrecognized organic disease, although the possibility that alterations of GI motility may be a consequence of prescribed drug therapy or even of self-medication must also be recognized. Psychiatric

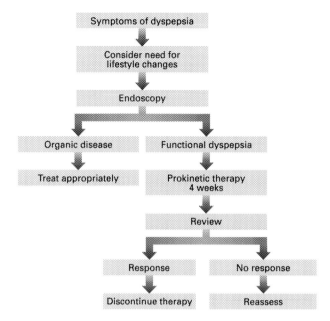

Fig. 7.7 Proposed flow chart for the management of dyspeptic patients according to information now available.

disease and psychopathology will also need to be considered. Physicians likely to be referred patients with 'difficult' dyspepsia are wise to have close working relationships with psychiatrists familiar with behavioral abnormalities and somatization as a response to psychological pressures.

These patients are difficult to manage, but the thrust must be to help them come to terms with their feelings and symptoms, rather than pursue an endless sequence of futile investigations of GI function. Fortunately, such patients are few. Nevertheless, they probably do require the attention of a major gastroenterologic referral center, where physicians not only have access to sophisticated diagnostic investigations but, hopefully, also have the wisdom to know when they should and should not be used.

References

1 Talley NJ, Piper DW. Comparison of the clinical features and illness behaviour of patients presenting with dyspepsia of unknown cause (essential dyspepsia) and organic disease. *Aust N Z J Med* 1986;**16**:352–9.
2 Talley NJ, Phillips SF. Non-ulcer dyspepsia: potential causes and pathophysiology. *Ann Intern Med* 1988;**108**:865–79.
3 Colin-Jones DG, Bloom B, Bodemar G *et al.* Management of dyspepsia: report of a working party. *Lancet* 1988;**1**:576–9.

4 Barbara L, Camilleri M, Corinaldesi R *et al.* Definition and investigation of dyspepsia: consensus of an international ad hoc working party. *Dig Dis Sci* 1989;**34**:1272–6.

5 Jones RH, Lydeard SE, Hobbs FDR *et al.* Dyspepsia in England and Scotland. *Gut* 1990;**31**:401–5.

6 Heading RC. Definitions of dyspepsia. *Scand J Gastroenterol* 1991;**26**(Suppl.182):1–6.

7 Talley NJ, Colin-Jones D, Koch KL, Koch M, Nyren O, Stanghellini V. Functional dyspepsia: a classification with guidelines for diagnosis and management. *Gastroenterol Int* 1991;**4**:145–60.

8 Schlemper RJ, van der Werf SDJ, Vandenbroucke JP, Biemond I, Lamers CBHW. Peptic ulcer, non-ulcer dyspepsia and irritable bowel syndrome in The Netherlands and Japan. *Scand J Gastroenterol* 1993;**28**(Suppl.200):33–41.

9 Crean GP, Holden RJ, Knill-Jones RP *et al.* A database on dyspepsia. *Gut* 1994:**35**:191–202.

10 Nyren O, Adami H-O, Gustavsson S, Lindgren PG, Loof L, Nyberg A. The 'epigastric distress syndrome': a possible disease entity identified by history and endoscopy in patients with nonulcer dyspepsia. *J Clin Gastroenterol* 1987;**9**:303–9.

11 Drossman DA, Thompson WG, Talley NJ, Funch-Jensen P, Janssens J, Whitehead WE. Identification of sub-groups of functional gastrointestinal disorders: working team report. *Gastroenterol Int* 1990;**3**:159–72.

12 Knill-Jones RP. Geographical differences in the prevalence of dyspepsia. *Scand J Gastroenterol* 1991;**26**(Suppl.182):17–24.

13 Talley NJ, Zinsmeister AR, Schleck CD, Melton LJ III. Dyspepsia and dyspepsia subgroups: a population-based study. *Gastroenterology* 1992;**102**:1259–68.

14 Holtmann G, Goebell H, Talley NJ. Dyspepsia in consulters and non-consulters: prevalence, health-care seeking behaviour and risk factors. *Eur J Gastroenterol Hepatol* 1994;**6**:917–24.

15 Doll R, Avery Jones F, Buckatzsch MM. Occupational factors in the aetiology of gastric and duodenal ulcers, with an estimate of their incidence in the general population. *Medical Research Council Special Report Series No 276*. London: HMSO, 1951.

16 Inoue M, Sekiguchi T, Harasawa S, Miwa T, Miyoshi A. Dyspepsia and dyspepsia subgroups in Japan: symptom profiles and experience with cisapride. *Scand J Gastroenterol* 1993;**28**(Suppl.195):36–9.

17 Jones R, Lydeard S. Prevalence of symptoms of dyspepsia in the community. *BMJ* 1989;**298**:30–2.

18 Lydeard S, Jones R. Factors affecting the decision to consult with dyspepsia: comparison of consulters and non-consulters. *J R Coll Gen Pract* 1989;**39**:495–8.

19 Jones R, Lydeard S. Dyspepsia in the community: a follow-up study. *Br J Clin Pract* 1992;**46**:95–7.

20 Edwards FC, Coghill NF. Clinical manifestations in patients with chronic atrophic gastritis, gastric ulcer and duodenal ulcer. *QJM* 1968;**37**:337–60.

21 Horrocks JC, De Dombal FT. Clinical presentation of patients with 'dyspepsia': detailed symptomatic study of 360 patients. *Gut*;**19**:19–26.

22 Talley NJ, McNeil D, Piper DW. Discriminant value of dyspeptic symptoms: a study of the clinical presentation of 221 patients with dyspepsia of unknown cause, peptic ulceration, and cholelithiasis. *Gut* 1987;**28**:40–6.

23 Dunbar F. Presentation and treatment of dyspepsia. *Curr Ther Res* 1992;**52**:349–53.

24 Talley NJ, Weaver AL, Tesmer DL, Zinsmeister AR. Lack of discriminant value of dyspepsia subgroups in patients referred for upper endoscopy. *Gastroenterology* 1993;**105**:1378–86.

25 Klauser AG, Voderholzer WA, Knesewitsch PA, Schindlbeck NE, Muller-Lissner SA. What is behind dyspepsia? *Dig Dis Sci* 1993;**38**:147–54.

26 Talley NJ, Zinsmeister AR, Schleck CD, Melton LJ III. Smoking, alcohol, and analgesics in dyspepsia and among dyspepsia subgroups: lack of an association in a community. *Gut* 1994;**35**:619–24.

27 Trespi E, Broglia F, Villani L, Luinetti O, Fiocca R, Solcia E. Distinct profiles of gastritis in dyspepsia subgroups: their different clinical responses to gastritis healing after *Helicobacter pylori* eradication. *Scand J Gastroenterol* 1994;**29**:884–8.

28 Heading RC and the Dyspepsia Study Group. Upper gastrointestinal symptoms in general practice: a multicentre UK study. *J Drug Dev Clin Pract* 1995;**7**:109–17.

29 Tytgat GNJ, Heading RC, Knill-Jones RP *et al.* Towards understanding dyspepsia. *Scand J Gastroenterol* 1991;**26**(Suppl.182):1–74.

30 Galmiche J-P, Jian R, Mignon M, Ruszniewski Ph, ed. *Non-ulcer Dyspepsia: Pathophysiological and Therapeutic Approaches.* Paris: John Libbey Eurotext, 1991.

31 Nyren O. Secretory abnormalities in functional dyspepsia. *Scand J Gastroenterol* 1991;**26**(Suppl.182):25–8.

32 Joffe SN, Primrose JN. Pain provocation test in peptic duodenitis. *Gastrointest Endosc* 1983;**29**:282–4.

33 George AA, Tsuchiyose M, Dooley CP. Sensitivity of the gastric mucosa to acid and duodenal contents in patients with nonulcer dyspepsia. *Gastroenterology* 1991;**101**:3–6.

34 Wienbeck M, Berges W. Esophageal disorders in the etiology and pathophysiology of dyspepsia. *Scand J Gastroenterol* 1985;**20**(Suppl.109): 133–7.

35 Waldron B, Cullen PT, Kumar R *et al.* Evidence for hypomotility in non-ulcer dyspepsia: a prospective multifactorial study. *Gut* 1991;**32**:246–51.

36 Small PK, Loudon MA, Waldron B, Smith D, Campbell FC. Importance of reflux symptoms in functional dyspepsia. *Gut* 1995;**36**:189–92.

37 Tytgat GNJ, Noach LA, Rauws EAJ. Is gastroduodenitis a cause of chronic dyspepsia? *Scand J Gastroenterol* 1991;**26**(Suppl.182):33–9.

38 Talley NJ. A relationship between *Helicobacter pylori* and non-ulcer dyspepsia: is there enough data to know? *Eur J Gastroenterol Hepatol* 1994;**6**:567–70.

39 Bernersen B, Johnsen R, Bostad L, Straume B, Sommer A-I, Burhol PG. Is *Helicobacter pylori* the cause of dyspepsia? *BMJ* 1992;**304**:1276–9.

40 Katelaris PH, Tippett GHK, Norbu P, Lowe DG, Brennan R, Farthing MJG. Dyspepsia, *Helicobacter pylori*, and peptic ulcer in a randomly selected population in India. *Gut* 1992;**33**:1462–6.

41 McCarthy C, Patchett S, Collins RM, Beattie S, Keane C, O'Morain C. Long-term prospective study of *Helicobacter pylori* in nonulcer dyspepsia. *Dig Dis Sci* 1995;**40**:114–19.

42 Malagelada J-R. Gastrointestinal motor disturbances in functional dyspepsia. *Scand J Gastroenterol* 1991;**26**(Suppl.182): 29–32.

43 Kerlin P. Postprandial antral hypomotility in patients with idiopathic nausea and vomiting. *Gut* 1989;**30**:54–9.

44 Camilleri M, Brown ML, Malagelada J-R. Relationship between impaired gastric emptying and abnormal gastrointestinal motility. *Gastroenterology* 1986;**91**:94–9.

45 Talley NJ, Shuter B, McCrudden G, Jones M, Hoschl R, Piper DW. Lack of association between gastric emptying of solids and symptoms in nonulcer dyspepsia. *J Clin Gastroenterol* 1989;**11**:625–30.

46 Jian R, Ducrot F, Ruskrone A *et al.* Symptomatic, radionuclide and therapeutic assessment of chronic idiopathic dyspepsia: a double-blind placebo-controlled evaluation of cisapride. *Dig Dis Sci* 1989;**34**:657–64.

47 Bolondi L. Bortolotti M, Santi V, Calletti T, Gaiani S, Labo G. Measurement of gastric emptying time by real-time ultrasonography. *Gastroenterology* 1985;**89**:752–9.

48 Ricci R, Bontempo I, La Bella A, De Tschudy A, Corazziari E. Dyspeptic symptoms and gastric antrum distension: an ultrasonographic study. *Ital J Gastroenterol* 1987;**19**:215–17.

49 Scott AM, Kellow JE, Shuter B *et al.* Intragastric distribution and gastric emptying of solids and liquids in functional dyspepsia: lack of influence of symptom subgroups and *H pylori*-associated gastritis. *Dig Dis Sci* 1993;**38**:2247–54.

50 Troncon LEA, Bennett RJM, Ahluwalia NK, Thompson DG. Gastric motility in functional dyspepsia. *Gut* 1994;**35**:327–32.

51 Jebbink RJ, vanBerge-Henegouwen GP, Akkermans LM, Smout AJ. Antroduodenal manometry: 24-hour ambulatory monitoring versus short-term stationary manometry in patient with functional dyspepsia. *Eur J Gastroenterol Hepatol* 1995;**7**:109–16.

52 Kellow JE, Phillips SF. Altered small bowel motility in irritable bowel syndrome is correlated with symptoms. *Gastroenterology* 1987;**92**:1885–93.

53 Tucci A, Corinaldesi R, Stanghellini V *et al. Helicobacter pylori* infection and gastric function in patients with chronic idiopathic dyspepsia. *Gastroenterology* 1992;**103**:768–74.

54 Pieramico O, Ditschuneit H, Malfertheiner P. Gastrointestinal motility in patients with non-ulcer dyspepsia: a role for *Helicobacter pylori* infection? *Am J Gastroenterol* 1993;**88**:364–8.

55 Mearin F, Cucala M, Azpiroz F, Malagelada J-R. The origin of symptoms on the brain–gut axis in functional dyspepsia. *Gastroenterology* 1991;**101**:999–1006.

56 Hertz AF. The sensibility of the alimentary tract in health and disease. *Lancet* 1911;**1**:1051–6.

57 Boyden EA, Rigler LG. Localization of pain accompanying faradic excitation of stomach and duodenum in healthy individuals. *J Clin Invest* 1934;**13**:833–51.

58 Lipkin M, Sleisenger MH. Studies of visceral pain: measurements of stimulus intensity and duration associated with the onset of pain in esophagus, ileum and colon. *J Clin Invest* 1958;**37**:28–34.

59 Ritchie J. Pain from distension of the pelvic colon by inflating a balloon in the irritable colon syndrome. *Gut* 1973;**14**:125–32.

60 Prior A, Sorial E, Sun WM, Read NW. Irritable bowel syndrome: differences between patients who show rectal sensitivity and those who do not. *Eur J Gastroenterol Hepatol* 1993;**5**:343–9.

61 Lemann M, Dederding JP, Flourie B, Franchisseur C, Rambaud JC, Jian R. Abnormal perception of visceral pain in response to gastric distension in chronic idiopathic dyspepsia: the irritable stomach syndrome. *Dig Dis Sci* 1991;**36**:1249–54.

62 Moragas G, Azpiroz F, Pavia J, Malagelada J-R. Relations among intragastric pressure, postcibal perception, and gastric emptying. *Am J Physiol* 1993;**264**:G1112–17.

63 Bradette M, Pare P, Douville P, Morin A. Visceral perception in health and functional dyspepsia: crossover study of gastric distension with placebo and domperidone. *Dig Dis Sci* 1991;**36**:52–8.

64 Mayer EA. The sensitive and reactive gut. *Eur J Gastroenterol Hepatol* 1994;**6**:470–7.

65 Mayer EA, Gebhart GF. Basic and clinical aspects of visceral hyperalgesia. *Gastroenterology* 1994;**107**:271–93.

66 Bouhassira D, Chollet R, Coffin B *et al.* Inhibition of a somatic nociceptive reflex by gastric distention in humans. *Gastroenterology* 1994;**107**:985–92.

67 Greydanus MP, Vassallo M, Camilleri M, Nelson DK, Hanson RB, Thomforde GM. Neurohormonal factors in functional dyspepsia: insights on pathophysiological mechanisms. *Gastroenterology* 1991;**100**:1311–18.

68 Enck P, Frieling T. Human gut–brain interactions. *J Gastrointest Mot* 1993;**5**:77–87.

69 Talley NJ, Fung LH, Gilligan IJ, McNeil D, Piper DW. Association of anxiety, neuroticism, and depression with dyspepsia of unknown cause. *Gastroenterology* 1986;**90**:886–92.

70 Watson RGP, Younge RJ, Lewis SA, Love AHG. Psychological aspects of flatulent dyspepsia. *Scand J Gastroenterol* 1987;**22**:821–6.

71 Magni G, di Mario F, Bernasconi G, Mastropaolo G. DSM-III diagnoses associated with dyspepsia of unknown cause. *Am J Psychiatry* 1987;**144**:1222–3.

72 Talley NJ, Phillips SF, Bruce B, Twomey CK, Zinsmeister AR, Melton LJ III. Relation among personality and symptoms in nonulcer dyspepsia and the irritable bowel syndrome. *Gastroenterology* 1990;**99**:327–33.

73 Morris C. Non-ulcer dyspepsia. *J Psychosom Res* 1991;**35**:129–40.

74 Langeluddecke P, Goulston K, Tennant C. Psychological factors in dyspepsia of unknown cause: a comparison with peptic ulcer disease. *J Psychosom Res* 1990;**34**:215–22.

75 Richter JE. Stress and psychologic and environmental factors in functional dyspepsia. *Scand J Gastroenterol* 1991;**26**(Suppl.182):40–6.

76 Talley NJ, Piper DW. Major life event stress and dyspepsia of unknown cause: a case control study. *Gut* 1986;**27**:127–34.

77 Bass C. Life events and gastrointestinal symptoms. *Gut* 1986;**27**:123–6.

78 Bennett E, Beaurepaire J, Langeluddecke P, Kellow J, Tennant C. Life stress and non-ulcer dyspepsia: a case-control study. *J Psychosom Res* 1991;**35**:579–90.

79 Hui WM, Shiu LP, Lam SK. The perception of life events and daily stress in nonulcer dyspepsia. *Am J Gastroenterol* 1991;**86**:292–6.

80 Talley NJ, Fett SL, Zinsmeister AR, Melton LJ III. Gastrointestinal tract symptoms and self-reported abuse: a population-based study. *Gastroenterology* 1994;**107**:1040–9.

81 Johnston BT, Lewis SA, Love AHG. Psychological factors in gastro-oesophageal reflux disease. *Gut* 1995;**36**:481–2.

82 Norrelund N, Helles A, Schmiegelow M. Ukaraktaristisk dyspepsi I almen praksis. En kontrolleret undersogelse med et antacidum (Aliminox®). *Ugeskr Laeger* 1980;**142**:1750–3.

83 Nyren O, Adami H-O, Bates S *et al*. Absence of therapeutic benefit from antacids or cimetidine in non-ulcer dyspepsia. *N Engl J Med* 1986;**314**:339–43.

84 Gotthard R, Bodemar G, Brodin U, Jonsson K-A. Treatment with cimetidine, antacid, or placebo in patients with dyspepsia of unknown origin. *Scand J Gastroenterol* 1988;**23**:7–18.

85 Talley NJ. Drug treatment of functional dyspepsia. *Scand J Gastroenterol* 1991;**26**(Suppl.182):47–60.

86 Holtz J, Plein K, Bunke R. Wirksamkeit von Ranitidine beim Reizmagensyndrom (functionelle dyspepsie) im vergleich zu einem antacidum. *Med Klin* 1994;**89**:73–80.

87 Misra SP, Dwivedi M, Misra V, Agarwal SK. Sucralfate versus ranitidine in non-ulcer dyspepsia: results of a prospective, randomized open controlled trial. *Indian J Gastroenterol* 1992;**11**:7–8.

88 Johannessen T, Petersen H, Kristensen P *et al*. Cimetidine on-demand in dyspepsia: experience with randomized controlled single subject trials. *Scand J Gastroenterol* 1992;**27**:189–95.

89 Galmiche J-P, Vallot T. Therapeutic strategy. In: Galmiche J-P, Jian R, Mignon M, Ruszniewski Ph, eds. *Non-ulcer Dyspepsia: Pathophysiological and Therapeutic Approaches.* Paris: John Libbey Eurotext, 1991:247–64.

90 Talley NJ. Functional dyspepsia: should treatment be targeted on disturbed physiology? *Aliment Pharmacol Ther* 1995;**9**:107–15.

91 Halter F, Miazza B, Brignoli R. Cisapride or cimetidine in the treatment of functional dyspepsia: results of a double-blind, randomized, Swiss multicentre study. *Scand J Gastroenterol* 1994;**29**:618–23.

92 Carvalhinhos A, Fidalgo P, Freire A, Matos L. Cisapride compared with ranitidine in the treatment of functional dyspepsia. *Eur J Gastroenterol Hepatol* 1995;**7**:411–17.

93 Talley NJ. 5-Hydroxytryptamine agonists and antagonists in the modulation of gastrointestinal motility and sensation: clinical implications. *Aliment Pharmacol Ther* 1992;**6**:273–89.

94 Prior A, Read NW. Reduction of rectal sensitivity and postprandial motility by granisetron, a $5HT_3$ receptor antagonist in patients with irritable bowel syndrome (IBS). *Aliment Pharmacol Ther* 1993;**7**:175–80.

95 Hammer J, Phillips SF, Talley NJ, Camilleri M. Effect of a $5HT_3$ antagonist (ondansetron) on rectal sensitivity and compliance in health and the irritable bowel syndrome. *Aliment Pharmacol Ther* 1993;**7**:543–51.

96 Maxton DG, Haigh CG, Whorwell PJ. $5HT_3$ antagonists: a role in irritable bowel syndrome and non-ulcer dyspepsia? *Gut* 1991;**32**:A1228.

97 Wilmer A, Tack J, Coremans G, Janssens J, Vantrappen G. Effect of ondansetron, a 5-HT_3-receptor antagonist, on perception of gastric distension and gastric compliance in healthy man. *Gastroenterology* 1993;**104**:A603.

98 Zerbib F, Bruley des Varannes S, Oriola RC *et al.* Alosetron does not affect the visceral perception of gastric distension in healthy subjects. *Aliment Pharmacol Ther* 1994;**8**:403–7.

99 Junien JL, Riviere P. Review article: the hypersensitive gut – peripheral kappa agonists as a new pharmacological approach. *Aliment Pharmacol Ther* 1995;**9**:117–126.

100 Coffin B, Lemann M, Fraitag B, Jian R. Effect of fedotozine on gastric visceral nociception in healthy subjects. *Dig Dis Sci* 1995;**40**:239.

101 Read NW, Bardhan KD, Whorwell PJ *et al.* Fedotozine in functional dyspepsia: results of a 6 week placebo-controlled multicenter therapeutic trial. *Dig Dis Sci* 1995;**40**:239.

102 Heatley RV, Rathbone BJ. Dyspepsia: a dilemma for doctors? *Lancet* 1987;**2**:779–82.

103 Brown C, Rees WDW. Dyspepsia in general practice. *BMJ* 1990;**300**:829–30.

104 Health and Public Policy Committee, American College of Physicians. Endoscopy in the evaluation of dyspepsia. *Ann Intern Med* 1985;**102**:266–9.

105 Colin-Jones DG. Practical guidelines for the management of dyspepsia. *Lancet* 1990;**336**:301–2.

106 Marton KI, Sox HC Jr, Wasson J, Duisenberg CE. The clinical value of the upper gastrointestinal tract roentgenogram series. *Arch Intern Med* 1980;**140**:191–5.

107 Davenport PM, Morgan AG, Darnborough A, De Dombal FT. Can preliminary screening of dyspeptic patients allow more effective use of investigational techniques? *BMJ* 1985;**290**:217–20.

108 Bytzer P, Hansen JM, Schaffalitzky de Muckadell OB. Empirical H_2-blocker therapy or prompt endoscopy in management of dyspepsia. *Lancet* 1994;**343**:811–16.

« 8 »
Intestinal Pseudo-obstruction
Eamonn M.M. Quigley

Introduction and basic physiology

'Intestinal pseudo-obstruction' refers to a number of clinical syndromes that are the clinical expression of profoundly disturbed intestinal motor function. The motor dysfunction may reflect a myopathic or neuropathic process, or both, the net effect of which is to severely disrupt the orderly transit of chyme along the gastrointestinal (GI) tract. To some extent, the pseudo-obstruction syndromes represent a prototype among motility disorders. Unlike with most disorders of motor function, pathologic correlates are available for many of the individual diseases that can cause these syndromes and their pathophysiology can be more clearly understood. These relatively rare disorders have attracted a great deal of attention because of their potential to enhance our understanding of the consequences of motor dysfunction and to provide models for the evaluation of correlations between symptoms, function, motility patterns, and pathologic findings. These disorders have also served as a template for the assessment of new therapeutic strategies. As both the pathophysiology of symptoms and the diagnostic studies are based on disturbed motor physiology, it stands to reason that before proceeding to a discussion of the pseudo-obstruction syndromes *per se*, we first review briefly the relevant physiology.

The organization of motor activity

Contractile activity at any level of the GI tract is based on fundamental electrophysiologic properties [1–3]. A consistent feature of GI myoelectric activity is an omnipresent, highly regular, recurring electrical pattern called the slow wave. Slow waves do not lead to contractions, which are related to the occurrence of action potentials, or spikes. Spikes occur only on the crest of slow waves; the frequency of spikes and, therefore, of contractions is phase-locked to slow waves. The maximal frequency of

171

contractile activity at a given site in the intestine is directly related to the slow-wave frequency in that region. Thus, the duodenal slow-wave frequency and the maximal frequency of phasic contractions are between 11 and 12 cycles per minute (cpm). These frequencies decline along the intestine to 9 cpm in the distal ileum. Small intestinal motility serves to mix an ingested meal with intestinal secretions and to propel digesta in an aborad direction when appropriate. Specialized muscles at the lower esophageal, pyloric, and ileocecal sphincters regulate transit across these regions and prevent orad reflux.

The patterns of motor activity along the length of the gut differ fundamentally during fasting and after ingestion of food. In the fasted state, motor activity is highly organized into a distinct, cyclically recurring sequence of events known as the migrating motor complex (MMC) [4–6]. The MMC consists of three distinct phases of motor activity that occur in sequence and migrate slowly along the length of the small intestine (Figure 8.1a). Each sequence begins with a period of motor quiescence (phase I), which is followed by a period of apparently random and irregular contractions (phase II), and culminates in a burst of uninterrupted phasic contractions (phase III, or the activity front). Individual cycles last 1–2 hours. Cycles originate in the proximal small intestine and migrate aborally; the velocity of propagation slows as the activity front progresses distally. Cyclic motor activity has also been identified in the lower esophageal sphincter (LES), stomach, gallbladder, and sphincter of Oddi.

As phase III develops in the proximal duodenum, associated motor events occur in the stomach. Basal tone in the LES is increased and there are superimposed phasic contractions, thereby preventing reflux of gastric contents during this time of intense gastric contractile activity. Tone increases in the proximal stomach, and superimposed phasic waves can be identified. At the same time, 1-cpm high-amplitude waves develop in the body of the stomach. True rhythmic activity occurs only in the distal antrum, where contractions at 3–5 cpm may be seen at the end of phase III. As phase III approaches and develops, antropyloroduodenal coordination increases and high-amplitude contractions propagate through the antrum, across the pylorus, and into the proximal duodenum, where they are associated with brief clusters of phasic contractions.

If food is ingested, the cyclic pattern is abolished and replaced by a band of random contractions, called the 'fed pattern' (Figure 8.1b), which may last 2.5–8.0 hours, after which the fasted pattern resumes if no more food has been ingested [7, 8].

In the small intestine the generation and propagation of the MMC appears to be independent of extrinsic nerves and is intrinsic to the gut. The ability to switch from the fasted to the fed state depends on extrinsic nerves, in particular on the vagus. While the integration of gastric events with the MMC is incompletely understood, both extrinsic nerves (the vagus, in particular) and hormonal factors (motilin, in particular) appear to be involved. In the stomach the gastric motor response to feeding is, in large part, mediated through the vagus.

Clinical features of intestinal pseudo-obstruction

The term 'intestinal pseudo-obstruction' refers to a diverse group of disorders with somewhat similar clinical features regardless of etiology [9–11]. Patients present with repeated episodes of nausea, vomiting, and abdominal pain and distention. On clinical grounds, they are often suspected initially of having a mechanical obstruction. Many patients are subjected to more than one diagnostic laparotomy before the correct diagnosis is even considered. Stasis may lead to bacterial colonization, with the subsequent development of diarrhea, steatorrhea, weight loss, and nutritional problems. In some individuals, constipation may be prominent, and in acute episodes, the abdominal distention may be striking. This syndrome may be the intestinal manifestation of a systemic disorder (secondary pseudo-obstruction) or may reflect a primary disorder of the intestinal musculature or its neural apparatus (primary chronic idiopathic intestinal pseudo-obstruction, or CIIP) (Table 8.1). Whether the disorder is primary or secondary, other parts of the GI tract may be involved, as well as extraintestinal organs, in particular the urinary tract.

Of the many causes of pseudo-obstruction (Table 8.2), scleroderma and other mixed connective-tissue diseases are by far the most common. In the earlier stages, sclerodermatous involvement of the small intestine results in motility changes indicative of a neuropathic process. In the later, more familiar stages, the predominant features are of a diffuse myopathic disorder [12]. Diagnosis is relatively easy to make in patients with the classic systemic features of scleroderma. The clinician must be alert, however, to the possibility of intestinal pseudo-obstruction in patients who present primarily with GI symptoms and in those with a less classic variant of scleroderma included under the category of mixed connective-tissue disease. In advanced scleroderma, bacterial overgrowth is common and should be diligently sought.

A pseudo-obstruction syndrome has been described in association with various muscular dystrophies and may also be a feature of such

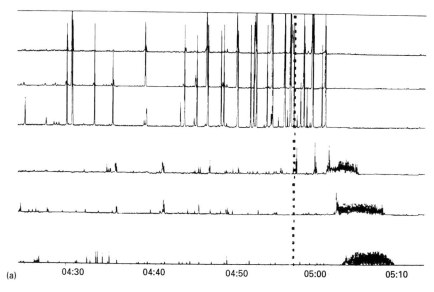

(a)   04:30   04:40   04:50   05:00   05:10

Fig. 8.1 Normal patterns of antroduodenal motor activity. (a) Fasting motor activity. Simultaneous recordings of motor activity from the antrum and duodenum demonstrate the three phases of the MMC. Shown in sequence, beginning on the extreme left, are phase I (motor quiescence), phase II (irregular activity), and phase III (a band of uninterrupted rhythmic contractions that migrate in an aboral direction). (b) Fed pattern. Following food administration, the fasting pattern is replaced by intense irregular activity. In (a) and (b), the top three tracings were obtained from sensors spaced 2-cm apart in the antrum and the lower three tracings from sensors 10-cm apart in the duodenum.

autonomic neuropathies as familial dysautonomia, ganglioneuromatosis, diabetic gastroenteropathy, and paraneoplastic neuropathy. There have been recent reports of the acute onset of a diffuse and profound gut dysmotility syndrome apparently in association with acute viral infections. This syndrome has perhaps been best described with cytomegalovirus (CMV) infection, especially in posttransplant patients, and with Epstein–Barr virus (EBV) infection, but may also result from enteric viral infections. These reports raise the intriguing possibility that some instances of idiopathic dysmotility may represent the aftermath of a viral infection. Endocrine and metabolic disorders represent another important subgroup, as do iatrogenic, or drug-induced, motor disorders. The importance of a careful drug history — in particular, a search for sur-reptitious opiate use — cannot be overemphasized.

Normal gastric acid secretion and motility are the most important factors in preventing bacterial overgrowth in the small intestine. It should come as no surprise, therefore, that dysmotility may be associated with

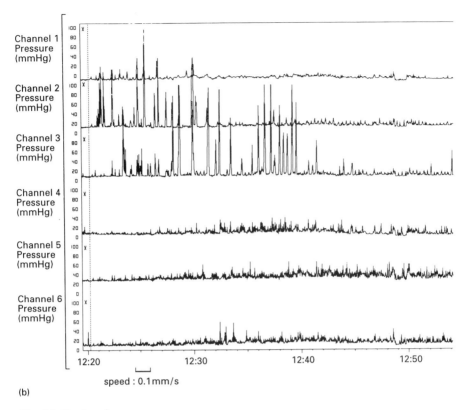

Channel 1 Pressure (mmHg)
Channel 2 Pressure (mmHg)
Channel 3 Pressure (mmHg)
Channel 4 Pressure (mmHg)
Channel 5 Pressure (mmHg)
Channel 6 Pressure (mmHg)

12:20   12:30   12:40   12:50

speed : 0.1mm/s

(b)

Fig. 8.1 *Continued*

bacterial overgrowth [13, 14]; indeed, the frequent occurrence of bacterial overgrowth in chronic pseudo-obstruction syndromes has already been alluded to.

Diagnosis

Perhaps the most crucial step in the diagnosis of pseudo-obstruction is to consider the possibility of such a diagnosis and thereby prevent yet another unnecessary laparotomy. Abdominal radiographs reveal marked dilatation of small intestinal loops (Figure 8.2) and a variable degree of colonic distention. Conventional contrast radiology may produce suggestive findings. In patients with myopathy, megaduodenum (Figure 8.3) and megacolon may occur, and the small intestine appears featureless, with a striking lack of haustral markings. The radiologic characteristics of scleroderma include close approximation of the valvulae conniventes (Figure 8.4), marked duodenal diverticulosis, and wide-mouthed diver-

Table 8.1 Classification of primary pseudo-obstruction syndromes.

I VISCERAL NEUROPATHY

A *Familial visceral neuropathy*
1   Recessive with intranuclear inclusions — diffuse pseudo-obstruction syndrome associated with autonomic insufficiency, pupillary denervation, and central nervous system abnormalities
2   Autosomal recessive — with mental retardation and calcification of the basal ganglia
3   Autosomal dominant

B *Sporadic visceral neuropathy*
1   Degenerative noninflammatory
2   Degenerative inflammatory — including paraneoplastic neuropathy, Chagas' disease, and cytomegalovirus infection; idiopathic varieties also have been described

C *Developmental visceral neuropathy* — including Hirschsprung's disease, diffuse aganglionosis, neurofibromatosis, and multiple endocrine adenomatosis type IIb

II VISCERAL MYOPATHY

A *Familial visceral myopathy*
1   Type I — autosomal dominant; features include esophageal dilatation, megaduodenum, redundant colon, and urinary tract involvement
2   Type II — autosomal recessive; features include dilatation of the stomach and small intestine, widespread diverticulosis, ptosis, and ophthalmoplegia

B *Sporadic visceral myopathy* — including scleroderma, polymyositis, myotonic dystrophy, progressive muscular dystrophy, amyloidosis, ceroidosis, and diffuse intestinal lymphoid infiltration

---

ticula throughout the colon. In patients with visceral neuropathy, in contrast, the main feature seen on a barium follow-through study or on enteroclysis is disordered motility.

Esophageal dysmotility is common in these disorders, reflecting their predilection for diffuse involvement of the GI tract. Esophageal manometry, a widely available and well-tolerated procedure, may provide direct evidence of dysmotility. Manometry is especially useful in the evaluation of patients with scleroderma and related disorders. A variety of esophageal manometric abnormalities have been described in other pseudo-obstruction syndromes, including an achalasia-like syndrome. In many situations, diagnosis may be more difficult and may not be apparent from either clinical features or the above-mentioned investigations. A number of methods that measure some aspect of intestinal motor function have been proposed to aid in the diagnosis at this stage.

Table 8.2 Etiology of intestinal pseudo-obstruction.

Primary CIIP	Secondary CIIP
Familial visceral neuropathy	Scleroderma
Sporadic visceral neuropathy	Mixed connective-tissue disease
	Systemic lupus erythematosus
Familial visceral myopathy	Dermatomyositis
(hollow visceral myopathy)	Sclerosing mesenteritis
Sporadic visceral myopathy	
	Muscular dystrophy
	Familial dysautonomia
	Parkinson's disease
	Chagas' disease
	Multiple endocrine neoplasia
	Ganglioneuromatosis
	Diabetes
	Hypothyroidism
	Hypoparathyroidism
	Amyloidosis
	Postviral
	Postischemic
	Paraneoplastic
	Posttransplant
	Drug induced
	Opiates
	Anticholinergics
	Antidepressants
	Calcium channel blockers
	Jejunal diverticulosis

CIIP, chronic idiopathic intestinal pseudo-obstruction.

The investigation of intestinal motor function

Intestinal transit

For many years, the sole technique for assessment of intestinal motor function was the radiologic observation of the passage of barium through the gut. Although fundamental to the definition of anatomic abnormalities, this technique was insensitive, subjective, and extremely difficult to quantify.

Hydrogen breath tests rely on the fact that carbohydrates, which pass through the small intestine undigested and unabsorbed, undergo fermentation by colonic bacterial flora on arrival at the cecum. The hydrogen produced is absorbed across the colonic mucosa, enters the splanchnic

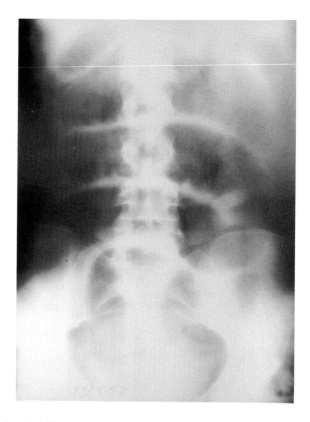

Fig. 8.2 Abdominal film appearance in pseudo-obstruction. Abdominal plain film from a patient with scleroderma demonstrates marked dilatation of small bowel loops.

circulation, and is exhaled in the breath [15]. The time from ingestion of a nonabsorbable carbohydrate to onset of a rise in breath hydrogen, therefore, is an index of the mouth-to-cecum transit time. Using either natural carbohydrate sources, such as potatoes, rice, or beans, or artificial compounds, such as lactulose, clinicians have estimated intestinal transit via exhaled breath hydrogen analysis. It should be remembered, however, that the transit time measured includes not only small intestinal transit, but also gastric emptying. This test provides information only about the arrival of the 'head' of the meal; its interpretation will be nearly impossible if small intestinal bacterial overgrowth is present, a common occurrence in pseudo-obstruction. A similar principle underlies the use of azulfidine to measure intestinal transit [16]. Following an oral dose of azulfidine, the sulfasalazine and sulfapyridine moieties are split by colonic bacteria; the detection of sulfapyridine in a venous blood sample indicates that the medication has traversed the small intestine. These techniques have not been evaluated prospectively in patients with pseudo-obstruction, but based on their reliance on bacterial metabolism, it seems unlikely that they will prove useful in this context.

Scintigraphic techniques, readily available in most hospitals, will detect gastroparesis in disorders involving the stomach and small intestine (see Figure 8.3b). Scintigraphy also has been used to measure small intestinal transit, but its use for this purpose has proved problematic for many reasons: the disassociation of some isotopes from food during digestion, an overlap between individual loops of intestine and between the intestine and other organs, and difficulty in defining the arrival of the meal in the cecum or right colon [17]. A recently described technique [18] involving the use of indium-111-labeled cation-exchange resin (Amberlite) pellets can accurately measure gastric emptying, small bowel transit and colonic filling in a single study. This technique has been evaluated in a wide variety of motility disorders, including pseudo-obstruction, and has been proposed as a sensitive screening test for dysmotility [19].

Electrical recordings from the small intestine

In the immediate postoperative period, small intestinal electrical activity can be recorded from electrodes implanted on the serosa at the time of surgery. These electrodes can subsequently be removed without the need for further abdominal exploration. In the more usual nonsurgical clinical setting, myoelectrical recordings obtained from electrodes mounted on intraluminal catheters have achieved limited success. The nature and significance of signals obtained from these systems remain the subject of considerable controversy.

Antroduodenal and small intestinal manometry

The direct measurement of pressure activity in the antrum, duodenum, and small intestine has now entered clinical practice, although it remains confined to specialized centers [6, 20]. Most institutions use a multilumen perfused catheter assembly, which is customized according to the intestinal site at which recordings are to be obtained. For example, for antroduodenal recordings the assembly includes an array of closely spaced sensors to straddle the pylorus, as well as recording sites in the duodenum and proximal jejunum. For small intestinal recordings, several widely spaced recording sites may be more appropriate. These assemblies are placed under fluoroscopic guidance, and recordings are typically

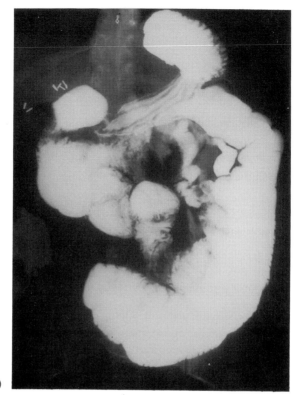

(a)

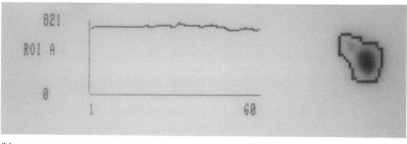

(b)

Fig. 8.3 Megaduodenum. (a) Upper GI barium study demonstrates dilatation of the duodenal bulb and second part of the duodenum. Note on the right mild dilatation of jejunal loops. (b) Gastric emptying study. Plot of radioactivity from region of interest in the fundus (shown on right) demonstrates no evidence of emptying over the first 60 minutes following meal ingestion (y-axis, count rate in counts; x-axis, time in minutes).

performed for several hours during fasting and following ingestion of a standardized liquid–solid meal. Recordings are analyzed for the various parameters of the MMC, for the presence and the nature of the motor response to the meal, and for abnormal patterns. Recently developed ambulatory systems combine solid-state miniaturized strain gauges, data

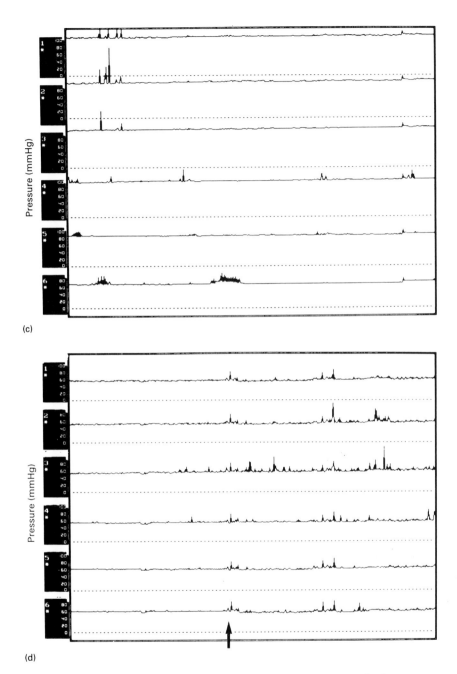

(c)

(d)

Fig. 8.3 *(continued)* Megaduodenum. (c) Antroduodenal manometry, fasting state. Note low-amplitude, infrequent phasic activity in the antrum (top three channels) and duodenum (lower three channels), suggesting a myopathic disorder. (d) Antro-duodenal manometry, fed pattern. Note poorly developed motor response in the antrum (top three channels) and duodenum (lower three channels) after meal ingestion (indicated by arrow); findings again are consistent with a myopathic process.

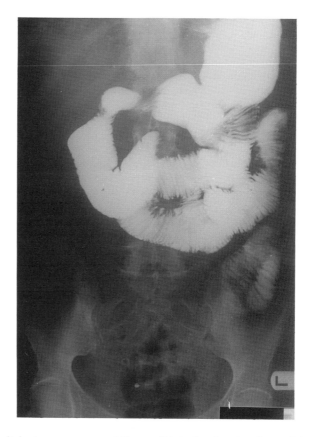

Fig. 8.4 Radiologic appearances of the small intestine in scleroderma (views from a barium upper GI series). Note duodenal and jejunal dilatation with prominence of the valvulae conniventes, giving rise to a 'coiled spring' appearance.

loggers similar to those used for 24-hour pH recordings, and appropriate computer software [21–23].

In patients with myopathy, manometry typically reveals hypomotility; in patients with advanced disease, virtually no contractile activity may be evident (see Figures 8.3c,d & 8.5a,b). In patients with a neuropathic disorder, individual contractions are of normal amplitude, but motor patterns are disorganized. The MMC is disrupted, with bursts of bizarre nonpropagating activity during fasting (Figure 8.6). Similarly, abnormal patterns may disrupt fed motility.

Intestinal biopsy

The current classification of primary pseudo-obstruction syndromes is based on a combination of clinical features and pathological findings (see

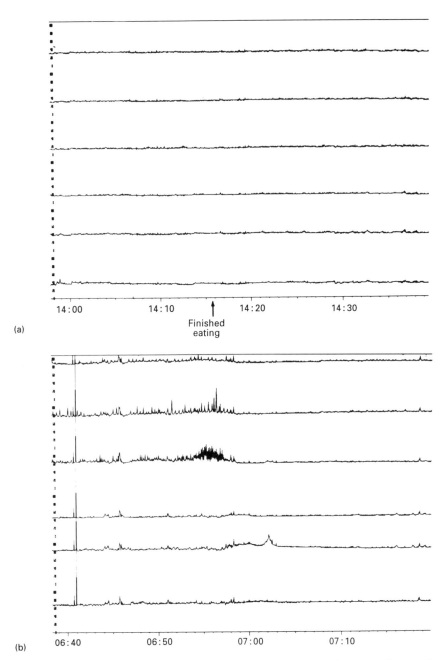

(a)

(b)

Fig. 8.5 Antroduodenal manometry in advanced scleroderma. (a) Complete absence of motor activity in the antrum and duodenum. (b) Phase III in scleroderma. Note rhythmic activity in the antrum (top two channels) and duodenum (lower four channels), which propagates in a normal fashion, but is of very low amplitude.

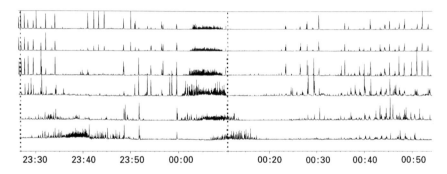

Fig. 8.6 Duodenal manometry in an enteric neuropathy. Note intense disorganized phasic activity. In the middle of the tracing is an abnormal phase III-like burst, featuring aberrant migration and preceded by a prolonged phasic burst in the lowest channel. This patient had symptomatic diabetic gastroenteropathy.

Table 8.1). While gross myopathic disorders may be detected with commonly available histologic techniques (Figure 8.7), a definitive pathologic evaluation of many of these disorders involves the highly specialized study of full-thickness intestinal biopsies [24]. For meaningful interpretation, biopsies or resection specimens must be sectioned in the plane of the myenteric plexus and stained using specific techniques, such as Wright's silver stain, to delineate the enteric nerves and ganglia.

Diagnostic dilemmas

Despite their fascination for clinical investigators and intestinal neuro-

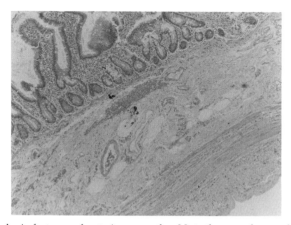

Fig. 8.7 Histologic features of enteric myopathy. Note the complete replacement of circular muscular layer by fibrosis.

pathologists, the pseudo-obstruction syndromes must be kept in clinical perspective. Individually and collectively, these are rare disorders. Functional disorders such as the irritable bowel syndrome (IBS) and nonulcer dyspepsia are many, many times more common, and, as already emphasized, an intestinal obstruction is a much more likely cause of dilated bowel loops than an intestinal neuropathy. Nevertheless, the diagnosis of intestinal pseudo-obstruction carries significant implications for the patient and for the physician in terms of prognosis and management. The importance of an accurate diagnosis comes into sharpest focus with the patient being considered for intestinal transplantation; an accurate diagnosis is imperative before total enterectomy and intestinal replacement is considered.

Three challenging diagnostic dilemmas may confront the physician in this context:

1   pseudo-obstruction versus obstruction;
2   pseudo-obstruction versus IBS or other functional bowel diseases;
3   pseudo-obstruction versus the narcotic bowel.

Pseudo-obstruction versus obstruction

The importance of a confident exclusion of obstruction cannot be over-stressed. In the patient who has not undergone surgery, localized Crohn's disease, intramural and extrinsic tumors, and such disorders as duplication and intussusception should be considered, and the patient should be evaluated by high-quality barium follow-through or enteroclysis studies, or both. In the patient who has undergone surgery, adhesion-related obstruction remains a possible cause of symptoms. Recently, Frank *et al.* [25] reported on the value of manometry in detecting obstructions missed by radiologic studies but confirmed at laparotomy. They contended that repetitive high-amplitude, nonpropagated contractions or clusters of contractions are highly suggestive of obstruction. Other investigators, however, have observed similar patterns in patients with functional disorders (Figure 8.8) and have failed to differentiate obstruction from pseudo-obstruction on the basis of manometric patterns. When manometric findings are inconclusive, there may be no alternative but to proceed to laparotomy. If no evidence of obstruction is discovered at laparotomy, a full-thickness intestinal biopsy should be obtained and examined histologically to investigate the possibility of myopathy or neuropathy.

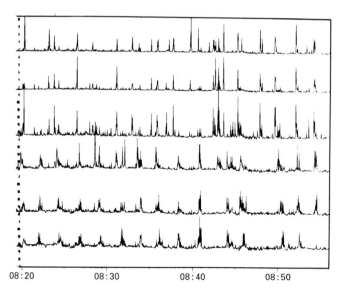

Fig. 8.8 Cluster activity (repetitive, high-amplitude, rapidly propagating pressure waves) in a patient with IBS.

Pseudo-obstruction versus functional bowel disease

By definition, patients with pseudo-obstruction should have clinical and radiologic features of intestinal obstruction that are incompatible with IBS. Problems in diagnosis have arisen owing to the expansion of the term 'pseudo-obstruction' to include patients with other manifestations of 'dysmotility,' such as gastroparesis or megacolon, or who manifest symptoms suggestive of small intestinal motor dysfunction in the absence of a true obstruction. This is a poorly defined area and a potential minefield. In the absence of a truly objective definition of an underlying motility disorder based on appropriate histologic studies, reports of 'pseudo-obstruction' based on manometry but without a compatible clinical picture (i.e. symptoms suggestive of obstruction and X-ray features) must remain speculative. While common sense dictates that degenerative disorders of intestinal muscle and nerve should have a 'preobstructive' phase, there is no agreement at present on the definition of this disorder or on its clinical or manometric features. In light of the reported overlap in manometric features between defined enteric neuromuscular disorders and functional syndromes, the use of manometry as the diagnostic 'gold standard' can lead to diagnostic error. For the moment, the main role of manometry in this clinical scenario is to define normality; normal findings on manometry render a diagnosis of pseudo-obstruction virtually untenable.

Pseudo-obstruction versus the narcotic bowel

The inappropriate attribution of symptoms — in particular, pain — to a primary motility disorder will, in some circumstances, lead to the dilemma of the narcotic bowel. While pain is a prominent symptom in pseudo-obstruction, the clinician should be alert to the possibility of a patient with functional visceral pain who has become dependent on narcotics and has developed gut motor dysfunction secondary to their long-term use. An inappropriate diagnosis of pseudo-obstruction in such patients will further delay the institution of appropriate therapy. The history should be carefully reviewed, and particular attention paid to the presenting features: are they truly compatible with motor dysfunction? A psychiatric consultation may help by revealing underlying depression or evidence of narcotic addiction. If a definitive diagnosis of pseudo-obstruction has not been established prior to narcotic use, the drugs should be withdrawn under appropriate supervision and the patient re-evaluated. Withdrawal symptoms have been successfully prevented in this context by the administration of clonidine [26].

Management

General principles

Dehydration and electrolyte abnormalities should be corrected by oral or intravenous administration of fluids and electrolytes, as appropriate. In the acute stage, gastric and intestinal decompression by nasogastric suction remains an important component of management. Metabolic, electrolyte, or endocrine abnormalities that may play a primary role in the pathogenesis of the motility problem should be defined and treated appropriately. The possibility of bacterial overgrowth should be investigated and, if present, treated with appropriate antibiotic therapy. Pain management may present a formidable challenge in these patients. Pain is especially prevalent in those with a neuropathic disorder and can lead to narcotic dependence. The physician should assess diligently for the presence of precipitating or exacerbating factors, which can be addressed by such measures as gastric or intestinal decompression. Hyman *et al.* [27, 28], who have considerable experience with pain management in children with pseudo-obstruction, stress the importance of two mechanisms in the pathogenesis of pain in these patients: visceral hyperalgesia and centrally mediated pain. They also emphasize the unsuitability of opiates, not only because of the risk of dependence, but also because of their lack of efficacy in addressing these mechanisms. To treat visceral hyperalgesia, they suggested the use of nonsteroidal anti-inflammatory drugs, clonidine, tricyclic antidepressants, local capsaicin, and epidural anesthesia. For centrally mediated pain, they recommended hypnosis and other psychological therapies.

Nutrition

Many patients with chronic intestinal motility problems develop malnutrition because of inadequate oral intake, vomiting, and malabsorption. Therefore, the identification and correction of nutritional deficiencies is an important component of management.

Several physiologic principles can guide appropriate nutritional management. Liquids are more readily emptied than solids, and the emptying of solids can be significantly accelerated by prior homogenization. Of the major dietary components, fat delays emptying significantly more than carbohydrate or protein; low-fat diets are, therefore, useful. Similarly, the indigestible component of meals should be reduced to a minimum because of the likelihood of poor emptying and transit and of bezoar formation. Diabetic patients with gastroparesis commonly present with bezoars, which are related to the loss of gastric MMC activity. With appropriate attention to detail, dietary support, and tailoring of the diet to the individual patient, a satisfactory oral regimen can be achieved in most patients. A number of alternatives can be considered for patients with more severe motility problems in whom oral nutrition may not be possible [29–32]. In patients who cannot tolerate a conventional diet, elemental diets administered either as the sole source of nutrition or as supplements may permit adequate dietary intake. When any type of oral intake cannot be tolerated, gastrostomy and jejunostomy feedings are available. When gastroparesis is the sole or dominant problem, percutaneous placement of a combined gastrostomy/jejunostomy tube simultaneously decompresses the stomach and permits enteral nutrition. Owing to a tendency of small intestinal catheters placed via a gastrostomy to displace proximally, some clinicians prefer direct surgical placement of a jejunostomy, either by open procedure or by laparoscopy [30].

A major limiting factor with any form of enteral nutrition in patients with pseudo-obstruction is pain exacerbation. For those with diffuse disorders in whom enteral nutrition in any form is impossible, total parenteral nutrition (TPN) may be the only reasonable route.

Prokinetic drugs (Table 8.3)

While enteric neurophysiologists and pharmacologists have made tremendous progress in the study of enteric receptors and neurotransmitters in *in vitro* models, the application of this knowledge to human disease is, given the complexity of regulation of motility in the intact animal, far from simple [33–35]. Clinicians must, therefore, be cautious when extrapolating *in vitro* data to clinical pharmacology and must be mindful that many pharmacologic studies of promotility agents have concentrated on the drug's effect on motor patterns, without attempting to assess any

Table 8.3 Prokinetic agents.

Cholinergic agonists	*5-HT agonists/antagonists*
Bethanechol*	Ondansetron*
Prostigmine*	(Cisapride*)
	(Clebopride)
Dopamine antagonists	(Metoclopramide*)
Metoclopramide*	(Renzapride)
Domperidone	
	CCK antagonist
Substituted benzamides	Loxiglumide
Cisapride*	
Renzapride	*Macrolides*
Zacopride	Erythromycin*
(Metoclopramide*)	New derivatives such as EM523
(Clebopride)	
	Opioid agonists
Somatostatin analog	Fedotozine
Octreotide*	Trimebutine
GnRH analog	*Opiate antagonist*
Leuprolide*	Naloxone*
Prostaglandin	
Misoprostol*	

*Approved for use in the USA but not necessarily for their motility effects.
( ) Inclusion of drugs listed in parentheses in this group remains controversial.
CCK, cholecystokinin; GnRH, gonadotropin-releasing hormone; 5-HT, 5-hydroxytryptamine.

related change in gut function. It tends to be forgotten that improved function — not more pressure 'waves' or different motor patterns — is the goal of therapy; functional correlates of motor effects should be sought whenever possible.

A number of common themes emerge from a review of the pharmacology of motility. Given the ubiquity of many of these receptors in various neuronal systems, it is not surprising that the usefulness of several prokinetic agents has been limited by central nervous system (CNS) and cardiovascular side effects. With many agents, tolerance has been a problem and long-term efficacy often proves elusive. Several agents are somewhat site specific, and we may be entering an era in which drugs are developed that are targeted to specific organs. Another significant obstacle to progress is that GI dysmotility syndromes are, in general, poorly defined, with definitions based on symptom patterns rather than on a histopathologic abnormality. Available data on prokinetics are derived from studies in patients with functional GI disorders, who are hardly an ideal population, given the poor definition of these syndromes and the likely multifactorial etiology of symptoms in these patients.

Cholinergic agonists

Cholinergic agonists are the original promotility agents. Their promotility effects rely primarily on stimulation of muscarinic M2-type receptors on the smooth muscle cell. Evidence of their effectiveness in motility disorders is, in general, inconsistent, although benefits in gastroesophageal reflux disease and gastroparesis have been claimed [36]. Not surprisingly, given their nonspecificity, cholinergic agonists are associated with a significant incidence of side effects and their use has virtually disappeared with the advent of newer agents.

Dopamine antagonists

Until recently, the most widely used prokinetic agent was metoclopramide, a dopamine antagonist with central and peripheral effects. In normal subjects and in disease states, metoclopramide has been shown [33, 36] to promote esophageal peristalsis, increase LES pressure, and accelerate gastric emptying. Unfortunately, the efficacy of metoclopramide in diseases has been far from consistent; several studies have demonstrated some efficacy in gastroesophageal reflux disease and gastroparesis [33, 36]. Long-term use has been complicated by a trend toward tolerance and a troubling incidence of CNS side effects. There is little evidence for its efficacy in pseudo-obstruction.

Recently, domperidone, a dopamine antagonist that operates primarily through peripheral (DA2) receptors, has become available for use throughout Europe, Canada, and South America but is as yet unavailable in the USA [37, 38]. Because it does not cross the blood–brain barrier, domperidone is free from the troublesome CNS side effects associated with metoclopramide. It can, however, cause hyperprolactinemia and, therefore, gynecomastia and galactorrhea. In patients with Parkinson's disease, domperidone has proven useful in the prevention of nausea related to dopaminergic medications [39]. Because domperidone gains access to the vomiting center, it has significant antinausea effects. In general, its efficacy appears similar to that of metoclopramide. Beneficial effects on esophageal and gastric physiology have been demonstrated in normal subjects. Particular interest has been generated by its apparent ability in experimental models to promote coordinated antropyloro-duodenal motor activity. In clinical use, domperidone is associated with a trend toward tolerance, similar to that seen with metoclopramide.

Other agents with some dopamine antagonist effects include clebo-pride, cinitapride, and perhaps cisapride. It should be noted that meto-clopramide and clebopride may potentiate acetylcholine release.

Substituted benzamides

Cisapride, which is now available for use throughout most of the world, has been the focus of several experimental and clinical studies [40]. Its precise mode of action remains somewhat controversial, but it would appear that the final common pathway is the facilitation of acetylcholine release from myenteric neurons [41]. Considerable evidence suggests that this may be achieved through a 5-hydroxytryptamine-4 (5-HT$_4$) receptor-mediated effect. Cisapride has been shown to promote esophageal peristalsis, augment LES pressure, accelerate gastric emptying, and promote intestinal and colonic transit. Of the commonly available oral agents (including metoclopramide, domperidone, and erythromycin), cisapride appears to have the most diffuse GI effects. It also benefits from an apparently low incidence of side effects; neurologic and hormonal abnormalities are distinctly unusual, with mild diarrhea and abdominal cramping being the only problems consistently associated with its use. As to the development of tolerance with long-term therapy, the status of cisapride remains somewhat uncertain, although studies to date suggest that this may be less of a problem than with metoclopramide and domperidone. Some studies [42] have shown continuing efficacy for up to 1 year in patients with gastroparesis.

Cisapride has demonstrated benefits in patients with gastroparesis and pseudo-obstruction in several studies [43–46]. In both short-term and long-term trials, the Mayo Clinic group [42, 44] demonstrated improvements in gastric emptying and motility in patients with gastroparesis and chronic intestinal pseudo-obstruction treated with cisapride. However, the relationship between objective improvements in emptying and symptom relief was somewhat inconsistent. Camilleri *et al.* [47] recently suggested that aspects of autonomic function may influence the response to cisapride. At present, cisapride is approved in the USA only for the treatment of gastroesophageal reflux disease; the recommended dosage is 10 mg three or four times daily. Studies in patients with gastroparesis, however, suggest that 20 mg three or four times daily may be required to achieve therapeutic effects.

Octreotide

A most surprising finding has been the discovery of the prokinetic effect of octreotide. Originally used in gastroenterology as a potent inhibitor of many GI functions, octreotide in low doses has been shown to stimulate motility, primarily through the induction of MMCs [48, 49]. In normal individuals, octreotide stimulated MMC induction at dosages as low as 10 μg; in patients with scleroderma, a 100-μg dose induced MMCs. Daily subcutaneous injections of octreotide 50 μg for 3 weeks reduced bacterial overgrowth in patients with scleroderma [48]. Octreotide may, therefore, have a place as adjunctive therapy in patients with such severe dysmotility syndromes as CIIP. A limiting factor may be its potential to inhibit gallbladder motility. In patients administered higher doses of octreotide (300–600 μg/day) for the treatment of acromegaly, gallbladder stasis leading to the development of sludge and gallstones has been documented [50]. Whether similar changes will occur with lower prokinetic doses is not known.

Recently octreotide has been recognized to significantly affect sensory input. In a provocative study, Hasler *et al.* [51] demonstrated that octreotide reduces the sensation of rectal distention through inhibition of visceral afferent pathways.

Macrolides

Erythromycin is associated with significant GI side effects, but the possibility that these effects may be related to the stimulation of motility was not well recognized until recently. It is now clear that erythromycin exerts a dose-dependent stimulatory effect on foregut motility [52]. Intravenously administered erythromycin may also promote gastric emptying by inhibiting isolated pyloric pressure waves (IPPWs) and pyloric tone [53]. These direct effects on contractile activity translate into an acceleration of gastric emptying, an abolition of the lag phase of solid emptying, the emptying of nondigested solids, and the induction of 'dumping' [54–59]. While several studies have consistently demonstrated the efficacy of intravenously administered erythromycin, the efficacy of oral administration has remained controversial. Thus, not all studies have shown long-term benefits in patients with gastroparesis, postvagotomy gastric stasis, the Roux syndrome, and intestinal pseudo-obstruction [60]. In a recent comprehensive review, Camilleri [60] concluded that erythromycin was most useful in the acute setting and recommended a regimen of intravenous administration (3 mg/kg every 8 hours) followed by oral administration (250 mg three times daily) for 5–7 days. Other factors limiting the usefulness of erythromycin include the absence of activity outside the proximal small intestine and a significant incidence of side effects.

5-HT agonists/antagonists

Several 5-HT receptors have been identified in the GI tract [61], with interest focused primarily on $5-HT_3$ and $5-HT_4$ receptors. The $5-HT_3$ antagonists, such as ondansetron, have been shown to inhibit motilin-induced MMCs, delay colonic transit, increase colonic contractile activity, and modulate sensory traffic. In contrast, $5-HT_4$ agonists facilitate acetylcholine release. As already mentioned, agents such as cisapride, metoclopramide, and renzapride may act, in part, through a $5-HT_4$ agonist effect. More specific $5-HT_4$ agonists are in development.

Other agents

Single case reports or small clinical studies have documented benefits with the use of leuprolide [62–64], misoprostol [65, 66], naloxone [67], and fedotozine [68] in a variety of motility disorders. Their place in the overall management of foregut dysmotility remains to be defined, however.

Conclusions

These are exciting times in the pharmacology of GI motility and we can look forward to many new developments [35]. The efficacy of many available agents is far from excellent, with the result that several centers have turned to combination therapy. Although there is at present no evidence from controlled studies to support this strategy, it is, at the very least, theoretically attractive when the agents used act through different mechanisms.

As the pseudo-obstruction syndromes are individually rare, and experience with any given prokinetic agent in these disorders limited, it is difficult to develop strict guidelines for their use in this context. It seems unreasonable to expect a response to a prokinetic agent in patients with an advanced myopathic process. Nevertheless, anecdotal evidence suggests that some patients with severe scleroderma may obtain some sympto-matic improvement. These agents are certainly worth trying, although the clinician should approach the prokinetic therapy for pseudo-obstruction with, at best, guarded optimism. In patients in whom oral therapy is tolerated, cisapride would appear to be the best choice among available agents. When this fails, subcutaneously administered octreotide may be added or substituted; the use of leuprolide also has its advocates. In the acute setting, intravenously administered erythromycin may alleviate gastroparesis, but probably exerts little beneficial effect beyond the pylorus; parenterally administered metoclopramide may be tried, but convincing evidence of efficacy is at present lacking.

Surgery

Surgical therapy for gastroparesis and motility disorders has, in general, proved disappointing, and the temptation to proceed to bypass proce-dures, in particular, should be resisted. Results of resection in diabetic patients with gastroparesis also have been disappointing. However, for patients with postoperative gastroparesis unresponsive to medical man-agement, resection may be considered. A subtotal gastrectomy, rather than less extensive resections, appears to give the best result.

For the pseudo-obstruction syndromes, surgical intervention should be limited to the placement of venting enterostomies. The results of seg-mental resections and bypass procedures have been almost universally disappointing [11].

For patients with severe, persistent obstructive symptoms, some clinicians have recommended subtotal enterectomy and TPN. For patients with severe motility problems, TPN-related liver disease, difficulties with intravenous access, and persistent pseudo-obstructive symptoms, total enterectomy and small intestinal transplantation, with or without transplantation of the liver, may be considered and have been performed at some centers [69]. Although there are reports of long-term survivors sustained on oral nutrition following isolated intestinal grafts, this procedure continues to be regarded as experimental. Small intestinal transplantation is associated with major morbidity, and the long-term absorptive and motor function of these grafts remains to be defined [70]. Transplantation has been performed in patients with primary motility disorders. Other concerns in this population include the possibility of recurrence of the primary disease process and the need to define intact esophageal and gastric motor function prior to transplantation.

References

1 Quigley EMM. Small intestinal motor activity: its role in gut homeostasis in health and disease. *Q J Med* 1987;**65**:799–810.
2 Szurszewski JH. Electrical basis for gastrointestinal motility. In: Johnson LR, ed. *Physiology of the Gastrointestinal Tract*, Vol. 1, 2nd edn. New York: Raven Press, 1987;383–422.
3 Sanders KM, Publicover NG. Electrophysiology of the gastric musculature. In: Schultz SG, Wood JD, Rauner BB, eds. *Handbook of Physiology*, 2nd edn. Section 6. The Gastrointestinal System. Vol. 1, Motility and Circulation, Part 1. Bethesda: American Physiological Society, 1989:187–216.
4 Sarna SK. Cyclic motor activity; migrating motor complex: 1985. *Gastroenterology* 1985;**89**:894–913.
5 Kellow JE, Borody TJ, Phillips SF, Tucker RL, Haddad AC. Human interdigestive motility: variations in patterns from esophagus to colon. *Gastroenterology* 1986;**91**:386–95.
6 Quigley EMM. Antroduodenal manometry. In: Hinder RA, ed. *Problems in General Surgery: Tests of Foregut Function*. Philadelphia: JB Lippincott Co, 1992:152–71.
7 Quigley EMM. Intestinal manometry in man: a historical and clinical perspective. *Dig Dis* 1994;**12**:199–209.
8 Malagelada J-R, Azpiroz F. Determinants of gastric emptying and transit in the small intestine. In: Schultz SG, Wood JD, Rauner BB, eds. *Handbook of Physiology*, 2nd edn. Section 6. The Gastrointestinal System. Vol. 1, Motility and Circulation, Part 2. Bethesda: American Physiological Society, 1989:909–37.
9 Camilleri M. Disorders of gastrointestinal motility in neurologic diseases. *Mayo Clin Proc* 1990;**65**:825–46.
10 Krishnamurthy S, Schuffler MD. Pathology of neuromuscular disorders of the small intestine and colon. *Gastroenterology* 1987;**93**:610–39.
11 Colemont LJ, Camilleri M. Chronic intestinal pseudo-obstruction: diagnosis and treatment. *Mayo Clin Proc* 1989;**64**:60–70.
12 Greydanus MP, Camilleri M. Abnormal postcibal antral and small bowel motility

due to neuropathy or myopathy in systemic sclerosis. *Gastroenterology* 1989;**96**:110–15.

13 Krishnamurthy S, Kelly MM, Rohrmann CA, Schuffler MD. Jejunal diverticulosis: a heterogeneous disorder caused by a variety of abnormalities of smooth muscle or myenteric plexus. *Gastroenterology* 1983;**85**:538–47.

14 Vantrappen G, Janssens J, Hellemans J, Ghoos Y. The interdigestive motor complex of normal subjects and patients with bacterial overgrowth of the small intestine. *J Clin Invest* 1977;**59**:1158–66.

15 Thompson DG. The clinical application of exhaled breath hydrogen testing for the study of gastrointestinal motility. In: Read NW, ed. *Gastrointestinal Motility. Which Test?* Petersfield, UK: Wrightson Biomedical Publishing, 1989:163–7.

16 Kellow JE, Borody TJ, Phillips SF, Haddad AC, Brown ML. Sulfapyridine appearance in plasma after salicylazasulfapyridine: another simple measure of intestinal transit. *Gastroenterology* 1986;**91**:396–400.

17 Datz FL, Christian PE, Hutson WR, Moore JG, Morton KA. Physiological and pharmacological interventions in radionuclide imaging of the tubular gastrointestinal tract. *Semin Nucl Med* 1991;**21**:140–52.

18 Camilleri M, Zinsmeister AR, Greydanus MP, Brown ML, Proano M. Towards a less costly but accurate test of gastric emptying and small bowel transit. *Dig Dis Sci* 1991;**36**:609–15.

19 Charles F, Camilleri M, Phillips SF, Thomforde GM, Forstrom LA. Scintigraphy of the whole gut: clinical evaluation of transit disorders. *Mayo Clin Proc* 1995;**70**:113–18.

20 Quigley EMM. Intestinal manometry — technical advances, clinical limitations. *Dig Dis Sci* 1992;**37**:10–13.

21 Lindberg G, Iwarzon M, Stal P, Seensalu R. Digital ambulatory monitoring of small-bowel motility. *Scand J Gastroenterol* 1990;**25**:216–24.

22 Husebye E, Skar V, Aalen OO, Osnes M. Digital ambulatory manometry of the small intestine in healthy adults: estimates of variations within and between individuals and statistical management of incomplete MMC periods. *Dig Dis Sci* 1990;**35**:1057–65.

23 Wilson P, Perdikis G, Hinder RA, Redmond EJ, Anselmino M, Quigley EMM. Prolonged ambulatory antroduodenal manometry in humans. *Am J Gastroenterol* 1994;**89**:1489–95.

24 Krishnamurthy S, Heng Y, Schuffler MD. Chronic intestinal pseudo-obstruction in infants and children caused by diverse abnormalities of the myenteric plexus. *Gastroenterology* 1993;**104**:1398–408.

25 Frank JW, Sarr MG, Camilleri M. Use of gastroduodenal manometry to differentiate mechanical and functional intestinal obstruction: an analysis of clinical outcome. *Am J Gastroenterol* 1994;**89**:339–44.

26 Sandgren JE, McPhee MS, Greenberger NJ. Narcotic bowel syndrome treated with clonidine. *Ann Intern Med* 1984;**101**:331–4.

27 Hyman PE. Chronic intestinal pseudo-obstruction. In: Hyman PE, ed. *Pediatric Gastrointestinal Motility Disorders*. New York: Academy Professional Information Services Inc, 1994:115–28.

28 Zeltzer LK, Arnoult S, Hamilton A, DeLaura S. Visceral pain in children. In: Hyman PE, ed. *Pediatric Gastrointestinal Motility Disorders*. New York: Academy Professional Information Services Inc, 1994: 155–76.

29 Basin WN. Advances in enteral nutrition techniques. *Am J Gastroenterol* 1992;**11**:1547–53.

30 Burtch GD, Shatney CH. Feeding jejunostomy (versus gastrostomy) passes the test of time. *Am Surg* 1987;**53**:54–7.

31 Matino JJ. Feeding jejunostomy in patients with neurologic disorders. *Arch Surg* 1981;**116**:169–71.

32 Ho C-S, Yee ACN, McPherson R. Complications of surgical and percutaneous nonendoscopic gastrostomy: review of 213 patients. *Gastroenterology* 1988;**95**:1206–10.

33 Ramirez B, Richter JE. Review article: promotility drugs in the treatment of gastro-oesophageal reflux disease. *Aliment Pharmacol Ther* 1993;**7**:5–20.

34 Dent J, ed. *Pharmacotherapy of Gastrointestinal Motor Disorders.* Sydney: Reed Healthcare Communications, 1991.

35 Quigley EMM. The clinical pharmacology of motility disorders: the perils (and pearls) of prokinesia. *Gastroenterology* 1994;**106**:1112–14.

36 Malagelada J-R, Rees WDW, Mazzotta LJ, Go VLW. Gastric motor abnormalities in diabetic and postvagotomy gastroparesis: effect of metoclopramide and bethanechol. *Gastroenterology* 1980;**78**:286–93.

37 Brogden RN, Carmine AA, Heel RC, Speight TM, Avery GS. Domperidone: a review of its pharmacological activity, pharmacokinetics and therapeutic efficacy in the symptomatic treatment of chronic dyspepsia and as an antiemetic. *Drugs* 1982;**24**:360–400.

38 Champion MC, Hartnett M, Yen M. Domperidone, a new dopamine antagonist. *Can Med Assoc J* 1986;**135**:457–61.

39 Parkes JD. Domperidone and Parkinson's disease. *Clin Neuropharmacol* 1986;**9**:517–32.

40 Hawkey CJ. The place of cisapride in therapeutics: an interim verdict. *Aliment Pharmacol Ther* 1991;**5**:351–6.

41 Heading RC, Wood JD. *Gastrointestinal Dysmotility: Focus on Cisapride.* New York: Raven Health Care Communications, 1992.

42 Abell TL, Camilleri M, DiMagno EP, Hench VS, Zinsmeister AR, Malagelada J-R. Long-term efficacy of oral cisapride in symptomatic upper gut dysmotility. *Dig Dis Sci* 1991;**36**:616–20.

43 Wehrmann T, Lembcke B, Caspary WF. Influence of cisapride on antroduodenal motor function in healthy subjects and diabetics with autonomic neuropathy. *Aliment Pharmacol Ther* 1991;**5**:599–608.

44 Camilleri M, Malagelada J-R, Abell TL, Brown ML, Hench V, Zinsmeister AR. Effect of six weeks of treatment with cisapride in gastroparesis and intestinal pseudo-obstruction. *Gastroenterology* 1989;**96**:704–12.

45 McHugh S, Lico S, Diamant NE. Cisapride versus metoclopramide: an acute study in diabetic gastroparesis. *Dig Dis Sci* 1992;**37**:997–1001.

46 Richards RD, Valenzuela GA, Davenport KS, Fisher KLK, McCallum RW. Objective and subjective results of a randomized, double-blind, placebo-controlled trial using cisapride to treat gastroparesis. *Dig Dis Sci* 1993;**38**:811–16.

47 Camilleri M, Balm RK, Zinsmeister AR. Determinants of response to a prokinetic agent in neuropathic chronic intestinal motility disorders. *Gastroenterology* 1994;**106**:916–23.

48 Soudah HC, Hasler WL, Owyang C. Effect of octreotide on intestinal motility and bacterial overgrowth in scleroderma. *N Engl J Med* 1991;**325**:1461–7.

49 O'Donnell LJ, Watson AJ, Cameron D, Farthing MJ. Effect of octreotide on mouth-to-caecum transit time in healthy subjects and in the irritable bowel syndrome. *Aliment Pharmacol Ther* 1990;**4**:177–81.

50 Ewins DL, Javaid A, Coskeran PB *et al.* Assessment of gall bladder dynamics, cholecystokinin release and the development of gallstones during octreotide treatment for acromegaly. *Q J Med* 1992;**83**:295–306.

51 Hasler WL, Soudah HC, Owyang C. A somatostatin analogue inhibits afferent pathways mediating perception of rectal distension. *Gastroenterology* 1993;**104**:1390–7.

52 Tack J, Janssens J, Vantrappen G *et al.* Effect of erythromycin on gastric motility in controls and in diabetic gastroparesis. *Gastroenterology* 1992;**103**:72–9.

53 Fraser R, Shearer T, Fuller J, Horowitz M, Dent J. Intravenous erythromycin overcomes small intestinal feedback on antral, pyloric and duodenal motility. *Gastroenterology* 1992;**103**:114–19.

54 Janssens, J. Peeters TL, Vantrappen G *et al.* Improvement of gastric emptying in diabetic gastroparesis by erythromycin. *N Engl J Med* 1990;**322**:1028–31.

55 Weber FH, Richards RD, McCallum RW. Erythromycin: a motilin agonist and gastrointestinal prokinetic agent. *Am J Gastroenterol* 1993;**88**:485–90.

56 Keshavarzian A, Isaac RM. Erythromycin accelerates gastric emptying of indigestible solids and transpyloric migration of the tip of an enteral feeding tube in fasting and fed states. *Am J Gastroenterol* 1993;**88**:193–7.

57 Mantides A, Xynos E, Chrysos E, Georgopoulos N, Vassilakis JS. The effect of erythromycin in gastric emptying of solids and hypertonic liquids in healthy subjects. *Am J Gastroenterol* 1993;**88**:198–202.

58 Richards RD, Davenport K, McCallum RW. The treatment of idiopathic and diabetic gastroparesis with acute intravenous and chronic oral erythromycin. *Am J Gastroenterol* 1993;**88**:203–7.

59 Fiorucci S, Distrutti E, Bassotti G *et al.* Effect of erythromycin administration on upper gastrointestinal motility in scleroderma patients. *Scand J Gastroenterol* 1994;**29**:807–13.

60 Camilleri M. The current role of erythromycin in the clinical management of gastric emptying disorders. *Am J Gastroenterol* 1993;**88**:169–71.

61 Talley NJ. Review article: 5-hydroxytryptamine agonists and antagonists in the modulation of gastrointestinal motility and sensation — clinical implications. *Aliment Pharmacol Ther* 1992;**6**:273–89.

62 Mathias JR, Ferguson KL, Clench MH. Debilitating 'functional' bowel disease controlled by leuprolide acetate, gonadotropin-releasing hormone (GnRH) analog. *Dig Dis Sci* 1989;**34**:761–6.

63 Mathias JR, Baskin GS, Reeves-Darby VG, Clench MH, Smith LL, Calhoon JH. Chronic intestinal pseudoobstruction in a patient with a heart–lung transplant: therapeutic effect of leuprolide acetate. *Dig Dis Sci* 1992;**37**:1761–8.

64 Mathias JR, Clench MH, Reeves-Darby VG *et al.* Effect of leuprolide acetate in patients with moderate to severe functional bowel disease: double-blind, placebo-controlled study. *Dig Dis Sci* 1994;**39**:1155–62.

65 Rutgeerts P, Vantrappen G, Hiele M, Ghoos Y, Onkelin XC. Effects on bowel motility of misoprostol administered before and after meals. *Aliment Pharmacol Ther* 1991;**5**:533–42.

66 Soffer EE, Launspach J. Effect of misoprostol on postprandial intestinal motility and orocecal transit time in humans. *Dig Dis Sci* 1993;**38**:851–5.

67 Kreek M-J, Schaefer RA, Hahn EF, Fishman J. Naloxone, a specific opioid antagonist, reverses chronic idiopathic constipation. *Lancet* 1983;**1**:261–2.

68 Fraitag B, Homerin M, Hecketsweiler P. Double-blind dose–response multicenter comparison of fedotozine and placebo in treatment of non-ulcer dyspepsia. *Dig Dis Sci* 1994;**39**:1072–7.

69 Vanderhoof JA, Langnas AN, Pinch LW, Thompson JS, Kaufman SS. Short bowel
    syndrome and intestinal transplantation. *J Pediatr Gastroenterol Nutr* 1991;**14**:359–70.
70 MacGilchrist AJ, Quigley EMM. Transplantation. In: Sherman D, Finlayson NDC,
    Carter D, Camilleri M, eds. *Diseases of the Gastrointestinal Tract and Liver.* London:
    Churchill Livingstone, 1996 (in press).

« 9 »

Pathogenesis and Management of the Irritable Bowel Syndrome

W. Grant Thompson

There is no pathophysiologic marker for the functional gastrointestinal (GI) syndromes. Therefore, we must rely on symptoms for their definition and classification. A series of international working teams [1–3] meeting in Rome developed a classification of these disorders and offered definitions and research criteria for each syndrome (Table 9.1). The irritable bowel syndrome (IBS) is distinct from other functional bowel disorders such as functional constipation and functional diarrhea (Table 9.2). The symptom criteria for the IBS are known as the Rome criteria and are shown in Table 9.3. Subjects with functional bowel symptoms that are insufficient to be classified as the IBS or as one of the other syndromes listed in Table 9.2 are said to have an unspecified functional bowel disorder. These disparate syndromes are likely to have different causes and require different tests and treatments.

Table 9.1 Definitions. (From Thompson *et al.* [3].)

A functional gastrointestinal disorder
'A variable combination of persistent or recurrent gastrointestinal symptoms not explained by structural or biochemical abnormalities. These may include symptoms attributable to the oropharynx, oesophagus, stomach, biliary tree, small or large intestine or anus.'

A functional bowel disorder
'A functional gastrointestinal disorder with symptoms attributable to the mid or lower intestinal tract. The symptoms include abdominal pain, bloating or distension and various symptoms of disordered defecation.'

The irritable bowel syndrome
'A functional bowel disorder in which abdominal pain is associated with defecation or a change in bowel habit, and with features of disordered defecation and with distension.'

Table 9.2 The functional bowel disorders. (From Thompson *et al.* [3].)

C	*Functional bowel disorders*
C1	**Irritable bowel syndrome**
C2	Functional abdominal bloating
C3	Functional constipation
C4	Functional diarrhea
C5	Unspecified functional bowel disorder

Table 9.3 Symptom criteria for IBS. (From Thompson *et al.* [3].)

At least 3 months of continuous or recurrent symptoms of:
- abdominal pain or discomfort that is:
  - (a)   relieved with defecation, and/or
  - (b)   associated with a change in frequency of stool, and/or
  - (c)   associated with a change in consistency of stools

and:

- two or more of the following, during at least a quarter of occasions or days:
  - (a)   altered stool frequency (defined here as more than three bowel movements per day or less than three per week)
  - (b)   altered stool form (lumpy/hard or loose/watery stool)
  - (c)   altered stool passage (straining, urgency, or feeling of incomplete evacuation)
  - (d)   passage of mucus
  - (e)   bloating or feeling of abdominal distention

Epidemiology

The IBS is very common. We [4] showed it to be present in 14% of British adults. Subsequent studies in the USA [5, 6], France [7], New Zealand [8], Denmark [9], and even China [10] indicate that such a prevalence rate is worldwide. Employing the Rome criteria, Drossman *et al.* [11] found the IBS to be present in 11.6% of respondents in a random sample of more than 8000 USA households. This study and a study [12] done in England indicate that IBS is twice as common in women as in men, but reports [9, 13] conflict as to a decreasing prevalence with age. These figures are sensitive to the definitions of IBS that are employed. In one instance [9], prevalence rates of 5–65% were found using different definitions. In a population survey [14], 38% of individuals who had had IBS by Manning and Rome criteria did not have it when surveyed 1 year later. However, about 9% who did not have IBS initially had acquired it. An even greater turnover was found over 5 years in that 95% had experienced some symptoms during that period [9].

Epidemiologic studies are hampered by a dependence on recall, which is notoriously flawed. For example, almost 40% of 961 adults with a previous fracture on their medical record had forgotten it when questioned 15 years later [15]. Most evidence suggests that IBS is a chronic relapsing disorder that probably occurs in most adults during their lifetime.

Most individuals reporting the IBS in population surveys do not seek medical help. Nevertheless, patients with the IBS constitute about 50% of those seen in Western [16] and Asian [17] clinics. Among Western clinic patients, women outnumber men by 3:1 or 4:1 [18, 19]. Curiously, in India and Sri Lanka, this ratio is reversed [20, 21]. Even though most IBS sufferers in the community do not consult a physician for their symptoms those who do present an important and costly health problem [4]. A management strategy must be developed with these facts in mind. There are indications that IBS patients seen by specialists are a subgroup of the whole, with psychosocial characteristics that are distinct from individuals with the same symptoms who do not seek medical care [22, 23] and probably distinct from IBS patients seen in primary care.

Prognosis

In terms of life expectancy, the prognosis of IBS is excellent. The symptoms are themselves benign, and there is no evidence that they predispose an individual to any other disorder. However, in terms of cure of symptoms, the outlook is not so good. Many studies [14, 24–28] confirm that despite a variety of treatments, most patients who receive a diagnosis of IBS still have symptoms when interviewed 1–10 years later. Given the fickleness of human memory, it is unlikely that many achieve a complete cure. In one survey [9], only 5% of IBS subjects interviewed at 5 years were completely free of symptoms. On the bright side, very few of these individuals had acquired an organic GI disease, and none seems to represent an original misdiagnosis.

Pathogenesis

Is IBS *'a qualitative or merely a quantitative departure from the psycho-physiological reactions of healthy persons?'* Thomas Almy [29].

The cause of IBS has confounded physicians for almost two centuries. Despite much research, we cannot even today offer a convincing explanation. Many hold strong beliefs. Some declare it is caused by something in the diet. Others cite evidence to suggest that it is an infection, or are convinced that it is a motility disorder. Still others believe that it is due to altered perception, a psychological disorder, psychophysiologic phenomena, or even abnormal illness behavior. Perhaps all of these are true, or none are true, or some are true some of the time. Keep Professor Almy's question in mind. A condition affecting at least 11% of a physically healthy population may be no disease at all. Rather, the IBS may represent a normal response of the gut to its environment, made more or less prominent in an individual's consciousness by his or her fears or psychological state.

A dietary disorder?

Burkitt and his medical missionary colleagues [30] in East Africa noted that IBS, constipation, and other 'Western' bowel disorders were uncommon in natives consuming an indigenous high-fiber diet. In a 1972 study [30] of rural African and Westernized populations, they noted that the greater the dietary fiber content, the greater the daily stool weight and the shorter the whole-gut transit time. These facts led to the 'fiber hypothesis,' the concept that many diseases of the colon and other organs result from the ingestion of a Western, refined, low-fiber diet. By implication, IBS is one such disease.

Subsequent studies [31] confirm that a high-fiber diet increases stool bulk and shortens gut transit time. Many studies [32] attest to the value of bran, psyllium, and other bulking materials in the treatment of constipation. However, the presence of IBS has not been linked to an individual's fiber intake, and its presence in countries such as China [10] raises doubt that a single dietary factor such as fiber deficiency is at fault. A more telling source of doubt is the lack of success of dietary fiber supplements, such as bran and psyllium, in the treatment of IBS, as measured by double-blind trials [33]. Fiber may be a safe, cheap placebo, but it is not a cure. The fiber story is made even more confusing by the report [34] that among 'healthy' volunteers, an outgoing personality and a positive self-image predict a larger stool output. Nevertheless, there is evidence [35] that if at least 30 g of dietary fiber is taken daily, constipation and some other symptoms may improve.

Some patients are certain that a food substance is the culprit, if only that food could be identified. This pervasive idea has spawned irrational diets that defy science, cause much inconvenience, and even compromise nutrition. A true food allergy, such as to shellfish, affects systems beyond the gut and is more likely to cause vomiting and diarrhea than IBS symptoms. Nonimmunoglobulin E (IgE)-mediated intolerances to wheat, dairy products, or beef are claimed to cause diarrhea in some cases, but not the IBS as strictly defined. Very few individuals with IBS can be confirmed by double-blind feedings to have a true food sensitivity [36]. It appears that this approach is likely to be useful only if the patient is suffering from diarrhea, but even that is disputed [36].

Certainly, a careful medical history should seek out evidence of lactose intolerance, excessive caffeine intake, use of sorbitol-containing gum, or other drug or dietary habits that may affect the gut [37]. Although a dietary factory may be involved in IBS in some individuals, it is unlikely to be the sole cause.

An infection or inflammation?

The IBS frequently follows an enteric infection [24, 28, 38]. Could IBS be, after all, an infection or an inflammation set up by an infection? Collins [39] suggests that cytokines emitted from submucosal mast cells or other inflammatory cells might cause the motility disturbances thought to occur in the IBS. Ileal mast-cell counts have been found to be greater in IBS patients than in controls [40]. On the other hand, rectal biopsies performed on 89 patients with the IBS as determined by established criteria and examined by blinded pathologists revealed no histologic difference between IBS patients and controls [41].

A motility disorder?

'[T]he bowels are at one time constipated, at another lax, in the same person. . . . How the disease has two such different symptoms I do not profess to explain. . .' W. Cumming [42].

Cumming's dilemma persists. Colon motility studies [43] in the 1960s suggested that in constipation, the motility index (frequency of contraction multiplied by amplitude of contraction) is increased. This holds up the passage of stool and causes abdominal pain. Conversely, this line of reasoning suggests that in those with diarrhea, the motility index is decreased. Here, the lax sigmoid permits liquid feces to trickle into the rectum, prematurely triggering defecation. But these observations have not turned out to be reliable features of constipation and diarrhea. Furthermore, it is now believed that the proximal colon and the small intestine are also dysfunctional in IBS [44–46]. In the 1970s, investigators

[47] reported that a 3-cycle per minute (cpm) myoelectric rhythm is more common in IBS patients than in controls. However, the specificity of this observation is doubted. Using a different technology, European workers [48] associated the recording of electrical short bursts in the colon with constipation and the lack of these bursts with diarrhea. In the 1980s, attention was drawn to the small bowel, where the secretory and motor responses to stress seem to be different in IBS patients than in normal individuals [44–46]. However, none of these phenomena is sufficiently specific to permit its use as a diagnostic test of IBS, nor indeed do any of them explain how the symptoms are generated.

Balloons inflated sequentially throughout the gut can identify trigger points that reproduce the abdominal pain experienced by most individuals with IBS [49, 50]. Even here, it is not certain to what extent the pain of IBS is a normal perception of abnormal physiology or an abnormal perception of normal physiology [51]. In IBS there is a tendency for both the small and large bowel to overreact to a variety of stimuli, such as drugs, stress, balloon distention, and even eating [47, 52, 53]. The last may represent an exaggerated gastrocolonic response [47]. Abnormalities in gut motility have yet to explain the diverse features of IBS.

A perception disorder?

The failure of motility observations to adequately explain IBS symptoms has led many to study the sensory or afferent connections between the gut and the brain. IBS patients appreciate pain at lower levels of rectal distention than do other individuals [53, 54], but they do not simply have a generalized low threshold for pain. Pain sensitivity as measured during electrocutaneous stimulation was similar in patients with either IBS or Crohn's disease, and both groups were less sensitive than were controls [55]. The autonomic connections between the enteric nervous system (ENS) and the central nervous system (CNS) are well known, and it is of further interest that the vagus and sympathetic nerves carry more afferent than efferent nerve fibers. 5-Hydroxytryptamine-3 (5-HT_3) and 5-HT_4 receptors may play an important role in transmitting impulses from the ENS to the CNS. Attempts are being made to develop antagonists to these receptors and thereby decrease gut sensitivity.

An individual's experience of pain may be greatly influenced by emotion, memory, culture, and psychosocial situation [56]. It is useful to distinguish acute pain from chronic pain [57]. Acute pain is linked to tissue pathology or organ dysfunction and, in the case of the gut, is associated with eating, defecation, and vomiting. Chronic pain is continuous and unassociated with physiologic responses to pain, such as sweating and tachycardia. The patient with chronic pain is often depressed, and there may be secondary gain or prior adverse experiences such as sexual abuse and threatening life events.

The perception of pain varies from patient to patient. Acute, function-related pain is primarily sensory or peripheral and may lend itself to treatment with analgesics directed at the organ involved. Chronic pain, which is influenced more by CNS controlling activity, may require treatment directed at behavior that is influenced by emotion or cognition. Drugs such as the tricyclic antidepressants enhance the production of 5-HT and inhibit pain impulses, thereby reducing the perception of noxious stimuli [58]. They may also enhance endorphin release. In contrast, benzodiazepines carry a risk of habituation, and via gamma-aminobutyric acid (GABA) production, they may inhibit the production of 5-HT and increase pain perception [59].

It is not only pain that may be misperceived by patients. They often misinterpret their bowel action as well [60]. Although stool frequency in the population ranges from three movements per week to three per day, many consider variations within this range to be abnormal. Others misinterpret frequent but hard, fragmented, or lumpy stool as diarrhea when, in fact, gut transit is prolonged. Heaton and O'Donnell [61] have termed this 'pseudodiarrhea.' Patients often complain of symptoms such as borborygmi, flatus, and distention, giving little indication that these symptoms are objectively different from those in noncomplainers. Lasser *et al.* [62] found that patients complaining of 'gas' or 'bloating' had no excess intestinal gas.

Clearly, how sensory input is perceived is an important determinant of the IBS. Acute, function-related symptoms need to be treated differently from symptoms that are chronic, continuous, and associated with psychosocial distress [56]. Nonetheless, perception alone does not explain the altered gut function, nor does it seem important in those with IBS symptoms who do not seek medical care.

A psychological disorder?

The notion that IBS symptoms are interrelated with, perhaps even caused by, an individual's psychological state is as old as the concept of IBS itself. Many studies [22, 23, 63, 64] attest that anxiety, depression, and other forms of psychological distress are more likely in IBS patients than in patients with organic disease. However, the patients in these studies were in a tertiary care setting and thus unlikely to be representative of all persons experiencing IBS symptoms. Whitehead *et al.* [23] and Drossman *et al.* [22] found that the psychosocial makeup of IBS sufferers in the community who do not see doctors is the same as that of normal individuals. It also appears that IBS and psychosocial distress, when they do occur in the same patient, are not necessarily concurrent [65, 66]. In one British clinic, chronic attendees with IBS were compared with newly referred patients [67]. Although psychological morbidity was similar in the two groups, the social consequences in the chronic attendees were more severe. There are no studies of the psychological state of IBS patients seen in primary care, but these patients are likely to represent an intermediate population.

The foregoing data do not support the notion that psychopathology *causes* the IBS. Indeed, antidepressants are most effective in IBS patients without psychopathology [68]. Perhaps a psychopathological condition worsens IBS symptoms or elevates them to the status of a medical problem in a person's consciousness (a perception disorder?). Could psychological distress be a determinant of health-care seeking? For the emotionally troubled person, IBS symptoms provide a socially acceptable vehicle for care.

These arguments are reinforced by observations [69] that IBS patients tend to seek medical care after a stressful or threatening life event. At the simplest level, a man with IBS who has ignored his symptoms for years may become acutely aware of them when a close relative succumbs to cancer. Compared with age- and less sex-matched controls, IBS patients commonly express concerns about cancer to their doctor [70]. Here, treatment is obvious. Reassure the patient that he or she does not have cancer; further treatment is usually unnecessary.

The management of patients whose visits appear to be precipitated by depression, job loss, marital breakup, or other personal catastrophe may be much more complicated. Many tertiary care patients are polysymptomatic, complaining of fatigue and headache [71, 72]. Others have suffered sexual or physical abuse [73]. In such situations, treatment that focuses on the gut symptoms may be misplaced.

A psychophysiologic disorder?

It is the common experience that emotion affects gut function. Who has not suffered some gut upset before an exam, a marriage, a death, or another stressful or emotional event? In the early 1950s, Almy [74] demonstrated that stress could alter gut motility but that the changes were not specific to the stress. One person may have 'butterflies,' another diarrhea, another vomiting, and yet another a migraine. It seems that a given emotion may elicit different responses at different times in different persons. Perhaps these responses can be learned in early childhood [75]. In the IBS the relationship of symptoms to stress is more subtle. Changes in stress may be important. Some even notice that symptoms improve during a crisis, only to return later.

In IBS patients, the gut appears to be more reactive to a variety of stimuli when compared with controls. Drugs [76], hormones [77], food [52], distention [53, 78], and emotional stress [79] elicit exaggerated motor responses. An air insufflation test has been suggested [80] for IBS. Using radiotelemetry equipment, Valori *et al.* [79] observed that motility of the small bowel was altered in a different manner in IBS patients than in controls. He and his colleagues employed such stressors as heavy metal music, nocturnal arousal, and parking in London traffic to challenge the small bowel. It seems certain that stresses may nonspecifically alter gut function, and the alterations seem to be different in IBS patients. What determines these reactions? Are they clues to the cause of IBS, or are they merely epiphenomena?

A behavioral disorder?

Compared with persons with peptic ulcer, those with IBS have more somatic symptoms, view colds and flu more seriously, and consult physicians more frequently for minor complaints [75]. As children, they also were more likely than others to have received gifts or remained home from school when ill. These data support the notions that persons with IBS are prone to chronic illness behavior and that this behavior is learned.

Health-care seeking in the IBS, particularly at tertiary care centers, may be due as much to a person's cultural and psychosocial states as to the IBS symptoms themselves. How else can one explain why women are more likely than men to take their IBS symptoms to a doctor in Western cultures, while the opposite is true in India [4]? Why do only a minority of those with the IBS seek medical attention? The concurrence of threatening life events and psychosocial distress may partially explain these phenomena.

An integrated view

It must be evident from the foregoing that purely mechanistic or purely psychological explanations of IBS are inadequate reconciliations of the available facts. The physician should weigh all the considerations presented here as he or she interviews a patient (Figure 9.1). Evaluation of the relative importance of diet, disordered physiology, misperceptions, psychosocial maladaptations, and altered behavior in a patient may be as important to management as the establishment of a correct diagnosis. Past experience with diagnosing and treating peptic ulcers should make us cautious about accepting any of the current hypotheses. There, the focus on either acid secretion or psychosomatics as the cause blinded us to other possibilities and made it difficult to accept the role of *Helicobacter pylori.*

Noone's gut functions perfectly all the time, and variation in the population is great. Whatever the underlying pathophysiology, some people ignore the symptoms, while others permit the symptoms to dominate their lives. This variability is undoubtedly influenced by the emotions and life events that buffet us all. Further complicating the matter are human behavior, subtly learned in early childhood, and the negative incentives of Western social welfare systems. Since cure is elusive and we can do little to change life situations, the objective of IBS treatment should be improved functioning.

A therapeutic approach

Despite the reality that the pathogenesis of IBS is unknown, we have learned much about its epidemiology, prognosis, and diagnosis. The task

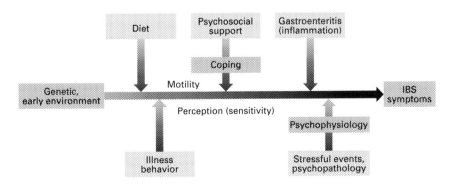

Fig. 9.1 Pathogenesis of IBS.

is to develop a strategy of management based on the known facts. Such a strategy should rely on six principles:

1 a positive diagnosis;
2 consideration of the patient's agenda;
3 critical appraisal of drugs and placebos;
4 the use of dietary fiber;
5 continuing care;
6 a graded therapeutic response.

A positive diagnosis

A careful history and physical examination permit a confident diagnosis that stands up over time. Physicians who consider the IBS a diagnosis of exclusion feel compelled to exclude all organic disease. This approach is expensive, especially if extrapolated to the many patients who seek medical care. The physician should attempt to establish a positive diagnosis at the first clinical encounter [3, 37, 56]. This is usually possible using the criteria shown in Table 9.3. A condition that affects up to 20% of the population is bound to coexist with organic disease in some. Therefore, one should inquire about symptoms such as anemia, bleeding, fever, weight loss, or a recent change in bowel habit.

If such symptoms and physical findings are absent, the investigation should be minimal. A sigmoidoscopy should be performed, but biopsy in search of microscopic colitis in the absence of continuous diarrhea is an unnecessary expense [41]. If the patient is older than 40 years of age or has risk factors for colon carcinoma, a barium enema is prudent. Even though the symptoms of the IBS are not those of polyp or cancer, a 'clean colon' is a reassuring start for all concerned. Other tests should be avoided unless indicated. An early, confident diagnosis permits tests to be minimized and reassures the patient that there is no mortal disease. Especially since fear of cancer is so common among IBS patients [70], such reassurance may be the physician's most effective therapeutic weapon.

The patient's agenda

Most persons with the IBS do not consult doctors. Those who do may have reasons for the visit beyond the gut. Severity of symptoms may be important, but psychosocial factors must also affect the decision. The answer to the question 'Why has this patient come to see the doctor now?' may be an important therapeutic clue. Fear of serious disease should be met by firm reassurance that none exists. Threatening life events, whether they precipitate the IBS or the consultation, should be discussed. Some patients may require psychological help or stress management expertise, but simple supportive psychotherapy by the attending physician may be salutary. In a Swedish study [81], IBS patients treated with eight sessions of supportive psychotherapy, which could be performed in any physician's office, had fewer symptoms and less psychological and physical disability, compared to a control group, when they were seen 3 months later. The improvement was even more marked 1 year later. This supports the notion that early, careful attention to the patient's psychosocial concerns has effective and lasting benefit. Such an approach is supported by an English study [82], which also noted that improvement is most likely if psychopathology is recognized and dealt with and the pain is not constant.

Drugs and placebos

'[N]ot a single study has been published that provides compelling evidence that any therapeutic agent is efficacious in the global treatment of IBS.' K.B. Klein [83].

There are too many clinical trials of drugs in IBS to report here. The reader is referred to Klein [83], who reviewed controlled trials conducted over a 20-year period and found them all flawed. The entry criteria are usually unclear, and the symptom criteria of Manning [84], Kruis [85], and the Rome teams [3] are recent innovations. Many studies are too small or too short, or have too many dropouts. Others have an inappropriate trial design or use improper statistics. Thus, no drug has been proven to be globally effective in treating IBS.

Although trial methodology is improving, studies subsequent to Klein's critique are still inadequate. An international working team [86] agreed with and updated Klein's conclusions and set out suggested standards for clinical trials. One meta-analysis [87] examined randomized controlled trials of smooth-muscle relaxants and concluded that five such drugs showed 27% and 19% improvements over placebo in global assessment and pain, respectively. However, only 26 of 148 known trials were selected, and abstracts and letters were discarded. Since it is likely that some trials failed to appear at all, a publication bias must be suspected. Even with negative studies possibly excluded, the benefits seem marginal at most. IBS is a benign disorder that affects up to 20% of adults through long periods of their lives. Physicians should discourage the chronic use of costly, systemic drugs of doubtful benefit, which in some cases may have unwanted consequences that can be more troublesome than the IBS itself.

Nevertheless, amid the rigors of science, there is a place for common sense in the use of drugs to treat the symptoms of IBS (Table 9.4). If diarrhea is the dominant symptom, with urgency, even incontinence, loperamide (Imodium®) may be helpful. This drug not only slows gut motility and decreases small bowel secretion but also increases anal sphincter strength [88]. Unlike other opiates, it does not enter the brain. Provided the diarrhea is genuine and not pseudodiarrhea [61], and reactive constipation does not result, such a drug can target the most troublesome symptom for a few patients. Other examples of such targeted therapy include bran or psyllium for constipation [33], avoidance of vegetables in the cabbage family, and perhaps use of alpha-D-galactosi-dase (Beano®) for excessive flatus, and a preprandial anticholinergic agent for abdominal pain that occurs after meals [47].

Anxiety and depression must be treated on their own merits. Treatment of psychological distress may permit a patient to cope better with IBS symptoms. In some pain-dominant IBS patients, tricyclic antidepressants may be helpful even if depression is not obvious [65, 66, 89). These drugs have proven effective in other chronic pain syndromes [90] and may act via central pathways that influence the perception of pain. They seem to be effective at low doses and before any change in mood

Table 9.4 Drugs useful for certain difficult IBS symptoms. (From Thompson [37].)

Indication	Drug	Maximum dose
Diarrhea-dominant IBS	Loperamide (Imodium®) Cholestyramine (Questran®)	1–2 tablets three times daily 1 teaspoonful (4 g) three times daily

Pain-dominant IBS
  Postmeal pain [47]
  Chronic pain syndrome
  [68]
	Dicyclomine (Bentyl®)
	Amitriptyline (Elavil®)
		10–20 mg before meals
		25 mg at bedtime, with
		increments to 100 mg

Constipation	Bran or psyllium	1 tablespoonful three times daily with meals, and adjust
Gas/bloat/flatus	Alpha-D-galactosidase (Beano®) Simethicone	— 1–2 tablets three times daily

occurs. A recommended starting dose of amitriptyline (Elavil®) is 25 mg at bedtime, with increments every 4–5 days until benefit is achieved. The dose seldom exceeds 100 mg, but anticholinergic or sedating side effects may necessitate switching to another drug, such as doxepin (Sinequan®).

An important feature of IBS symptoms is the tendency to improve with placebo. In existing therapeutic trials, the placebo response ranges from 40 to 70% [37]. There are lessons to be learned from this placebo response.

1   It demonstrates the variability of the disease, which tends to improve with time.

2   It supports the contention that no drug is generally acceptable for IBS patients without convincing demonstration of efficacy in defined-entry, randomized, placebo-controlled, double-blind clinical trials.

3   Placebos may be useful in certain circumstances. It is said that if a placebo is to have a therapeutic effect, the patient must believe that it will. Nevertheless, in a group of neurotic patients, placebo was effective even when they knew the pills were inert [91]. It seems that the symbolic giving of medication has a therapeutic value. Logical placebos that have a plausible rationale, yet are inexpensive and safe, may exploit these phenomena.

4   The most important implication of the placebo response is that it demonstrates the beneficial effect of a successful physician–patient encounter.

Dietary fiber

Although bran, psyllium, and dietary fiber are not proven effective in the treatment of IBS [33, 92, 93], they should still be tried by the primary care doctor. Fiber is effective in constipation and pseudodiarrhea. Ingestion of sufficient fiber has a visible effect on stool form and is a cheap, safe method of eliciting the placebo response. It also involves the patient in his or her own care in a way that passive ingestion of a pill may not. Fiber needs to be taken in sufficient doses. To encourage compliance and more easily titrate the dose of fiber, the author prefers to have the patient take three tablespoonsful three times a day with meals and adjust the amount according to its effect on the stool. There are reports of intolerance to bran in patients at tertiary care centers, but such patients have usually tried bran and failed [94, 95]. Specialists are less likely to achieve success with fiber in their selected patients than a primary care physician encountering a patient for the first time. If bran works, referral becomes redundant.

Continuing care

Cure, or even acceptance of the diagnosis, is an unrealistic goal for some troubled IBS patients. Unsatisfied with their doctor, they are prone to turn to practitioners of alternative medicine [96, 97]. Some diets and remedies recommended by these sources are inappropriate, even harmful, and important intervening disease may be overlooked. It is, therefore, important that the physician assure the patient of the availability of continuing care.

Emotionally disturbed patients benefit from regular, brief visits. These visits offer reassurance, and control 'doctor-shopping' and inappropriate ordering of tests and treatments. Through such visits, the doctor can be vigilant for a change in symptoms. Assistance may be sought from psychologists, psychiatrists, or other services if needed. Some patients may benefit from a stress management program. Patients with severe symptoms may require the multidisciplinary services of a pain clinic. Although biofeedback [98] and hypnosis [99] seem to benefit some patients, such services are not available in many cities. If the physician seems to lose the confidence of a patient, referral to an esteemed colleague may help by confirming the diagnosis and reinforcing the management plan.

A graded therapeutic response [56]

The therapeutic response must be tailored to the individual needs of IBS sufferers if we are to use our resources economically and effectively. Most individuals with the IBS do not seek medical attention. Many who do consult a primary care physician are worried about the meaning of their symptoms and will likely respond to explanation and reassurance. Those who return with the same symptoms or who are referred to specialists may require more attention. Those who chronically seek help from subspecialists are a small, unhappy, but costly subgroup in whom psychosocial factors may be more disabling than the gut symptoms themselves.

The primary care physician should emphasize the positive diagnosis, the chronic yet benign nature of the symptoms, the role of stress, and the inutility of drugs. Bulk, such as bran, improves constipation and is otherwise a safe, cheap placebo. For nonresponders, once the foregoing items have been dealt with satisfactorily, supportive psychotherapy and drugs for specific indications may be added. Overinvestigation or repeated testing and referral without substantial indication may undermine the patient's confidence in the doctor's conclusions. The emphasis should be directed toward improved daily functioning. There may be a role for special treatments such as stress management, psychotherapy, behavioral modification, or a psychotherapeutic agent such as amitriptyline. In the end, there is no substitute for the ongoing support of a caring family doctor.

Summary

The cause of the IBS is unknown, but it is very common in the community. Most sufferers do not see doctors. There is evidence that factors other than symptoms contribute to the decision to seek medical care. Examination of these factors not only suggests that the cause is multifactorial, but also offers clues for the management of individual patients. There is either some evidence for, or strong belief in, the importance of diet, inflammation, disordered motility, psychophysiology, or psychopathology in the genesis of the IBS. It seems that severe life events and an altered perception of symptoms may also be important and that several factors may act in concert to induce illness behavior. In some patients, all factors may be present; in others, apparently none. But the more factors are at work, the more complex the treatment.

Management should take advantage of the known features of the disease. Its prevalence, recognizable symptoms, and benign nature indicate the reassurance value of a positive diagnosis. The tendency of patients, especially chronic complainers, to have psychopathology or antecedent stressful life events may indicate important management issues. Although drugs are unproved in the global treatment of IBS, certain agents may benefit specific symptoms and may also employ the placebo response to advantage. Insecure patients or chronic complainers need continuing care. Different levels of disability require a graded treatment response to IBS complaints. This implies reassurance and drug-free management at the primary care level, with increments of psychosocial support and specific use of drugs in nonresponders. The goal of therapy in severe, intractable cases should be improved functioning rather than cure.

References

1 Drossman DA, Funch-Jensen P, Janssens J, Talley NJ, Thompson WG, Whitehead WE. Identification of subgroups of functional bowel disorders. *Gastroenterol Int* 1990;**3**:159–72.

2 Thompson WG, Working Team for Functional Bowel Disorders. C. Functional bowel disorders and D. functional abdominal pain. In: Drossman DA, ed. *The Functional Gastrointestinal Disorders.* Boston: Little, Brown, 1944:115–73.

3 Thompson WG, Creed F, Drossman DA, Heaton KW, Mazzacca G. Functional bowel disorders and functional abdominal pain. *Gastroenterol Int* 1992;**5**:75–91.

4 Thompson WG. Irritable bowel syndrome: prevalence, prognosis and consequences. *Can Med Assoc J* 1986;**134**:111–13.

5 Drossman DA, Sandler RS, McKee DC, Lovitz AJ. Bowel patterns among subjects not seeking health care: use of a questionnaire to identify a population with bowel dysfunction. *Gastroenterology* 1982;**83**:529–34.

6 Longstreth GF, Wolde-Tsadik G. Irritable bowel-type symptoms in HMO examinees: prevalence, demographics and clinical correlates. *Dig Dis Sci* 1993;**38**:1581–9.

7 Bommelaer G, Rouch M, Dapoigny M *et al.* Epidemiology of intestinal functional disorders in an apparently healthy population. *Gastroenterol Clin Biol* 1986;**10**:7–12.

8 Welch GW, Pomare EW. Functional gastrointestinal symptoms in a Wellington community sample. *N Z Med J* 1990;**103**:418–20.

9 Kay L, Jørgensen T, Jensen KH. The epidemiology of irritable bowel syndrome in a random population: prevalence, incidence, natural history and risk factors. *J Intern Med* 1994;**236**:23–30.

10 Wen B-Z, Pan Q-Y. Functional bowel disorders in apparently healthy Chinese people. *Chin J Epidemiol* 1988;**9**:345–9.

11 Drossman DA, Li Z, Andruzzi E *et al.* US householder survey of functional gastrointestinal disorders: prevalence, sociodemography and health impact. *Dig Dis Sci* 1993;**38**:1569–80.

12 Heaton KW, O'Donnell LJD, Bradden FEM, Mountford RA, Hughes AO, Cripps PJ. Symptoms of irritable bowel syndrome in a British urban community: consulters and nonconsulters. *Gastroenterology* 1992;**102**:1962–7.

13 Argreus L, Svardsudd K, Nyren O, Tibblin G. The epidemiology of abdominal symptoms: prevalence and demographic characteristics in a Swedish adult population: a report from the Abdominal Symptom Study. *Scand J Gastroenterol* 1994;**29**:102–9.

14 Talley NJ, Weaver AL, Zinsmeister AR, Melton LJ III. Onset and disappearance of gastrointestinal symptoms and functional gastrointestinal disorders. *Am J Epidemiol* 1992;**136**:165–77.

15 Jonsson B, Gardsell P, Johnell O, Redlund-Johnell I, Sernbo I. Remembering fractures: fracture registration and proband recall. *J Epidemiol Community Health* 1995;**48**:489–90.

16 Switz DM. What the gastroenterologist does all day: a survey of a state society's practice. *Gastroenterology* 1976;**70**:1048–50.

17 Kang JY, Yap I, Gwee KA. The pattern of functional and organic disorders in an Asian gastroenterological clinic. *J Gastroenterol Hepatol* 1994;**9**:124–7.

18 Thompson WG. Gastrointestinal symptoms in the irritable bowel compared with peptic ulcer and inflammatory bowel disease. *Gut* 1984;**25**:1089–92.

19 Harvey RF, Salih SY, Read AE. Organic and functional disorders in 2000 gastroenterology outpatients. *Lancet* 1983;**1**:632–4.

20 Mendis BLJ, Wijesiriwardena BC, Sheriff MHR, Dharmadasa K. Irritable bowel syndrome. *Ceylon Med J* 1982;**27**:171–81.

21 Mathur AK, Tandon BN, Prakash OM. Irritable colon syndrome. *J Indian Med Assoc* 1966;**46**:651–5.

22 Drossman DA, McKee DC, Sandler RS *et al*. Psychosocial factors in the irritable bowel syndrome: a multivariate study of patients and nonpatients with irritable bowel syndrome. *Gastroenterology* 1988;**95**:701–8.

23 Whitehead WE, Bosmajian L, Zonderman AB, Costa PT Jr, Schuster MM. Symptoms of psychologic distress associated with irritable bowel syndrome: comparison of community and medical clinic samples. *Gastroenterology* 1988;**95**:709–14.

24 Chaudhary NA, Truelove SC. The irritable colon syndrome. *Q J Med* 1962;**31**:307–22.

25 Waller SL, Misiewicz JJ. Prognosis in the irritable-bowel syndrome. *Lancet* 1969;**2**:753–6.

26 Holmes KM, Salter RH. Irritable bowel syndrome: a safe diagnosis. *BMJ* 1982;**285**:1533–4.

27 Svendsen JH, Munck LK, Andersen JR. Irritable bowel syndrome — prognosis and diagnostic safety: a 5-year follow-up study. *Scand J Gastroenterol* 1985;**20**:415–18.

28 Harvey RF, Mauad EC, Brown AM. Prognosis in the irritable bowel syndrome: a five-year prospective study. *Lancet* 1987;**1**:963–5.

29 Almy TP. The irritable bowel syndrome: back to square one? *Dig Dis Sci* 1980;**25**:401–3.

30 Burkitt DP, Walker ARP, Painter NS. Effect of dietary fibre on stools and transit times, and its role in the causation of disease. *Lancet* 1972;**2**:1408–12.

31 Müller-Lissner SA. Effect of wheat bran on weight of stool and gastrointestinal transit time: a meta analysis. *BMJ* 1988;**296**:615–17.

32 Taylor R. Management of constipation, I: high fibre diets work. *BMJ* 1900;**300**:1063–4.

33 Heaton KW. Role of dietary fibre in irritable bowel syndrome. In: Read NW, ed. *Irritable Bowel Syndrome*. London: Grune & Stratton Ltd, 1985:203–22.

34 Tucker DM, Sandstead HH, Logan GM Jr *et al*. Dietary fiber and personality factors as determinants of stool output. *Gastroenterology* 1981;**81**:879–83.

35 Lambert JP, Brunt PW, Mowat NAG *et al*. The value of prescribed 'high-fibre' diets for the treatment of the irritable bowel syndrome. *Eur J Clin Nutr* 1991;**45**:601–9.

36 Pearson DJ. Pseudo food allergy. *BMJ* 1986;**292**:221–2.

37 Thompson WG. *Gut Reactions*. New York: Plenum Medical Book Co, 1989.

38 White WH. A study of 60 cases of membranous colitis. *Lancet* 1905;**2**:1229–35.

39 Collins SM. Is the irritable gut an inflamed gut? *Scand J Gastroenterol* 1992;**192**(Suppl.):102–5.

40 Weston AP, Biddle, WL, Bhatia PS, Miner PB Jr. Terminal ileal mucosal mast cells in irritable bowel syndrome. *Dig Dis Sci* 1993;**38**:1590–5.

41 McIntosh D, Thompson WG, Patel D, Barr JR, Guindi M. Is rectal biopsy necessary in irritable bowel syndrome? *Am J Gastroenterol* 1992;**87**:1407–9.

42 Cumming W. Electro-galvanism in a peculiar affection of the mucous membrane of the bowels. *Lond Med Gazette* 1849;**NS9**:969–73.

43 Connell AM. The motility of the pelvic colon, II: paradoxical motility in diarrhoea and constipation. *Gut* 1962;**3**:342–8.

44 Kellow JE, Phillips SF. Altered small bowel motility in irritable bowel syndrome is correlated with symptoms. *Gastroenterology* 1987;**92**:1885–93.

45 Kellow JE, Phillips SF, Miller LJ, Zinsmeister AR. Dysmotility of the small intestine in irritable bowel syndrome. *Gut* 1988;**29**:1236–43.

46 Kumar D, Wingate DL. The irritable bowel syndrome: a paroxysmal motor disorder. *Lancet* 1985;**2**:973–7.

47 Sullivan MA, Cohen S, Snape WJ Jr. Colonic myoelectrical activity in irritable-bowel syndrome: effect of eating and anticholinergics. *N Engl J Med* 1978;**298**:878–83.

48 Bueno L, Fioramonti J, Ruckebusch Y, Frexinos J, Coulom P. Evaluation of colonic myoelectrical activity in health and functional disorders. *Gut* 1980;**21**:480–5.

49 Swarbrick ET, Hegarty JE, Bat L, Williams CB, Dawson AM. Site of pain from the irritable bowel. *Lancet* 1980;**2**:443–6.

50 Moriarty KJ, Dawson AM. Functional abdominal pain: further evidence that whole gut is affected *BMJ* 1982;**284**:1670–2.

51 Ford MJ. The irritable bowel syndrome. *J Psychosom Res* 1986;**30**:399–410.

52 Wright SH, Snape WJ Jr, Battle W, Cohen S, London RL. Effect of dietary components on gastrocolonic response. *Am J Physiol* 1980;**238**:G228–32.

53 Whitehead WE, Holtkotter B, Enck P *et al.* Tolerance for rectosigmoid distention in irritable bowel syndrome. *Gastroenterology* 1990;**98**:1187–92.

54 Ritchie J. Pain from distension of the pelvic colon by inflating a balloon in the irritable bowel syndrome. *Gut* 1973;**14**:125–32.

55 Cook IJ, van Eeden A, Collins SM. Patients with irritable bowel syndrome have greater pain tolerance than normal subjects. *Gastroenterology* 1987;**93**:727–33.

56 Drossman DA, Thompson WG. The irritable bowel syndrome: review and a graduated multicomponent treatment approach. *Ann Intern Med* 1992;**116**:1009–16.

57 Buccini R, Drossman DA. Chronic idiopathic abdominal pain. *Curr Concepts Gastroenterol* 1988;**12**:3–11.

58 Peters JL, Large RG. A randomised control trial evaluating in- and outpatient pain management programmes. *Pain* 1990;**41**:283–93.

59 Melzack R, Wall P. Gate-control and other mechanisms. In: Melzack R, Wall P, eds. *The Challenge of Pain*, 2nd edn. London: Pelican Books, 1988:165–93.

60 O'Donnell LJD, Virjee J, Heaton KW. Detection of pseudodiarrhoea by simple clinical assessment of intestinal transit rate. *BMJ* 1990;**300**:439–40.

61 Heaton KW, O'Donnell LJD. An office guide to whole gut transit time: patients' recollection of their stool form. *J Clin Gastroenterol* 1994;**19**:28–30.

62 Lasser RB, Bond JH, Levitt MD. The role of intestinal gas in functional abdominal pain. *N Engl J Med* 1975;**293**:524–6.

63 Hislop IG. Psychological significance of the irritable colon syndrome. *Gut* 1971;**12**:452–7.

64 Clouse RE. Anxiety and gastrointestinal illness. *Psychiatr Clin North Am* 1988;**11**:399–417.

65 Clouse RE, Lustman PJ, Geisman RA, Alpers DH. Antidepressant therapy in 138 patients with irritable bowel syndrome: a five-year clinical experience. *Aliment Pharmacol Ther* 1994;**8**:409–16.

66 Walker EA, Roy-Byrne PP, Katon WJ. Irritable bowel syndrome and psychiatric illness. *Am J Psychiatry* 1990;**147**:567–72.

67 Guthrie EA, Creed FH, Whorwell PJ, Tomenson B. Outpatients with irritable bowel syndrome: a comparison of first time and chronic attenders. *Gut* 1992;**33**:361–3.

68 Clouse RE. Antidepressants for functional gastrointestinal syndromes. *Dig Dis Sci* 1994;**39**:2352–63.

69 Creed F, Craig T, Farmer R. Functional abdominal pain, psychiatric illness, and life events. *Gut* 1988;**29**:235–42.

70 Kettell J, Jones R, Lydeard S. Reasons for consultation in irritable bowel syndrome: symptoms and patient characteristics. *Br J Gen Pract* 1992;**42**:459–61.

71 Whorwell PJ, McCallum M, Creed FH, Roberts CT. Non-colonic features of irritable bowel syndrome. *Gut* 1986;**27**:37–40.

72 Maxton DG, Morris JA, Whorwell PJ. Ranking of symptoms by patients with the irritable bowel syndrome. *BMJ* 1989;**299**:1138.

73 Drossman DA, Leserman J, Nachman G *et al.* Sexual and physical abuse in women with functional or organic gastrointestinal disorders. *Ann Intern Med* 1990;**113**:828–33.

74 Almy TP. Experimental studies on the irritable colon. *Am J Med* 1951;**10**:60–7.

75 Whitehead WE, Winget C, Fedoravicius AS, Wooley S, Blackwell B. Learned illness behavior in patients with irritable bowel syndrome and peptic ulcer. *Dig Dis Sci* 1982;**27**:202–8.

76 Wangel AG, Deller DJ. Intestinal motility in man, III: mechanisms of constipation and diarrhea with particular reference to the irritable colon syndrome. *Gastroenterology* 1965;**48**:69–84.

77 Harvey RF, Read AE. Effect of cholecystokinin on colon motility and symptoms in patients with the irritable bowel syndrome. *Lancet* 1973;**1**:1–3.

78 Bradette M, Delvaux M, Staumont G, Fioramonti J, Bueno L, Flexinos J. Evaluation of colonic sensory thresholds in IBS patients using a barostat: definition of optimal conditions and comparison with healthy subjects. *Dig Dis Sci* 1994;**39**:449–57.

79 Valori RM, Kumar D, Wingate DL. Effects of different types of stress and of 'prokinetic' drugs on the control of the fasting motor complex in humans. *Gastroenterology* 1986;**90**:1890–900.

80 Kang JY, Gwee KA, Yap I. The colonic air insufflation test indicates a colonic cause of abdominal pain: an aid in the management of irritable bowel syndrome. *J Clin Gastroenterol* 1994;**18**:19–22.

81 Svedlund J, Sjödin I, Ottosson J-O, Dotevall G. Controlled study of psychotherapy in irritable bowel syndrome. *Lancet* 1983;**2**:589–92.

82 Guthrie E, Creed F, Dawson D, Tomenson B. A controlled trial of psychological treatment for the irritable bowel syndrome. *Gastroenterology* 1991;**100**:450–7.

83 Klein KB. Controlled treatment trials in the irritable bowel syndrome: a critique. *Gastroenterology* 1988;**95**:232–41.

84 Manning AP, Thompson WG, Heaton KW, Morris AF. Towards positive diagnosis of the irritable bowel. *BMJ* 1978;**2**:653–4.

85 Kruis W, Thieme CH, Weinzierl M, Schussler P, Holl J, Paulus W. A diagnostic score for the irritable bowel syndrome: its value in the exclusion of organic disease. *Gastroenterology* 1984;**87**:1–7.

86 Talley NJ, Nyren O, Drossman DA *et al.* The irritable bowel syndrome: toward optimal design of controlled treatment trials. *Gastroenterol Int* 1994;**6**:189–211.

87 Poynard T, Naveau S, Mory B, Chaput JC. Meta-analysis of smooth muscle relaxants in the treatment of irritable bowel syndrome. *Aliment Pharmacol Ther* 1994;**8**:499–510.

88 Read M, Read NW. Anal sphincter function in diarrhoea: influence of loperamide. *Clin Res Rev* 1981;**1**:219–24.

89 Lancaster-Smith MJ, Prout BJ, Pinto T, Anderson JA, Schiff AA. Influence of drug treatment on the irritable bowel syndrome and its interaction with psychoneurotic morbidity. *Acta Psychiatr Scand* 1982;**66**:33–41.

90 Tura B, Tura SM. The analgesic effect of tricyclic antidepressants. *Brain Res* 1990;**518**:19–22.

91 Brody H. The lie that heals: the ethics of giving placebos. *Ann Intern Med* 1982;**97**:112–18.

92 Heaton KW. Effect of diet on intestinal function and dysfunction. In: Snape WJ Jr, ed. *Pathogenesis of Functional Bowel Disease*. New York: Plenum Medical Book Co, 1989:79–99.

93 Snook J, Shepherd HA. Bran supplementation in the treatment of irritable bowel syndrome. *Aliment Pharmacol Ther* 1994;**8**:511–14.

94 Francis CY, Whorwell PJ. Bran and irritable bowel syndrome: time for reappraisal. *Lancet* 1994;**344**:39–40.

95 Thompson WG. Doubts about bran. *Lancet* 1994;**344**:3.

96 Smart HL, Mayberry JF, Atkinson M. Alternative medicine consultations and remedies in patients with the irritable bowel syndrome. *Gut* 1986;**27**:826–8.

97 Verhoef MJ, Sutherland LR, Brkich L. Use of alternative medicine by patients attending a gastroenterology clinic. *Can Med Assoc J* 1990;**142**:121–5.

98 Schwarz SP, Blanchard EB, Neff DF. Behavioral treatment of irritable bowel syndrome: a 1-year follow-up study. *Biofeedback Self Regul* 1986;**11**:189–98.

99 Whorwell PJ, Prior A, Colgan SM. Hypnotherapy in severe irritable bowel syndrome: further experience. *Gut* 1987;**28**:423–5.

Chronic Constipation: Pathogenesis, Diagnosis, Treatment

Lawrence R. Schiller

Introduction and definitions

Constipation is a symptom, not a disease, and may be caused by many different conditions. Patients may describe as constipation any of three aspects of dysfunctional defecation: infrequency, dyschezia, or excessive stool hardness. The extent to which these three symptoms coexist in an individual patient is variable. Some patients may complain of constipation even when stool is evacuated daily, while others describe infrequent, but easily passed stools as constipation. This variability can confound the results of research studies when standardized definitions are not used.

Of the symptoms of constipation, only stool frequency has been quantified in a large number of individuals. Normal stool frequency varies from twice daily to three times weekly; thus, infrequency is defined as the passage of fewer than three stools per week. Dyschezia, or excessive straining during evacuation, is a subjective symptom. Since some straining is necessary to initiate evacuation, the threshold for excessive straining is blurry and self-defined. Lestar *et al.* [1] have suggested that measurement of the work needed to initiate defecation correlates with straining, but this type of measurement has not been widely performed. The degree of stool deformability during straining may be a measure of stood hardness, but this has not been studied systematically in patients complaining of constipation.

Physiology of normal bowel function

Approximately 1000 ml of ileal effluent enters the colon daily. Over the course of 24 hours, 90% of the water and salt is absorbed by the mucosa as the fluid traverses the colon. Carbohydrates delivered to the colon are fermented by bacteria into short-chain fatty acids, which are partly absorbed. Dietary fiber, bacteria, and other nonfermented solids accumulate as fluid is absorbed, forming the matrix for solid stool. The hydration of stool delivered to the rectum depends on the interaction of two factors: the ability of the mucosa to absorb water from luminal contents (absorption rate multiplied by time) and the physicochemical retention of water by stool solids due to adsorption and osmotic forces. Stools do not begin to solidify until they reach the sigmoid colon. Remarkably, stool consistency and water content show little variation in healthy individuals, despite substantial differences in diet, stool frequency, and daily stool weight.

The movement of material through the colon has been studied with the use of radio-opaque and radioactive markers. Flow through the colon tends to be sluggish compared with flow through the small intestine. Movements of the right colon contribute primarily to the mixing of luminal contents and tend to be slow and nonpropulsive. Scintigraphy has shown that material stays in the right colon for up to 8 hours before moving distally. Movements of the left colon are more phasic and are involved in the propulsion of luminal contents distally. Episodic 'mass movements' rapidly propel stool to the rectosigmoid area. The luminal contents remain in the descending colon for a relatively short time, but tend to be retained in the sigmoid colon.

Contractions in the sigmoid colon increase after meals and propel stool into the rectum, distending it. Rectal distention results in relaxation of the internal anal sphincter via intramural descending neurons. This relaxation allows the stool to come into contact with the sensitive lining of the upper anal canal. The combined sensations of rectal distention and contact are perceived as the need to defecate. After infancy, rectal distention also leads to contraction of the external anal sphincter and increased contraction of the puborectalis muscle (by a learned response), which prevents immediate defecation and allows time for the rectum to relax, reducing intrarectal pressure. This reduces the likelihood of precipitate defecation, permitting an individual to choose a place to evacuate or to defer defecation until later (Figure 10.1) [2].

When a person is ready to defecate, he or she sits or squats, moving the anal sphincter anteriorly, thus causing some straightening of the rectoanal angle. Tonic contraction of the external anal sphincter and puborectalis muscles is inhibited and a Valsalva maneuver is performed, increasing intra-abdominal pressure and pushing the stool into the anal canal. This process triggers reflex defecation organized in the spinal cord, resulting in contraction of the rectum and inhibition of tonic contraction of the internal anal sphincter. Stool is propelled through the anus by the large pressure differential. The puborectalis and internal and external sphincter muscles

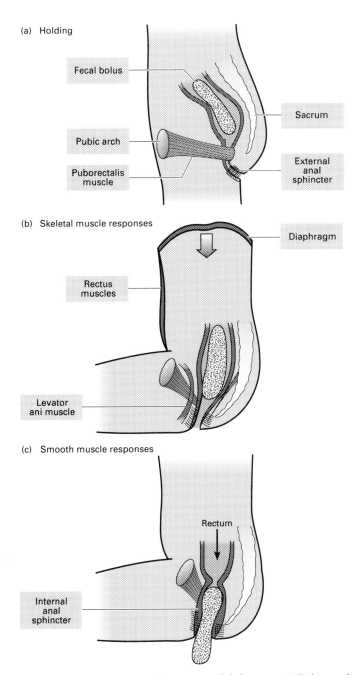

(a) Holding

Fecal bolus

Sacrum

Pubic arch

Puborectalis muscle

External anal sphincter

(b) Skeletal muscle responses

Diaphragm

Rectus muscles

Levator ani muscle

(c) Smooth muscle responses

Rectum

Internal anal sphincter

Fig. 10.1 Schematic representation of the process of defecation. (a) Puborectalis and external anal sphincter contract. (b) Puborectalis and external anal sphincter relax; levator ani and rectus muscles and diaphragm contract. (c) Internal anal sphincter relaxes; there is a rectal contraction. (From Schiller [2], with permission.)

then resume their normal resting tone. This complex mechanism ordinarily enables easy evacuation and maintenance of continence at other times.

Pathophysiology of constipation

Secondary constipation

The complexity of the mechanism of normal bowel function sets the stage for the many malfunctions that can cause the symptom of constipation. Problems that affect the functions of smooth or striated muscle, that disable the autonomic or somatic nerves, or that alter the colorectal anatomy or luminal contents may all produce constipation.

Prominent among the disorders producing secondary constipation are systemic endocrine and metabolic diseases, including diabetes mellitus, hypercalcemia, hypokalemia, porphyria, hypothyroidism, panhypopituitarism, hyperparathyroidism, pseudohypoparathyroidism, pheochromocytoma, and glucagonoma. Diabetes and porphyria are believed to produce constipation by altering nerve function. For example, a recent study [3] showed that the substance P content in rectal mucosa was reduced in diabetic patients with constipation compared to those without, suggesting that the lack of this excitatory neurotransmitter was related to constipation. The other metabolic and endocrine conditions mentioned above are believed to produce secondary constipation primarily by influencing smooth-muscle function.

Neurologic diseases are also associated with constipation. An epidemiologic survey [4] of hospitalized Medicare patients in the USA has suggested that central nervous system (CNS) disorders account for most of that association and that disruption of neural regulation is responsible for constipation. CNS lesions that have been linked with constipation include spinal cord injury, cauda equina tumor, lumbar disc disease, tabes dorsalis, multiple sclerosis, Parkinson's disease, stroke, and brain tumor. Paraplegia is associated with slow transit, particularly in the left colon [5]. Parkinson's disease may produce outlet obstruction by promoting paradoxical contraction of the external anal sphincter [6]. A large survey [7] found constipation in 43% of patients with multiple sclerosis. Studies [8, 9] in smaller groups of patients have shown that multiple sclerosis is associated with dysfunction of the external anal sphincter and pelvic floor, which may cause constipation. Peripheral nervous system conditions, such as autonomic neuropathy, neurofibromatosis, and ganglioneuromatosis, have also been associated with constipation.

Disorders of the enteric nervous system (ENS) can also cause constipation. The best described is Hirschsprung's disease, in which the normal development of the ENS is interrupted and a variable length of distal colon has no ganglion cells. The lack of these cells in the myenteric plexus prevents normal peristalsis and the reflex relaxation of the internal anal sphincter in response to rectal distention. The aganglionic distal segment creates an obstruction and is responsible for the proximal dilatation of the colon that is characteristic of this disorder. Neurogenic chronic intestinal pseudo-obstruction and chronic laxative abuse are also thought to cause constipation by damaging the ENS.

A number of organic disorders affecting the structures of the anus, rectum, and colon can cause constipation, including stenotic or obstructing lesions (such as tumors), diverticular disease, inflammatory bowel disease, ischemia, volvulus, endometriosis, and postoperative strictures. Painful lesions, such as anal fissures, thrombosed hemorrhoids, mucosal prolapse, and ulcerative proctitis, can also induce constipation. Smooth-muscle diseases, such as smooth-muscle myopathy, myotonic dystrophy, and progressive systemic sclerosis, produce constipation by altering colonic transit or the function of the rectum and internal anal sphincter [10–12].

Iatrogenic constipation is receiving increasing recognition. Constipation is associated with a number of drugs from different therapeutic categories, including drugs interacting with neurons in the CNS or ENS (e.g. opiates), drugs with direct effects on smooth muscle (e.g. calcium channel antagonists), and those altering luminal contents (e.g. cholestyramine) (Table 10.1) [13, 14]. Surgery can also result in or worsen constipation. For example, rectopexy for rectal prolapse has been associated with constipation in some patients [15, 16].

Dietary factors may also be responsible for constipation. Habitual ingestion of a low-residue diet may result in infrequent stools and the complaint of constipation. The prevalence of this problem varies from country to country, depending on the amount of fiber in the typical diet. In the USA, insufficient fiber intake may no longer be as common as it once was because of increased popular awareness of the health advantages of fiber consumption.

Idiopathic constipation

If none of the preceding problems is present, constipation is considered to be idiopathic. Physiologic studies have categorized patients with idio-

Table 10.1 Drugs associated with constipation.

Analgesics
    Nonsteroidal anti-inflammatory agents
    Opiates and related narcotics

Anticholinergic drugs
    Atropine and related antispasmodics
    Antidepressants
    Neuroleptic drugs (antipsychotic agents, antiemetics)
    Agents used to treat Parkinson's disease

Anticonvulsants

Antihistamines

Antihypertensive drugs
    Calcium channel antagonists
    Clonidine
    Hydralazine
    Monoamine oxidase (MAO) inhibitors
    Methyldopa

Chemotherapeutic agents
    Vinca derivatives

Diuretics

Metal ions and minerals
    Aluminum (antacids, sucralfate)
    Barium sulfate
    Calcium (antacids, dietary supplements)
    Iron supplements
    Heavy metals (arsenic, lead, mercury)

Resins
    Cholestyramine
    Sodium polystyrene sulfonate (Kayexalate)

pathic constipation into three groups based on pathophysiology: (i) patients with slow transit ('colonic inertia'); (ii) patients with functional outlet obstruction of various types; and (iii) patients with a combination of slow transit and functional outlet obstruction.

Colonic inertia

Slow transit through the colon is the most common finding in large series of patients with idiopathic constipation. Manometric studies [17–22] have shown convincingly that reduced motility is the cause of slow transit in these patients. Furthermore, these patients do not demonstrate the normal increase in colonic motility induced by feeding [22–24], or by cholinergic stimulation with edrophonium [25]. The colonic abnormality may be part of a more widespread autonomic process: some patients also demonstrate prolonged gastric and small-bowel transit [26, 27], as well as abnormal results on cholinergic cutaneous and cardiac tests [28, 29].

The structural basis of this autonomic neuropathy has been explored using sophisticated microscopic techniques. Abnormalities in the myenteric plexus [30,31] and changes in enteric neurotransmitters [32–36] have been described, but no coherent picture or etiology has emerged. Indeed, it is not known whether these changes are primary or secondary to constipation or its treatment.

Because most patients with colonic inertia are women, investigators have studied the potential influence of sex hormones on colon function. Half of the women in one study [37] reported some improvement in symptoms just before or during menstruation; in another study [38], circulating concentrations of all steroid hormones were lower in constipated women than in healthy women. The implications of these findings are not clear.

Functional outlet obstruction

A key insight gained from the array of physiologic techniques developed in the 1980s was that many patients complaining of constipation had abnormal expulsion of stool from the rectum [39–43]. Investigators [39, 40, 44–46] soon related this phenomenon to failure to inhibit the activity of the external anal sphincter and pelvic floor when attempting to defecate, although some authors [47, 48] did not find this correlation. This condition has been called *anismus* or *spastic pelvic floor syndrome*.

It has become clear that a variety of abnormalities that can be classified under the rubric of 'functional outlet obstruction constipation' can cause obstructed defecation (Table 10.2), including striated muscle dysfunction, problems with the dynamics of the smooth muscle of the rectum [49, 50], impaired rectal sensation [51–55], internal anal sphincter dysfunction [56], and even transient anatomic obstruction due to mucosal or rectal prolapse or intussusception.

With so many potential contributing factors to functional outlet obstruction, it is difficult to determine which problems cause constipation and which ones result from constipation. For example, some patients with chronic constipation show evidence of central neurogenic problems [51, 52] or pudendal neuropathy [45, 57, 58]. Do these problems result from

Table 10.2 Causes of functional outlet obstruction.

Abnormal nervous function
CNS dysfunction
   Spinal cord or cauda equina lesions
   Multiple sclerosis
   Parkinson's disease
   Stroke
   Brain tumor
Peripheral nervous system dysfunction
   Autonomic neuropathy (diabetes)
   Neurofibromatosis and ganglioneuromatosis
   Hirschsprung's disease and variants

Smooth-muscle dysfunction
Megarectum

Failure to open outlet
Anismus (striated-muscle dysfunction)
   Inappropriate puborectalis and anal sphincter contraction
   Spastic puborectalis muscle
Internal anal sphincter (smooth-muscle) dysfunction
   Hypertonic internal anal sphincter
   Incomplete internal anal sphincter relaxation

Transient anatomic obstruction
Rectal mucosal intussusception
Rectal prolapse
Solitary rectal ulcer syndrome
Enterocele

chronic straining [59], or do they reflect an independent process, perhaps related to the pathogenesis of the original process responsible for constipation [60]? There is a similar problem with rectocele and anismus: is the rectocele due to anismus, or does it contribute to excessive straining by making rectal emptying less efficient [61, 62]?

It is likely that the significant factors in the pathogenesis of functional outlet obstruction vary from patient to patient. It is also likely that no single defect will prove to be the underlying explanation for all, or even most, cases of functional outlet obstruction constipation. A detailed analysis of the physiologic studies [46, 63–68] that have examined multiple factors is needed to understand the basis for constipation in individual patients. In such an analysis [69] of patients with chronic constipation, many were found to have both colonic inertia and functional outlet obstruction. A provocative study [70] has suggested that normal men can voluntarily suppress defecation, resulting in changes in segmental colonic transit; the implication is that colonic inertia may be the consequence of functional outlet obstruction. Clinically, patients often present with a long history of infrequent defecation without dyschezia (suggesting colonic inertia), followed by the development of dyschezia. This pattern raises the question whether colonic inertia can result in functional outlet obstruction, perhaps by producing dysfunctional defecation habits.

Clinical observations and studies of voluntary suppression of defecation have also raised the question of a psychological basis for constipation, especially when the underlying disorder is a dysfunction of striated muscle. An epidemiologic study [71] of US military veterans showed that constipation was more common than expected in those with schizophrenia or major depression. However, it was not possible to separate the possible effects of medications used to treat the psychiatric illnesses on bowel function. Psychological testing of small groups of patients has shown [72–76] that constipation, especially with normal colonic transit, is associated with higher scores for hypochondriasis, depression, and global psychological distress, even when medical attention has been sought for constipation. A recent study [77] has suggested that women with the irritable bowel syndrome (IBS) often have a history of sexual abuse. It would not be surprising to find a similar finding in women with chronic constipation.

Evaluation of patients with constipation

Constipation is a common complaint, accounting for more than 2.5 million patient visits in the USA. An even greater number of individuals have this symptom but self-treat with over-the-counter (OTC) laxatives. The task of the physician is to identify the large number of patients who do not need an extensive evaluation and the small group of patients who require more intensive efforts. Several recent reviews [78–82] deal with various aspects of this task.

Symptom analysis

It is essential to understand exactly what the patient means by constipation. The physician should elicit information about the duration of symptoms, frequency of evacuation, stool characteristics (bulk, size, consistency, presence of blood), awareness of the need to defecate, ease of defecation, extent of straining, and the presence of pain with defecation. Associated symptoms, such as abdominal pain, bloating, distention, and gaseousness, should be recorded. The physician should also ask about any methods used by the patient to treat constipation, such as laxative and enema use, adaptations in posture when defecating, use of digital manipulation to encourage evacuation, and dietary changes. A list of all medications, both prescription and OTC, should be drawn up and reviewed. The physician should also explore evidence of previous or current symptoms compatible with endocrine, metabolic, neurologic, and local anorectal problems that may cause constipation. It is also useful to investigate any psychological factors that may have prompted the patient to seek medical attention. Psychological factors not only may influence the course of the disease (e.g. childhood encopresis, depression, anismus), but invariably color the patients' perceptions of their symptoms and their responsiveness to diagnostic and therapeutic recommendations.

Physicians should try to differentiate chronic constipation from constipation-predominant IBS. IBS is characterized by marked abdominal pain, usually relieved by defecation. Some variation in bowel symptoms is typical in IBS patients. In contrast, patients with chronic constipation tend to have less severe abdominal pain and less weekly variation in symptoms. In addition, although symptoms suggestive of functional outlet obstruction (e.g. dyschezia, incomplete evacuation) are sometimes included in the criteria for IBS, they are more typical of chronic constipation. Nevertheless, most patients with chronic constipation will have some symptoms suggestive of IBS [83].

Special attention should be paid to the history in individuals presenting with constipation in childhood, young adulthood, and old age. Patients in these age groups have unique problems that need to be considered when formulating a differential diagnosis (Table 10.3) [78, 84–86].

Physical examination

Patients should be examined for evidence of systemic conditions that can cause constipation. An unusual dermatoglyphic (fingerprint) pattern, consisting of an increased frequency of digital arches, is present in some patients with early-onset constipation [87]. The abdomen should be examined carefully for distention, tympany, tenderness, and evidence of fecal loading.

Assessment of the perineum, anus, and rectum should include inspection and a thoughtful digital examination. The examiner should

Table 10.3 Age-related special considerations.

Childhood	Congenital anomalies
	Hirschsprung's disease and variants
	Childhood encopresis
Young adulthood	Eating disorder
	Laxative abuse
	Anismus
Old age	Pelvic floor dysfunction
	Chronic laxative abuse
	Poor diet
	Neurogenic constipation
	Hypothyroidism
	Side effects associated with drugs

look for evidence of soft-tissue deformities, external hemorrhoids, and perianal dermatitis, which may indicate concomitant fecal incontinence. The perianal skin should be stroked gently with a pin to elicit the cutaneoanal reflex ('anal wink'). This reflex can be lost if the afferent or efferent nerves or the sacral spinal cord is damaged. The bulk and tone of the anal sphincter should be assessed by digital examination. To evaluate contraction of the external anal sphincter and puborectalis muscles, the patient should be asked to squeeze as if to prevent defecation. The examiner should palpate all quadrants of the anal canal, looking for tenderness, fluctuation, and tumor. The patient should then be requested to simulate defecation by bearing down. The examiner should assess the puborectalis muscle and anal sphincter for paradoxical contractions suggestive of functional outlet obstruction and should watch for descent of the pelvic floor. The amount and consistency of stool within the rectum should be noted. Finally, a careful neurologic examination, with attention to the lower extremities, should be conducted.

Diagnostic testing

A complete history and physical examination, as outlined above, are indicated in all patients complaining of constipation, but further tests should be performed selectively. Some patients, particularly young individuals with a long history of relatively minor problems and a normal physical examination, may require no further studies; an empiric trial of fiber supplementation may be sufficient. However, young people with complicated or disabling symptoms and older patients with a short history or abnormal physical findings require further studies to arrive at a definitive diagnosis of the primary disease in cases of secondary constipation. In addition, studies can reveal the physiologic basis of symptoms in patients with idiopathic constipation so that treatment can proceed on a rational basis.

Clinical laboratory tests

Laboratory tests can detect a primary process causing constipation, such as hypercalcemia, hypokalemia, diabetes, or hypothyroidism. These tests should be ordered only when indicated by the history and physical examination.

Anoscopy and sigmoidoscopy

Inspection of the anal canal and rectum should be considered in patients with rectal bleeding or obstructive symptoms and in patients over 40 years of age to exclude the possibility of a tumor or other lesions. The presence of erythema or ulceration, particularly on the anterior rectal wall, may indicate mucosal prolapse. A biopsy of the mucosa in this area may show pathognomonic changes associated with this condition.

Routine radiographic studies

In patients complaining of abdominal distention or bloating, plain radiograms of the abdomen should be obtained to distinguish between fecal loading of the colon and gaseous distention. Radiographic evidence of fecal loading, especially in the left colon, can be correlated with abnormal colonic transit [88]. In patients with marked abdominal pain, radiograms can exclude the possibility of obstruction. A barium enema is more useful than colonoscopy for evaluation of the constipated patient, especially when pain is present. The barium enema can exclude the possibility of mechanical obstruction, define megacolon, and permit analysis of the pattern of haustral folds. Although a long or redundant colon is present in many constipated patients, there is no evidence that this is responsible for constipation or any of its symptoms. Redundancy is not an indication for resection unless volvulus is present.

Functional studies

When primary causes of constipation have been excluded and an empiric trial of dietary fiber supplementation has failed, the physician should consider the possibility of idiopathic constipation. At this point, patho-physiologic studies may provide pertinent information and help to identify a rational course of therapy. Such studies are mandatory when surgery is contemplated because clinical criteria are inexact for predicting pathophysiology, and the failure to identify functional outlet obstruction preoperatively may lead to an unsuccessful colectomy for colonic inertia. To ensure reproducible results, physiologic studies should be performed in facilities that evaluate an adequate number of such patients.

Colon transit studies

Tests quantifying transit through the colon are simple in concept, but need to be executed carefully. Ingestion of radio-opaque markers, either as a bolus or on a daily basis, is followed by interval radiography of the abdomen. Transit time can be calculated by a number of methods based on this technique; segmental transit time can also be determined [89]. The use of laxatives to prepare the bowel does not seem to change the overall retention of markers, but may alter their distribution in the colon [90]. Colonic transit is unaffected by the phase of the menstrual cycle, and transit time does not differ sufficiently between men and women to warrant a sex-based adjustment of normal limits [91]. Transit may be slowed in the presence of functional outlet obstruction; therefore, pro-longed transit time should not necessarily be equated with colonic inertia [92]. However, a normal transit time in a patient complaining of con-stipation indicates the presence of either outlet obstruction or factitious constipation.

Scintigraphic techniques have also been devised to measure global and segmental colon transit [93–95]. With these techniques, a radioisotope is delivered to the colon in particulate form after ingestion with a mixed meal. A gamma camera is used to image the radioactivity as the isotope passes through regions of interest defined by the operator. The results of scintigraphic techniques correlate well with results obtained with radio-opaque markers if a 'geometric center' method of analysis is used. The main advantage of scintigraphy over the use of radio-opaque markers is limited exposure to radiation.

Colon motility studies

Colonoscopy has been used to introduce manometric catheters as far as the right colon, making it possible to obtain motility tracings from the colon [17, 18, 24, 64, 65]. These studies have shown reductions in the amplitude and frequency of contractions in some patients with colonic inertia and an insensitivity to physiologic stimulation induced by feeding and pharmacologic stimulation with bisacodyl. While this information is valuable in research, at present it has relatively little value in the evaluation of patients with constipation.

Anorectal manometry

Anorectal manometry has proven to be useful for the evaluation of abnormalities in rectal sensation or compliance, anal sphincter hypertonicity, and abnormal relaxation of the anal sphincter. The results of standard and ambulatory manometry are reproducible and of help in the evaluation of patients with constipation [22, 96–98]. However, manometry is less helpful for the diagnosis of anismus and needs to be used in concert with other techniques [99]. Manometry can screen constipated patients for Hirschsprung's disease; loss of the rectoanal relaxation reflex in response to rectal distention has been used as the criterion for biopsy, which is required for a definitive diagnosis. In one study [100], manometry had a positive predictive value of 0.94 and a negative predictive value of 0.88 for detection of Hirschsprung's disease, suggesting that reliance solely on manometric findings could lead to misdiagnosis in a substantial number of patients.

Defecography and expulsion testing

Defecography (proctography), in which the rectum and anus are imaged while the patient strains and then expels barium inserted into the rectum, is valuable for the evaluation of patients with suspected functional outlet obstruction [101–104]. Defecography is the best technique available for visualizing pelvic floor and rectal wall motions during rectal emptying. It is helpful for the diagnosis of internal (mucosal) intussusception, solitary rectal ulcer syndrome, rectocele, and anismus.

  Defecography is not a flawless test, however. Some individuals with no history of trouble with defecation may have abnormal findings, and some patients with normal anatomy may have poor rectal emptying. The most difficult situation arises when defecation problems are present and the results of defecography are abnormal; the question then is whether the finding explains the symptom. The question can often be resolved by considering the patient's history or clinical findings. Defecography should be performed to exclude functional outlet obstruction when a subtotal colectomy is planned for the treatment of colonic inertia.

Isotope proctography, a scintigraphic test, is designed to quantify rectal emptying [105, 106] and can also be used to visualize the rectum and examine movements of the pelvic floor and rectoanal angle. This method does not detect rectal wall abnormalities, such as intussusception, and is therefore less useful than defecography.

Simpler techniques for measuring the ability to evacuate stool include placing a given volume of material (either liquid or paste) into the rectum, asking the patient to defecate into a container on a scale, and then plotting the mass defecated against time [107, 108]. Another technique is the balloon expulsion test, in which the patient is asked to defecate a balloon that had been placed in the rectum and then was filled with a given volume of liquid [109–111]. This test is subject to the willingness of the patient to cooperate and has been less useful in practice than initially anticipated.

Other tests

Electromyography (EMG) is useful for the evaluation of skeletal muscle activation and denervation. It can detect paradoxical, abnormal activity of the external anal sphincter and puborectalis muscles during defecation and thus is useful for the diagnosis of anismus [112, 113]. Technique is important. Because needle-electrode EMG may produce artifacts due to pain, the thin-wire technique or the anal plug method is preferable [114].

Balloon sphincterography, in which a cylindrical latex balloon is placed across the anal canal, filled with barium under pressure, and then fluoroscoped, was introduced as a simple test to measure anal sphincter pressure and the anorectal angle [115]. It has proven to be more difficult to interpret than defecography, although it yields reproducible measurements [116].

Which tests to order?

When evaluating a patient with difficult constipation, the key clinical question involves the relative contributions of colonic inertia and functional outlet obstruction to symptoms. In most settings, a radio-opaque marker study of colonic transit is readily available and can be used to identify patients with colonic inertia. The possibility of functional outlet obstruction can be explored with anorectal manometry and defecography. These studies are becoming more readily available as centers interested in gastrointestinal problems establish motility laboratories and radiologists become more adept at defecography. The other tests mentioned above may be useful in research settings, but add relatively little to the recommended studies.

Treatment

The goals of therapy for chronic constipation are to: (i) relieve symptoms; (ii) treat the underlying disorders when constipation is a secondary symptom; (iii) educate patients on the long term nature of idiopathic constipation and the lifestyle changes required for its successful management; and (iv) warn patients about the dangers of some OTC treatments and chronic straining.

It is essential to clarify exactly what the patient's symptoms are. The cardinal symptoms of constipation — infrequency of evacuation, difficulty in defecation, and passage of hard stools — do not respond uniformly to laxatives or other measures. Other symptoms such as abdominal bloating and distention may also fail to respond to these treatments and may need individualized management. Failure to appreciate these issues may lead to a loss of confidence in the doctor when the patient continues to suffer from 'constipation'.

Patients need to be educated about the expected course of constipation. For many patients, lifestyle changes, such as dietary modifications, will have to be lifetime commitments. Patients should be informed that their problem may not be curable in the sense of an acute illness and that it will need continuing attention. Patients also should know that effective therapy may produce incidental symptoms that are unpleasant.

Dietary modification

A recent retrospective review [117] of self-reported constipation and dietary history in the USA found that constipated subjects consumed fewer calories overall than nonconstipated individuals as well as smaller amounts of the following foods: cheese; beans and peas; milk, meat, and poultry; beverages; fruits and vegetables. These findings suggest that the physician could rationally prescribe greater intake of these foods for patients with constipation, but the efficacy of such an approach has not been evaluated in a controlled study.

Most experts recommend that patients with idiopathic constipation first increase their intake of dietary fiber to 20–30 g/day before any extensive evaluation is undertaken. Fiber intake may be increased by altering the composition of the diet or by adding medicinal fiber or fiber-like drugs, such as psyllium, methylcellulose, and polycarbophil, to the diet. Although increasing dietary fiber can increase stool frequency and bulk, it may lead to increased bloating due to fermentation of the fiber by colonic bacteria. Psyllium and the other medicinal fiber products may be less fermentable than dietary sources and thus less likely to produce excess gas. The dose of fiber may also be critical: the amount of gas produced is roughly proportional to the amount of the substrate consumed. Fiber supplementation may be unhelpful in patients with dyschezia or severe colonic inertia, in whom increased fiber intake may just produce more stool to evacuate. Such patients may require a low-residue diet for optimal symptom improvement.

Retraining and biofeedback

Defecation is automatic and uninhibited in infants. Toddlers undergo toilet training and learn by trial and error to inhibit defecation until a socially convenient time. This process involves learning to use the skeletal muscles of the pelvic floor and the anal sphincter. Once children learn to contract these muscles to preserve continence, they must also learn how to inhibit the contraction of these muscles to allow defecation to proceed when it is appropriate.

Many chronically constipated children fail to inhibit contraction of the skeletal muscles of the pelvic floor when attempting to defecate. This produces a form of functional outlet obstruction that is often complicated by fecal impaction and 'overflow' incontinence (encopresis). Retraining (habit training) has been advocated as a corrective measure [118]. It involves disimpaction followed by scheduled attempts to defecate after a meal (when the gastrocolic reflex is active) and the use of enemas or suppositories as salvage therapy for failure to evacuate. This approach has been found to improve encopresis in a substantial proportion of children and to increase stool frequency. Biofeedback techniques have also been used [119–122]: the EMG activity of the external anal sphincter or the pelvic floor is demonstrated to the child, and he or she is asked to minimize this activity during defecation. The initial results of biofeedback are often satisfactory. In nonresponders, an inadequate rectoanal response to rectal distention may be responsible for the failure to relax the external anal sphincter [122].

Biofeedback training has been used in adults to treat anismus, which also involves paradoxical responses of the pelvic floor and external anal sphincter [123–125]. Biofeedback not only improves symptoms in up to 90% of patients, but also improves objective measures of defecation dynamics [124]. Although controlled prospective trials are lacking, the technique is innocuous enough to be tried in cooperative patients with anismus. In brief, surface or plug electrodes are used to pick up the EMG signal from the external anal sphincter. Patients are asked to minimize the EMG voltage while attempting to strain. Most programs include use of simulated stool for practicing defecation once inhibition of contraction of the external anal sphincter is learned.

Drug therapy with neuromuscular agents

Patients with colonic inertia might be expected to respond to drugs that alter enteric nerve or colonic smooth-muscle function. Results of studies with these agents have been variable, with some success reported with bethanechol, naloxone, cisapride, and misoprostol.

Bethanechol is of limited use because of generalized cholinergic effects (e.g. abdominal cramps, hypersalivation); its main indication is constipation due to the anticholinergic side effects of drugs that cannot be discontinued.

Naloxone, an opiate antagonist, has produced improvement in some constipated patients, suggesting that excessive endogenous opiate activity may be responsible for constipation in these individuals. Orally effective opiate antagonists are being investigated for this indication.

Cisapride, a prokinetic drug, has been assessed in several published trials [126–129] and seems to be more effective than placebo in relieving symptoms of constipation. In doses ranging from 5 mg three times daily to 20 mg twice daily, there were few reported side effects. Unfortunately, the participants in these studies were not stratified according to the pathophysiology of their constipation — potentially an important omission. In an acute study [130] using a scintigraphic transit technique, cisapride was most effective in patients with colonic inertia, while those with functional outlet obstruction showed much less improvement in transit. Larger, randomized studies of patients with colonic inertia are needed to demonstrate the effectiveness of cisapride in chronic constipation. At present, dosages of 10–20 mg three times daily can be tried as empiric therapy in patients with colonic inertia.

Misoprostol, a prostaglandin analog, was introduced clinically as a prophylactic agent for nonsteroidal anti-inflammatory drug-induced gastric ulcers. A side effect is diarrhea, attributed to prostaglandin-induced inhibition of intestinal absorption and stimulation of intestinal motility. Anecdotal experience suggests that misoprostol may have some efficacy in constipation. A double-blind, placebo-controlled trial [131] demonstrated short-term benefit in patients with severe constipation.

Laxatives

A variety of vegetable and chemical agents induce diarrhea when ingested; several have gained acceptance as therapeutic agents for patients with constipation (Table 10.4). In general, laxatives produce their effects by osmotically retaining water, inhibiting intestinal absorption of

Table 10.4 Therapeutic use of laxatives.

Category/agent	Typical adult dose
Laxatives that modify luminal contents	
Psyllium preparations	10–20 g*
Polycarbophil	4–6 g*
Methylcellulose	4 g*
Mineral oil	15–30 ml
Osmotic agents	
Magnesium hydroxide (8.1 g/100 ml)	15–60 ml
Sodium phosphate solution	
(66 g/100 ml)	20–40 ml orally
(22 g/100 ml)	120 ml rectally
Lactulose syrup (10 g/15 ml)	15–60 ml
Sorbitol syrup (10.5 g/15 ml)	15–60 ml
Polyethylene glycol–electrolyte solution	240–360 ml
Stimulant laxatives	
Castor oil	30–60 ml
Cascara fluid extract	5 ml
Senna (standardized concentrate)	15–60 mg
Phenolphthalein	30–200 mg
Bisacodyl	10–20 mg orally or rectally

* In divided doses.

water and electrolytes, stimulating intestinal motility, or altering the luminal contents.

Osmotic agents, such as magnesium, sulfate, and phosphate salts, are poorly absorbed and induce intraluminal retention of water, bringing additional fluid into the rectum and thus increasing the water content of stool and softening stools. Osmotic agents can be ingested orally or administered as an enema or suppository. Absorption of these ions limits their effectiveness as laxatives; prolonged use can lead to reduced efficacy. Absorption can also lead to hypermagnesemia, hyperphosphatemia, and hypocalcemia. Congestive heart failure may result as a result of sodium overload, especially if large doses are used or if renal function is impaired. The efficacy of fermentable osmotic agents, such as lactulose and sorbitol, may decrease over time as these agents are fermented into short-chain organic acids and absorption of these acids reduces the amount of osmotically active substances remaining in the lumen. These agents are also likely to produce bloating and gaseousness because fermentation produces carbon dioxide and hydrogen as by-products. These side effects may limit the acceptance of these agents by patients who are already suffering from these symptoms.

A new approach to osmotic laxation is the use of poorly absorbed, nonfermentable polyethylene glycol–electrolyte solutions. These solutions were initially designed to prepare the colon for colonoscopy. Rapid ingestion results in the delivery of a large volume of fluid to the rectum. Ingestion of a smaller volume on a daily basis may produce effective laxation in patients with chronic constipation [132]. The original solutions relied largely on the osmotic activity of sodium sulfate. However, when these solutions are ingested slowly, sufficient sulfate can be absorbed to limit the laxative effect. Use of improved lavage solutions, containing higher concentrations of polyethylene glycol and no sodium sulfate, may be more effective for treatment of constipation [133].

Since osmotic laxatives are nonsystemic and safe when used appropriately, they are often the agents of choice when long-term therapy is required. The effect of osmotic laxatives generally increases linearly with the dose. Thus, the dose can be reduced if stools become too loose and increased if the laxative effect is insufficient. Recommended starting doses for adults are shown in Table 10.4.

Many laxatives produce their effects by inhibiting water and electrolyte absorption or by stimulating secretion through interaction with epithelial, nerve, or smooth-muscle cells. Most of these agents also alter motility and are known as stimulant laxatives. This category includes:

surfactant agents, such as docusate; diphenylmethane derivatives, such as phenolphthalein and bisacodyl; ricinoleic acid (castor oil); and anthraquinones, such as senna and cascara. Details of the mechanisms of action of these agents in humans are still sparse. Interactions with enterocyte transport proteins, stimulation of cyclic adenosine monophosphate (cAMP), and induction of prostaglandin release have been postulated as mechanisms for their laxative effects. Direct or indirect effects on enteric nerves may also be responsible for the effects of some of these agents.

Some stimulant laxatives, such as castor oil, produce such strong effects that they are inappropriate for chronic use. Others, such as anthraquinone derivatives, may produce toxic effects on enteric nerves, perhaps producing a neurogenic pseudo-obstruction with chronic use, although the evidence is divided at present [134]. Potent stimulant laxatives should be avoided, whenever possible, because of their potential for long-term toxicity.

Another family of laxatives is composed of agents that modify luminal contents, including bulking or hydrophilic agents, such as psyllium, methylcellulose, and calcium polycarbophil, and the lubricating agent mineral oil. Bulking agents are large organic polymers that are not absorbed and not subject to digestion in the small intestine. These laxatives interact with water and cause retention of water in a gel phase. This action tends to increase the bulk of luminal contents, possibly stimulating peristalsis, and also tends to soften hard stools with which the gel becomes admixed. Mineral oil works through a different mechanism. It is poorly absorbed and tends to coat fecal pellets or to become emulsified with stool, inhibiting stool formation.

Bulking agents can sometimes exacerbate bloating. If fiber supplementation does not improve constipation, it should be discontinued. In patients with severe colonic inertia or outlet obstruction, bulking agents may fail to encourage defecation and may only create more stool to be evacuated. Mineral oil can usually be used safely, but it can cause severe pulmonary problems if aspirated, can reduce fat-soluble vitamin absorption, and can lead to anal leakage.

Laxatives are necessary in most chronically constipated patients if no specific therapy is available or effective. For chronic use, the least potent, best-tolerated agents should be used. Examples include: stool-modifying agents, such as fiber and mineral oil; drugs with minor effects on intestinal absorption, such as stool softeners like docusates; and osmotic agents. If these simple approaches do not work, more potent laxatives may be required, but these should be used with great caution.

Surgery

Patients with refractory colonic inertia may best be treated with subtotal colectomy with ileorectal anastomosis [135–138], which can restore regular bowel movements and reduce symptoms such as bloating and abdominal distention. Patients need to be selected carefully with the help of physiologic and psychological evaluations [139–145]. Surgery is not as successful in patients with severe abdominal pain, major depression, or

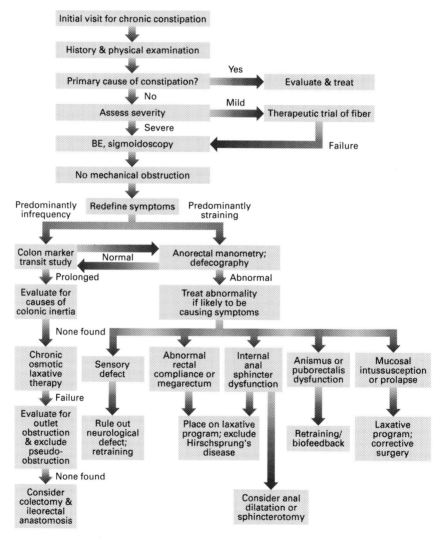

Fig. 10.2 Algorithm for a clinical approach to patients with chronic constipation. BE, barium enema.

evidence of functional outlet obstruction as in patients without these features.

Summary and future directions

A clinical algorithm depicting the approach to chronic constipation based on current concepts and readily available tests is provided in Figure 10.2.

Investigation of the pathophysiology of constipation has provided insights into some of the mechanisms underlying this symptom. Further study may elucidate the etiology of these abnormalities and provide better modalities of treatment (Table 10.5).

Table 10.5 Future directions in the study of constipation.

Classification
- More precise clinical classification of individual patients by pathophysiologic or etiologic categories

Diagnosis
- Improved tests (more precise, less expensive, less radiation exposure)
- Formal studies of the utility of tests in clinical decision making

Etiology
- Testable hypotheses to explain the etiology of colonic inertia and functional outlet obstruction

Therapy
- Safer laxatives (reduced toxicity, fewer side effects)
- More effective drugs with specific effects on enteric nerves
- Improved biofeedback techniques for skeletal-muscle dysfunction
- More reliable surgical intervention for refractory cases

Prevention
- Better understanding of the potential hazards of laxative therapy
- Improved primary toilet training
- Lay education as to the diversity of stool habits

References

1 Lestar B, Penninckx FM, Kerremans RP. Defecometry: a new method for determining the parameters of rectal evacuation. *Dis Colon Rectum* 1989;**32**:197–201.
2 Schiller LR. Fecal incontinence. In: Sleisenger MH, Fordtran JS, eds. *Gastrointestinal Disease: Pathophysiology/Diagnosis/Management*, 5th edn. Philadelphia: WB Saunders Co, 1993:934–53.

3 Lysy J, Karmeli F, Goldin E. Substance P levels in the rectal mucosa of diabetic patients with normal bowel function and constipation. *Scand J Gastroenterol* 1993;**28**:49–52.

4 Johanson JF, Sonnenberg A, Koch TR, McCarty DJ. Association of constipation with neurologic diseases. *Dig Dis Sci* 1992;**37**:179–86.

5 Menardo G, Bausano G, Corazziari E *et al.* Large-bowel transit in paraplegic patients. *Dis Colon Rectum* 1987;**30**:924–8.

6 Mathers SE, Kempster PA, Law PJ *et al.* Anal sphincter dysfunction in Parkinson's disease. *Arch Neurol* 1989;**46**:1061–4.

7 Hinds JP, Eidelman BH, Wald A. Prevalence of bowel dysfunction in multiple sclerosis: a population survey. *Gastroenterology* 1990;**98**:1538–42.

8 Waldron DJ, Horgan PG, Patel FR, Maguire R, Given HF. Multiple sclerosis: assessment of colonic and anorectal function in the presence of faecal incontinence. *Int J Colorectal Dis* 1993;**8**:220–4.

9 Gill KP, Chia YW, Henry MM, Shorvon PJ. Defecography in multiple sclerosis patients with severe constipation. *Radiology* 1994;**191**:553–6.

10 Eckardt VF, Nix W. The anal sphincter in patients with myotonic muscular dystrophy. *Gastroenterology* 1991;**100**:424–30.

11 Basilisco G, Barbera R, Vanoli M, Bianchi P. Anorectal dysfunction and delayed colonic transit in patients with progressive systemic sclerosis. *Dig Dis Sci* 1993;**38**:1525–9.

12 Kamm MA, Hoyle CHV, Burleigh DE *et al.* Hereditary internal anal sphincter myopathy causing proctalgia fugax and constipation: a newly defined condition. *Gastroenterology* 1991;**100**:805–10.

13 Krevsky B, Maurer AH, Niewiarowski T, Cohen S. Effect of verapamil on human intestinal transit. *Dig Dis Sci* 1992;**37**:919–24.

14 Monane M, Avorn J, Beers MH, Everitt DE. Anticholinergic drug use and bowel function in nursing home patients. *Arch Intern Med* 1993;**153**:633–8.

15 Madden MV, Kamm MA, Nicholls RJ, Santhanam AN, Cabot R, Speakman CT. Abdominal rectopexy for complete prolapse: prospective study evaluating changes in symptoms and anorectal function. *Dis Colon Rectum* 1992;**35**:48–55.

16 Siproudhis L, Ropert A, Gosselin A *et al.* Constipation after rectopexy for rectal prolapse. Where is the obstruction? *Dig Dis Sci* 1993;**38**:1801–8.

17 Bassotti G, Gaburri M, Imbimbo BP *et al.* Colonic mass movements in idiopathic chronic constipation. *Gut* 1988;**29**:1173–9.

18 Bazzocchi G, Ellis J, Villanueva-Meyer J *et al.* Postprandial colonic transit and motor activity in chronic constipation. *Gastroenterology* 1990;**98**:686–93.

19 Waldron DJ, Kumar D, Hallan RI, Wingate DL, Williams NS. Evidence for motor neuropathy and reduced filling of the rectum in chronic intractable constipation. *Gut* 1990;**31**:1284–8.

20 Bassotti G, Betti C, Pelli MA, Morelli A. Prolonged (24-hour) manometric recording of rectal contractile activity in patients with slow transit constipation. *Digestion* 1991;**49**:72–7.

21 Grotz RL, Pemberton JH, Levin KE, Bell AM, Hanson RB. Rectal wall contractility in healthy subjects and in patients with chronic severe constipation. *Ann Surg* 1993;**218**:761–8.

22 Ferrara A, Pemberton JH, Grotz RL, Hanson RB. Prolonged ambulatory recording of anorectal motility in patients with slow-transit constipation. *Am J Surg* 1994;**167**:73–9.

23 Bassotti G, Morelli A, Whitehead WE. Abnormal rectosigmoid myoelectric

response to eating in patients with severe idiopathic constipation (slow-transit type). *Dis Colon Rectum* 1992;**35**:753–6.

24 Bassotti G, Imbimbo BP, Betti C, Dozzini G, Morelli A. Impaired colonic motor response to eating in patients with slow-transit constipation. *Am J Gastroenterol* 1992;**87**:504–8.

25 Bassotti G, Chiarioni G, Imbimbo BP *et al*. Impaired colonic motor response to cholinergic stimulation in patients with severe chronic idiopathic (slow transit type) constipation. *Dig Dis Sci* 1993;**38**:1040–5.

26 van der Sijp JRM, Kamm MA, Nightingale JMD *et al*. Disturbed gastric and small bowel transit in severe idiopathic constipation. *Dig Dis Sci* 1993;**38**:837–44.

27 Marzio L, Del Bianco R, Donne MD, Pieramico O, Cuccurullo F. Mouth-to-cecum transit time in patients affected by chronic constipation: effect of glucomannan. *Am J Gastroenterol* 1989;**84**:888–91.

28 Altomare D, Pilot M-A, Scott M *et al*. Detection of subclinical autonomic neuropathy in constipated patients using a sweat test. *Gut* 1992;**33**:1539–43.

29 Aggarwal A, Cutts TF, Abell TL *et al*. Predominant symptoms in irritable bowel syndrome correlate with specific autonomic nervous system abnormalities. *Gastroenterology* 1994;**106**:945–50.

30 Krishnamurthy S, Schuffler MD, Rohrmann CA, Pope CE II. Severe idiopathic constipation is associated with a distinctive abnormality of the colonic myenteric plexus. *Gastroenterology* 1985;**88**:26–34.

31 Schouten WR, ten Kate FJ, de Graaf EJR, Gilberts ECAM, Simons JL, Kluck P. Visceral neuropathy in slow transit constipation: an immunohistochemical investigation with monoclonal antibodies against neurofilament. *Dis Colon Rectum* 1993;**36**:1112–7.

32 Koch TR, Carney JA, Go L, Go VLW. Idiopathic chronic constipation is associated with decreased colonic vasoactive intestinal peptide. *Gastroenterology* 1988;**94**:300–10.

33 Milner P, Crowe R, Kamm MA, Lennard-Jones JE, Burnstock G. Vasoactive intestinal polypeptide levels in sigmoid colon in idiopathic constipation and diverticular disease. *Gastroenterology* 1990;**99**:666–75.

34 Goldin E, Karmeli F, Selinger Z, Rachmilewitz D. Colonic substance P levels are increased in ulcerative colitis and decreased in chronic severe constipation. *Dig Dis Sci* 1989;**34**:754–7.

35 Lincoln J, Crowe R, Kamm MA, Burnstock G, Lennard-Jones JE. Serotonin and 5-hydroxyindoleacetic acid are increased in the sigmoid colon in severe idiopathic constipation. *Gastroenterology* 1990;**98**:1219–25.

36 Dolk A, Brodén G, Holmstrom B, Johansson C, Schultzberg M. Slow transit chronic constipation (Arbuthnot Lane's disease): an immunohistochemical study of neuropeptide-containing nerves in resected specimens from the large bowel. *Int J Colorectal Dis* 1990;**5**:181–7.

37 Turnbull GK, Thompson DG, Day S, Martin J, Walker E, Lennard-Jones JE. Relationships between symptoms, menstrual cycle and orocecal transit in normal and constipated women. *Gut* 1989;**30**:30–4.

38 Kamm MA, Farthing MJ, Lennard-Jones JE, Perry LA, Chard T. Steroid hormone abnormalities in women with severe idiopathic constipation. *Gut* 1991;**32**:80–4.

39 Preston DM, Lennard-Jones JE. Anismus in chronic constipation. *Dig Dis Sci* 1985;**30**:413–18.

40 Kuijpers HC, Bleijenberg G. The spastic pelvic floor syndrome: a cause of constipation. *Dis Colon Rectum* 1985;**28**:669–72.

41 Read NW, Abouzekry L, Read MG, Howell P, Ottewell D, Donnelly TC. Anorectal function in elderly patients with fecal impaction. *Gastroenterology* 1985;**89**:959–66.

42 Read NW, Timms JM, Barfield LJ, Donnelly TC, Bannister JJ. Impairment of defecation in young women with severe constipation. *Gastroenterology* 1986;**90**:53–60.

43 Bannister JJ, Davison P, Timms JM, Gibbons C, Read NW. Effect of stool size and consistency on defecation. *Gut* 1987;**28**:1246–50.

44 Barnes PR, Lennard-Jones JE. Function of the striated anal sphincter during straining in control subjects and constipated patients with a radiologically normal rectum or idiopathic megacolon. *Int J Colorectal Dis* 1988;**3**:207–9.

45 Johansson C, Nilsson BY, Mellgren A, Dolk A, Holmstrom B. Paradoxical sphincter reaction and associated colorectal disorders. *Int J Colorectal Dis* 1992;**7**:89–94.

46 Roberts JP, Womack NR, Hallan RI, Thorpe AC, Williams NS. Evidence from dynamic integrated proctography to redefine anismus. *Br J Surg* 1992;**79**:1213–15.

47 Jones PN, Lubowski DZ, Swash M, Henry MM. Is paradoxical contraction of puborectalis muscle of functional importance? *Dis Colon Rectum* 1987;**30**:667–70.

48 Miller R, Duthie GS, Bartolo DC, Roe AM, Locke-Edmunds J, Mortensen NJ. Anismus in patients with normal and slow transit constipation. *Br J Surg* 1991;**78**:690–2.

49 Verduron A, Devroede G, Bouchoucha M *et al.* Megarectum. *Dig Dis Sci* 1988;**33**:1164–74.

50 Bouchoucha M, Denis P, Arhan P *et al.* Morphology and rheology of the rectum in patients with chronic idiopathic constipation. *Dis Colon Rectum* 1989;**32**:788–92.

51 Varma JHS, Smith AN. Neurophysiological dysfunction in young women with intractable constipation. *Gut* 1988;**29**:963–8.

52 Kerrigan DD, Lucas MG, Sun WM, Donnelly TC, Read NW. Idiopathic constipation associated with impaired urethrovesical and sacral reflex function. *Br J Surg* 1989;**76**:748–51.

53 De Medici A, Badiali D, Corazziari E, Bausano G, Anzini F. Rectal sensitivity in chronic constipation. *Dig Dis Sci* 1989;**34**:747–53.

54 Kamm MA, Lennard-Jones JE. Rectal mucosal electrosensory testing: evidence for a rectal sensory neuropathy in idiopathic constipation. *Dis Colon Rectum* 1990;**33**:419–23.

55 Speakman CT, Kamm MA, Swash M. Rectal sensory evoked potentials: an assessment of their clinical value. *Int J Colorectal Dis* 1993;**8**:23–8.

56 Kamm MA, Lennard-Jones JE, Nicholls RJ. Evaluation of the intrinsic innervation of the internal anal sphincter using electrical stimulation. *Gut* 1989;**30**:935–8.

57 Kiff ES, Barnes PR, Swash M. Evidence of pudendal neuropathy in patients with perineal descent and chronic straining at stool. *Gut* 1984;**25**:1279–82.

58 Snooks SJ, Barnes PR, Swash M, Henry MM. Damage to the innervation of the pelvic floor musculature in chronic constipation. *Gastroenterology* 1985;**89**:977–81.

59 Engel AF, Kamm MA. The acute effect of straining on pelvic floor neurological function. *Int J Colorectal Dis* 1994;**9**:8–12.

60 Jorge JMN, Wexner SD, Ehrenpreis ED, Nogueras JJ, Jagelman DG. Does perineal descent correlate with pudendal neuropathy? *Dis Colon Rectum* 1993;**36**:475–83.

61 Johansson C, Nilsson BY, Holmstrom B, Dolk A, Mellgren A. Association between rectocele and paradoxical sphincter response. *Dis Colon Rectum* 1992;**35**:503–9.

62 Siproudhis L, Dautreme S, Ropert A *et al.* Dyschezia and rectocele: a marriage of convenience? Physiologic evaluation of the rectocele in a group of 52 women

complaining of difficulty in evacuation. *Dis Colon Rectum* 1993;**36**:1030–6.

63 Shouler P, Keighley MR. Changes in colorectal function in severe idiopathic chronic constipation. *Gastroenterology* 1986;**90**:414–20.

64 Reynolds JC, Ouyang A, Lee CA, Baker L, Sunshine AG, Cohen S. Chronic severe constipation: prospective motility studies in 25 consecutive patients. *Gastroenterology* 1987;**92**:414–20.

65 Varma JS, Bradnock J, Smith RG, Smith AN. Constipation in the elderly: a physiologic study. *Dis Colon Rectum* 1988;**31**:111–15.

66 Waldron D, Bowes KL, Kingma YJ, Cote KR. Colonic and anorectal motility in young women with severe idiopathic constipation. *Gastroenterology* 1988;**95**:1388–94.

67 Thorpe AC, Williams NS, Badenoch DF, Blandy JP, Grahn MF. Simultaneous dynamic electromyographic proctography and cystometrography. *Br J Surg* 1993;**80**:115–20.

68 Pezim ME, Pemberton JH, Levin KE, Litchy WJ, Phillips SF. Parameters of anorectal and colonic motility in health and in severe constipation. *Dis Colon Rectum* 1993;**36**:484–91.

69 Bassotti G, Chiarioni G, Vantini I *et al.* Anorectal manometric abnormalities and colonic propulsive impairment in patients with severe chronic idiopathic constipation. *Dig Dis Sci* 1994;**39**:1558–64.

70 Klauser AG, Voderholzer WA, Heinrich CA, Schindlbeck NE, Muller-Lissner SA. Behavioral modification of colonic function. Can constipation be learned? *Dig Dis Sci* 1990;**35**:1271–5.

71 Sonnenberg A, Tsou VT, Muller AD. The 'institutional colon': a frequent colonic dysmotility in psychiatric and neurologic disease. *Am J Gastroenterol* 1994;**89**:62–6.

72 Devroede G, Girard G, Bouchoucha M *et al.* Idiopathic constipation by colonic dysfunction: relationship with personality and anxiety. *Dig Dis Sci* 1989;**34**:1428–33.

73 Heymen S, Wexner SD, Gulledge AD. MMPI assessment of patients with functional bowel disorders. *Dis Colon Rectum* 1993;**36**:593–6.

74 Wald A, Hinds JP, Caruana BJ. Psychological and physiological characteristics of patients with severe idiopathic constipation. *Gastroenterology* 1989;**97**:932–7.

75 Merkel IS, Locher J, Burgio K, Towers A, Wald A. Physiologic and psychologic characteristics of an elderly population with chronic constipation. *Am J Gastroenterol* 1993;**88**:1854–9.

76 Grotz RL, Pemberton JH, Talley NJ, Rath DM, Zinsmeister AR. Discriminant value of psychological distress, symptom profiles, and segmental colonic dysfunction in outpatients with severe idiopathic constipation. *Gut* 1994;**35**:798–802.

77 Drossman DA, Leserman J, Nachman G *et al.* Sexual and physical abuse in women with functional or organic gastrointestinal disorders. *Ann Intern Med* 1990;**113**:828–33.

78 Wald A. Constipation and fecal incontinence in the elderly. *Gastroenterol Clin North Am* 1990;**19**:405–18.

79 Marshall JB. Chronic constipation in adults. How far should evaluation and treatment go? *Postgrad Med* 1990;**88**:49–63.

80 Gattuso JM, Kamm MA. Review article: the management of constipation in adults. *Aliment Pharmacol Ther* 1993;**7**:487–500.

81 Bartolo DC, Kamm MA, Kuijpers H, Lubowski DZ, Pemberton JH, Rothenberger D. Working party report: defecation disorders. *Am J Gastroenterol* 1994;**89**(Suppl.8):S154–9.

82 Camilleri M, Thompson WG, Fleshman JW, Pemberton JH. Clinical management of intractable constipation. *Ann Intern Med* 1994;**121**:520–8.

83 Marcus SN, Heaton KW. Irritable bowel-type symptoms in spontaneous and induced constipation. *Gut* 1987;**28**:156–9.

84 Stewart RB, Moore MT, Marks RG, Hale WE. Correlates of constipation in an ambulatory elderly population. *Am J Gastroenterol* 1992;**87**:859–64.

85 Preston DM, Lennard-Jones JE. Severe chronic constipation of young women: 'idiopathic slow transit constipation'. *Gut* 1986;**27**:41–8.

86 Loening-Baucke V. Chronic constipation in children. *Gastroenterology* 1993;**105**:1557–64.

87 Gottlieb SH, Schuster MM. Dermatoglyphic (fingerprint) evidence for a congenital syndrome of early onset constipation and abdominal pain. *Gastroenterology* 1986;**91**:428–32.

88 Starreveld JS, Pols MA, van Wijk HJ, Bogaard JW, Poen H, Smout AJ. The plain abdominal radiograph in the assessment of constipation. *Zeitschr Gastroenterol* 1990;**28**:335–8.

89 Bouchoucha M, Devroede G, Arhan P *et al.* What is the meaning of colorectal transit time measurement? *Dis Colon Rectum* 1992;**35**:773–82.

90 Bergin AJ, Read NW. The effect of preliminary bowel preparation on a simple test of colonic transit in constipated subjects. *Int J Colorectal Dis* 1993;**8**:75–7.

91 Hinds JP, Stoney B, Wald A. Does gender or the menstrual cycle affect colonic transit? *Am J Gastroenterol* 1989;**84**:123–6.

92 Kuijpers HC. Application of the colorectal laboratory in diagnosis and treatment of functional constipation. *Dis Colon Rectum* 1990;**33**:35–9.

93 Stivland T, Camilleri M, Vassallo M *et al.* Scintigraphic measurement of regional gut transit in idiopathic constipation. *Gastroenterology* 1991;**101**:107–15.

94 Roberts JP, Newell MS, Deeks JJ, Waldron DW, Garvie NW, Williams NS. Oral [^{111}In] DTPA scintigraphic assessment of colonic transit in constipated subjects. *Dig Dis Sci* 1993;**38**:1032–9.

95 van der Sijp JRM, Kamm MA, Nightingale JMD *et al.* Radioisotope determination of regional colonic transit in severe constipation: comparison with radioopaque markers. *Gut* 1993;**34**:402–8.

96 Meunier PD, Gallavardin D. Anorectal manometry: the state of the art. *Dig Dis* 1993;**11**:252–64.

97 Jorge JM, Wexner SD. Anorectal manometry: techniques and clinical applications. *South Med J* 1993;**86**:924–31.

98 Roberts JP, Williams NS. The role and technique of ambulatory anal manometry. *Baillières Clin Gastroenterol* 1992;**6**:163–78.

99 Ger GC, Wexner SD, Jorge JMN, Salanga VD. Anorectal manometry in the diagnosis of paradoxical puborectalis syndrome. *Dis Colon Rectum* 1993;**36**:816–25.

100 Low PS, Quak SH, Prabhakaran K, Joseph VT, Chiang GS, Aiyathurai EJ. Accuracy of anorectal manometry in the diagnosis of Hirschsprung's disease. *J Pediatr Gastroenterol Nutr* 1989;**9**:342–6.

101 Nielsen MB, Buron B, Christiansen J, Hegedus V. Defecographic findings in patients with anal incontinence and constipation and their relation to rectal emptying. *Dis Colon Rectum* 1993;**36**:806–9.

102 Mezwa DG, Feczko PJ, Bosanko C. Radiologic evaluation of constipation and anorectal disorders. *Radiol Clin North Am* 1993;**31**:1375–93.

103 Goei R. Anorectal function in patients with defecation disorders and asymptomatic subjects: evaluation with defecography. *Radiology* 1990;**174**:121–3.

104 Wald A, Caruana BJ, Freimanis MG, Bauman DH, Hinds JP. Contributions of evacuation proctography and anorectal manometry to evaluation of adults with constipation and defecatory difficulty. *Dig Dis Sci* 1990;**35**:481–7.

105 Wald A, Jafri F, Rehder J, Holeva K. Scintigraphic studies of rectal emptying in patients with constipation and defecatory difficulty. *Dig Dis Sci* 1993;**38**:353–8.

106 Papachrysostomou M, Stevenson AJ, Ferrington C, Merrick MV, Smith AN. Evaluation of isotope proctography in constipated subjects. *Int J Colorectal Dis* 1993;**8**:18–22.

107 Kamm MA, Bartram CI, Lennard-Jones JE. Rectodynamics: quantifying rectal evacuation. *Int J Colorectal Dis* 1989;**4**:161–3.

108 Shafik A, Abdel-Moneim K. Fecoflowmetry: a new parameter assessing rectal function in normal and constipated subjects. *Dis Colon Rectum* 1993;**36**:35–42.

109 Barnes PR, Lennard-Jones JE. Balloon expulsion from the rectum in constipation of different types. *Gut* 1985;**26**:1049–52.

110 Fleshman JW, Dreznik Z, Cohen E, Fry RD, Kodner IJ. Balloon expulsion test facilitates diagnosis of pelvic floor outlet obstruction due to nonrelaxing puborectalis muscle. *Dis Colon Rectum* 1992;**35**:1019–25.

111 Beck DE. Simplified balloon expulsion test. *Dis Colon Rectum* 1992;**35**:597–8.

112 Wexner SD, Marchetti F, Salanga VD, Corredor C, Jagelman DG. Neurophysiologic assessment of the anal sphincters. *Dis Colon Rectum* 1991;**34**:606–12.

113 Jorge JMN, Wexner SD, Ger GC, Salanga VD, Nogueras JJ, Jagelman DG. Cinedefecography and electromyography in the diagnosis of nonrelaxing puborectalis syndrome. *Dis Colon Rectum* 1993;**36**:668–76.

114 Johansson C, Nilsson BY, Holmstrom B, Dolk A. Is paradoxical sphincter reaction provoked by needle electrode electromyography? *Dis Colon Rectum* 1991;**34**:1109–12.

115 Lahr CJ, Cherry DA, Jensen LL, Rothenberger DA. Balloon sphincterography: clinical findings after 200 patients. *Dis Colon Rectum* 1988;**31**:347–51.

116 Jorge JMN, Wexner SD, Marchetti F, Rosato GO, Sullivan ML, Jagelman DG. How reliable are currently available methods of measuring the anorectal angle? *Dis Colon Rectum* 1992;**35**:332–8.

117 Sandler RS, Jordan MC, Shelton BJ. Demographic and dietary determinants of constipation in the US population. *Am J Public Health* 1990;**80**:185–9.

118 Lowery SP, Srour JW, Whitehead WE, Schuster MM. Habit training as treatment of encopresis secondary to chronic constipation. *J Pediatr Gastroenterol Nutr* 1985;**4**:397–401.

119 Keren S, Wagner Y, Heldenberg D, Golan M. Studies of manometric abnormalities of the rectoanal region during defecation in constipated and soiling children: modification through biofeedback therapy. *Am J Gastroenterol* 1988;**83**:827–31.

120 Loening-Baucke V. Modulation of abnormal defecation dynamics by biofeedback treatment in chronically constipated children with encopresis. *J Pediatr* 1990;**116**:214–22.

121 Bennings MA, Buller HA, Taminiau JA. Biofeedback training in chronic constipation. *Arch Dis Child* 1993;**68**:126–9.

122 Loening-Baucke V. Persistence of chronic constipation in children after biofeedback treatment. *Dig Dis Sci* 1991;**36**:153–60.

123 Wexner SD, Cheape JD, Jorge JMN, Heymen S, Jagelman DG. Prospective assessment of biofeedback for the treatment of paradoxical puborectalis contraction. *Dis Colon Rectum* 1992;**35**:145–50.

124 Papachrysostomou M, Smith AN. Effects of biofeedback on obstructive defecation: reconditioning of the defecation reflex? *Gut* 1994;**35**:252–6.

125 Bleijenberg G, Kuijpers HC. Biofeedback treatment of constipation: a comparison of two methods. *Am J Gastroenterol* 1994;**89**:1021–6.

126 Muller-Lissner SA. Treatment of chronic constipation with cisapride and placebo. *Gut* 1987;**28**:1033–8.

127 Murray RD, Li BU, McClung HJ, Heitlinger L, Rehm D. Cisapride for intractable constipation in children: observations from an open trial. *J Pediatr Gastroenterol Nutr* 1990;**11**:503–8.

128 van Outryve M, Milo R, Toussaint J, van Eeghem P. 'Prokinetic' treatment of constipation-predominant irritable bowel syndrome: a placebo-controlled study of cisapride. *J Clin Gastroenterol* 1991;**13**:49–57.

129 Staiano A, Cucchiara S, Andreotti MR, Minella R, Manzi G. Effect of cisapride on chronic idiopathic constipation in children. *Dig Dis Sci* 1991;**36**:733–6.

130 Krevsky B, Maurer AH, Malmud LS, Fisher RS. Cisapride accelerates colonic transit in constipated patients with colonic inertia. *Am J Gastroenterol* 1989;**84**: 882–7.

131 Soffer EE, Metcalf A, Launspach J. Misoprostol is effective treatment for patients with severe chronic constipation. *Dig Dis Sci* 1994;**39**:929–33.

132 Andorsky RI, Goldner F. Colonic lavage solution (polyethylene glycol electrolyte lavage solution) as a treatment for chronic constipation: a double-blind, placebo-controlled study. *Am J Gastroenterol* 1990;**85**:261–5.

133 Fordtran JS, Santa Ana CA, Cleveland MVB. A low-sodium solution for gastro-intestinal lavage. *Gastroenterology* 1990;**98**:11–16.

134 Riecken EO, Zeitz M, Emde C *et al.* The effect of an anthraquinone laxative on colonic nerve tissue: a controlled trial in constipated women. *Zeitschr Gastroenterol* 1990;**28**:660–4.

135 Beck DE, Jagelman DG, Fazio VW. The surgery of idiopathic constipation. *Gastroenterol Clin North Am* 1987;**16**:143–56.

136 Kamm MA, Hawley PR, Lennard-Jones JE. Outcome of colectomy for severe idiopathic constipation. *Gut* 1988;**29**:969–73.

137 Yoshioka K, Keighley MR. Clinical results of colectomy for severe constipation. *Br J Surg* 1989;**76**:600–4.

138 Stabile G, Kamm MA, Hawley PR, Lennard-Jones JE. Colectomy for idiopathic megarectum and megacolon. *Gut* 1991;**32**:1538–40.

139 Fisher SE, Breckon K, Andrews HA, Keighley MR. Psychiatric screening for patients with faecal incontinence or chronic constipation referred for surgical treatment. *Br J Surg* 1989;**76**:352–5.

140 Zenilman ME, Dunnegan DL, Soper NJ, Becker JM. Successful surgical treatment of idiopathic colonic dysmotility: the role of preoperative evaluation of coloanal motor function. *Arch Surg* 1989;**124**:947–51.

141 Wexner SD, Daniel N, Jagelman DG. Colectomy for constipation: physiologic investigation is the key to success. *Dis Colon Rectum* 1991;**34**:851–6.

142 Pemberton JH, Rath DM, Ilstrup DM. Evaluation and surgical treatment of severe chronic constipation. *Ann Surg* 1991;**214**:403–11.

143 Sunderland GT, Poon FW, Lauder J, Finlay IG. Videoproctography in selecting patients with constipation for colectomy. *Dis Colon Rectum* 1992;**35**:235–7.

144 Fleshman JW, Fry RD, Kodner IJ. The surgical management of constipation. *Baillières Clin Gastroenterol* 1992;**6**:145–62.

145 Rex DK, Lappas JC, Goulet RC, Madura JA. Selection of constipated patients as subtotal colectomy candidates. *J Clin Gastroenterol* 1992;**15**:212–17.

Visceral Sensation and Perception in Functional Bowel Disorders

Michael D. Crowell

Sensations arising from the viscera have intrigued philosophers, physicians, and scientists for most of recorded history. Only recently, though, have we begun to understand visceral sensation and perception and its role in gastrointestinal (GI) disorders. The amount of empirical data on somatosensory sensation and perception, in both basic science and clinical arenas, has grown tremendously over the past years, but our understanding of these mechanisms in the viscera has progressed much more slowly. Technological advances have intensified the efforts of investigators to understand visceral sensation and perception and its role in functional bowel disorders that are characterized by visceral pain. This chapter briefly reviews the neurophysiology of visceral afferents and theories of pain transmission, and then explores the role of viscoelastic properties of smooth muscle in sensation and perception, the dynamics of visceral sensation and perception, and finally methodologic issues that have arisen as a result of technological developments.

Neurophysiology of visceral sensation and perception

Visceral afferents

Visceral afferents can be grouped by the location of the sensory nerve endings, the type of sensation conveyed, and the pathways used to reach the central nervous system (CNS). Visceral pain is thought to be derived principally from receptors in the mesentery and within the smooth-muscle layers of the gut. These afferent fibers travel primarily with the sympathetic nerves into the dorsal horn of the spinal cord. Afferent fibers from the mucosa travel via vagal pathways, primarily serve vegetative functions, and are thought to have little effect on pain or pressure perception under normal conditions [1, 2]. These observations are based largely on early investigations [3] that showed pain to be produced by stimulation of the splanchnic nerves, but not by stimulation of the vagus nerve. Chronic visceral pain and experimentally induced pain can be blocked by sectioning the dorsal roots of the spinal nerves, while leaving the vagus intact [4, 5]. Recent data, however, show that electrical stimulation of the vagus inhibits some and facilitates other spinothalamic tract neurons associated with pain [6] and that vagotomy at the cervical level attenuates the antinociceptive effects of morphine [7]. These observations suggest that spinal visceral afferents interact with vagal afferents at the level of the brainstem, where more complex interactions between these innervations also are likely to occur.

Pain transmission and control

Two basic theories have been proposed to account for the transmission of pain from the periphery, and additional factors have been postulated as facilitators or inhibitors of the transmission of sensory information from the viscera. These topics were recently reviewed [8] and will be only briefly described in the following sections.

Intensity theory

The intensity theory of pain transmission states that the same receptors in the gut respond to both pressure and pain and that these receptors can be distinguished by the frequency of neuronal firing [9, 10]. Sengupta *et al.* [2] identified three types of afferent mechanoreceptors, which they classified according to their discharge frequency: low-threshold, high-threshold, and wide-dynamic range mechanoreceptors. Vagal mechanoreceptors are of the low-threshold type, while splanchnic afferents are a mixture of the wide-dynamic range and high-threshold types. Vagal fibers have been found to discharge maximally during both peristalsis and luminal distention, whereas only a small percentage of splanchnic afferents fire during contractile events. The wide dynamic range of the splanchnic mechanoreceptors lends support to the hypothesis that a homogeneous population of afferents is responsible for encoding both innocuous and noxious stimuli within the gut [1].

Specificity theory

The specificity theory proposes that there are specific populations of afferent fibers that respond only to noxious intensities of stimulation and may represent the recruitment of specific nociceptors. Electrophysiologic studies have identified a relatively large number of fibers that appear to respond only at distention levels associated with pain. These fibers make up approximately 30% of all distention-sensitive fibers [2, 11]. Recent evidence has led some proponents of the intensity theory to acknowledge the existence of these high-threshold fibers, and investigators have begun to incorporate them into more comprehensive theories of pain transmission.

Other factors influencing pain transmission and control

Mechanoreceptor sensitization

Mucosal mechanoreceptors may participate in the transmission of painful sensations under certain circumstances. Recruitment of 'hidden nociceptors' has been demonstrated during ischemia, chemical irritation, inflammation, and immune responses [12, 13]. More than 50% of mucosal mechanoreceptors associated with spinal afferents fall into this category. These spinal neurons are normally not excited by painful stimuli: they become responsive only after sensitization [9].

Parasympathetic fibers from the mucosa can also modulate pain transmission, but do not appear to mediate pain directly. Electrical stimulation of the abdominal vagus generally results in nausea and vomiting, but not in pain [1]. It has also been shown [7] that electrical stimulation of vagal afferents can activate descending pathways, which inhibit some and facilitate other spinothalamic tract neurons in the spinal cord. However, stimulation of vagal afferents is more likely to inhibit than to facilitate pain transmission [6].

Gating mechanisms

Gating mechanisms at the level of the brainstem and spinal cord (dorsal horn) may be responsible for presynaptic inhibition, resulting in stimulation-induced analgesia. Empiric findings suggest that all spinal cord neurons receiving afferents from the viscera also receive afferents from muscle or cutaneous somatic receptors. No exclusively visceral spinal afferent pathway has been identified. Studies [14] have shown that cutaneous stimulation has both facilitatory and inhibitory effects on visceral afferents at the neuronal level. Simultaneous stimulation of both receptive fields produces a greater response in spinal neurons, and sequential stimulation produces inhibition in both directions.

The activation of modulatory circuits by somatic stimuli may significantly influence reflex and visceral sensory responses to distention.
Coffin *et al.* [15] recently evaluated this hypothesis in eight healthy
volunteers. Graded isobaric distentions were performed in the stomach
and duodenum, while transcutaneous electrical stimulation was simultaneously applied to the hand at two different intensities. An intensity-
dependent reduction in the perception of gut distention was observed. No
significant effect on reflex gastric relaxation was observed in response to
duodenal distention. The investigators concluded that somatic stimulation reduces the perception of gut distention without interfering with
local reflex responses.

Thus, pain transmission may be facilitated or inhibited by gating
mechanisms at the level of the brainstem or spinal cord. Recent data [16]
have also identified inhibitory interneurons at this level capable of raising
the threshold for firing in primary pain afferents. Stimulation of the cortex
can activate these interneurons and may be the neurologic basis for CNS
modulation of pain. These observations may help to explain the
mechanisms responsible for the modulation of pain thresholds in patients
with anxiety disorders and depression.

Smooth-muscle tone

Sensory neurons respond as if they were 'in series' with smooth-muscle
fibers [17] and, therefore, many neurons in the brainstem that fire in
response to noxious stimuli also fire in response to spontaneous contractions [18]. Atropine reduces smooth-muscle tone in the gut and
increases the distention volume required to produce pain, but does not
significantly alter the pressure required to produce pain [19]. Therefore,
smooth-muscle tone and contractility may influence the threshold for
excitation of receptors responsible for pain transmission either directly or
indirectly.

These observations suggest that the role of smooth-muscle tone in pain
transmission is confounded by its interaction with smooth-muscle contractility. Pain reports may be associated with discrete contractile events
[20], and distention at the threshold levels associated with pain generally
results in increased contractile activity. Therefore, pain reported in
association with luminal distention may be the result of elicited contractile
events rather than a direct function of local distention. Additional evidence
for this hypothesis is provided by studies showing that pain is often
reported far from the actual site of the distending balloon. Ritchie [21]

suggested that this phenomenon may be due to contractile events that are initiated by the distention but which occur at more distant points within the bowel. These observations may, in part, explain the large variations noted in referred pain associated with visceral distention. However, high-amplitude propagated contractions in the colon are generally not associated with reports of abdominal pain [22, 23].

Influence of dynamic properties of smooth muscle on visceral sensation and perception

The most consistent finding in the irritable bowel syndrome (IBS) is a reduced tolerance for pain produced by intraluminal distention. In fact, the symptom that distinguishes the IBS from organic disease is abdominal pain associated with changes in bowel habits [24]. Empiric data have shown that patients with the IBS have a reduced tolerance for noxious colonic distention [25], as well as an increased sensitivity to nonpainful stimuli [26, 27]. This pattern does not appear to be limited to the colon and rectum; increased sensitivity to distention also has been reported in the esophagus [28], stomach [29], and distal ileum [30]. Increased smooth-muscle tone or decreased compliance may thus account for reduced sensory thresholds in patients with functional bowel disorders [31], although earlier studies generally did not support this hypothesis. For example, Ritchie [21] reported that intraluminal pressures at the pain threshold were lower in patients with IBS than in healthy controls, and Whitehead et al. [32] reported a poor correlation between compliance and sensory thresholds. These early results may have been limited by the measurement techniques used, however.

Adaptive relaxation of smooth muscle

The recent development of the computerized barostat/visceral stimulator has generated renewed interest in the clinical evaluation of visceral sensation and perception and has enabled investigators to begin to evaluate the influence of more dynamic properties of smooth muscle on visceral perception.

A recent study [33] showed that adaptive relaxation of smooth-muscle tone occurred in response to balloon distention of the rectum at a constant pressure. In seven healthy volunteers (31.3 ± 2.35 years) a 10 × 15-cm infinitely compliant polyethylene bag was positioned in the rectum with its base 10 cm from the anal verge. Individual rectal perception thresholds were determined using cumulative stepwise pressure distentions, administered in increments of 2 mmHg. Isobaric rectal distention was then performed over a 25-minute period using a computer-controlled barostat (Synectics Medical, Sweden) at the previously determined urge thresholds. The system patency was confirmed before and after each study. The volume required to maintain the preset pressure at the urge threshold increased significantly from minute 1 (268.7 ± 22.4 ml) to minute 5 (300.4 ± 22.5 ml) to minute 25 (342.1 ± 23.7 ml). The subjects reported no change in intensity of the urge to defecate during the distention period. These data suggest that in healthy controls the rectum displays adaptive relaxation in response to chronic stretching of the rectal wall, which is a critical response needed for the normal, short-term storage function of the rectum.

Impaired adaptive relaxation in IBS

Impairment of adaptive relaxation may contribute to symptoms in patients with chronic recurrent abdominal pain and urgency. We [34], therefore, compared changes in rectal volume in healthy controls and patients with the IBS during continuous rectal distention at pressures associated with the first sensation and moderate urge to defecate. Sensory thresholds were determined in six healthy volunteers (32.8 ± 9.6 years) and five patients with the IBS (32.2 ± 8.2 years) using the computerized visceral stimulator. The intrabag pressure was increased in increments of 2 mmHg in a cumulative stepwise fashion up to the urge threshold and tracked for 15 minutes. Continuous distentions were then performed for 10 minutes at the pressure associated with each individual's threshold for first sensation ($\bar{x} = 7.6 \pm 0.8$ mmHg) and moderate urge ($\bar{x} = 16.0 \pm 1.2$ mmHg). The order of experimental conditions was counterbalanced. Dependent measures were the minute means derived from the intrabag pressure and volume.

Rectal volume increased significantly over the 10-minute distention period (17% in controls and 12% in patients with the IBS) at the pressure associated with moderate urge. A significant volume–time interaction emerged due to differences in the rate of adaptation between controls (6.47 ml/min) and patients with the IBS (4.10 ml/min). Significant adaptive relaxation (a 16% decrease) was also noted at the pressure associated with first sensation (7.58 ± 0.78 mmHg). Adaptive relaxation of the rectum (a gradual decrease in rectal tone in response to chronic distention) was greater in healthy controls than in patients with the IBS and resulted in the need for larger intrabag volumes to maintain similar intrabag pressures. We concluded that symptoms of urgency and lower thresholds for abdominal pain in patients with the IBS may, in fact, be due to impaired adaptive relaxation of the rectum in response to chronic distention, resulting in greater stimulation of visceral mechanoreceptors with luminal distention.

Influence of adaptive relaxation on visceral perception

To evaluate the influence of this adaptive response on visceral perception more directly, we developed an electronic sliding potentiometer that provides a digitized signal from a 70-mm Likert-type scale (Synectics Medical, Sweden) and permits continual monitoring and recording of changes in the intensity of perception. We [35] evaluated changes in smooth-muscle tone and visceral perception in response to continuous pressure and continuous volume distention at each individual's thresholds for the moderate urge to defecate. In 14 volunteers (32.8 $\pm$ 9.6 years), sensory thresholds were determined following an overnight fast. Continuous rectal distentions were performed for 20 minutes at the predetermined pressure and, in a separate trial, at the volume associated with moderate urge. The order of experimental conditions was counterbalanced. The dependent measures were the minute means derived from the intrabag pressure and volume and the minute means for urge intensity.

During continuous pressure distention, the rectal volume increased by 66% from minute 1 (175 $\pm$ 68 ml) to minute 20 (291 $\pm$ 75 ml). Urge-intensity ratings showed a biphasic pattern, with a 36% increase from minute 1 to minute 10, followed by a 23% decline from minute 10 to minute 20, without further changes in volume or pressure (Figure 11.1). Continuous volume distention resulted in a 20% decrease in rectal pressure from minute 1 (26.1 $\pm$ 5.6 mmHg) to minute 20 (20.8 $\pm$ 4.1 mmHg). Urge intensity decreased by 28% from minute 1 to minute 20.

Thus, adaptive relaxation of the rectum was confirmed using both pressure and volume distention. Smooth-muscle relaxation in response to distention also had a significant impact on visceral perception. During isobaric distention, intensity ratings remained stable or increased over the distention period, while volume increased. During isovolumetric distention, the intensity rating and the intrarectal pressure decreased. Changes in visceral perception late in the distention period, when volume and pressure were relatively stable, suggest that perceptual adaptation

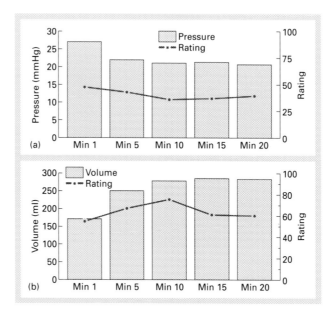

Fig. 11.1 Minute means for 20-minute volume distention (a) and pressure distention (b) at individual urge thresholds (average of 214.7 ml in (a), 26.6 mmHg in (b)). During continuous volume distention, pressure (bars) and pain-intensity ratings (lines) decreased progressively. During continuous pressure distention, volume and pain intensity increased progressively over the 20-minute period. Min, minute.

may also occur at the level of the CNS. These data also emphasize the significant individual differences in the patterns of change in intensity ratings during distention.

These investigations showed a consistent increase in volume with continuous isobaric rectal distention and a consistent decrease in pressure during continuous isovolumetric distention. Visceral perception was altered in relation to pressure changes associated with sustained distention. The simultaneous changes observed in volume, pressure, and intensity strongly support the role of adaptive relaxation of the rectum in response to distention, and suggest that this adaptive relaxation has a direct influence on perception. Furthermore, these findings [36, 37] suggest that continuous rectal distention over prolonged periods may have long-term effects on gut wall tension and perception, as previously suggested.

The observation that the rectal wall has adaptive abilities is not new [38, 39]. It has been difficult, however, to investigate changes in rectal tone during balloon distention because standard methodologies are based on isovolumetric distention [40–42]. Akervall *et al.* [43] and Crowell *et al.* [44] have suggested that isobaric distention, a method derived from measurement of intestinal tone [45–47], overcomes many of the problems associated with the more traditional stepwise procedures [40]. Determinations of rectal sensory thresholds via volumetric distention are confounded by the ability of the rectum to adapt when distended, resulting in progressive, uncontrolled changes in intraluminal pressure. Isobaric techniques, on the other hand, allow distention stimuli to be maintained at a constant rate in the presence of variations in volume. Nonetheless, even isobaric methods depend on the specific characteristics of the stimulus. Furthermore, anatomic variations may still cause great interindividual variability in intrarectal volumes.

Sensitization and habituation

Although the preceding data show that temporal changes in smooth muscle are important for an understanding of visceral sensation and perception, they do not specifically address the dynamic properties of sensation and perception. Sensitization and habituation are two well-known factors that affect somatosensory thresholds. To date, however, no studies have addressed their influence on the evaluation of visceral sensory thresholds. To assess the role of perceptual sensitization and habituation — increases or decreases in perception in response to repeated stimulation — we [48] investigated systematic changes in the volume and pressure profiles required to maintain a moderate pain rating over 30 consecutive distention trials. In 26 healthy subjects (33 ± 9 years) and 25 patients with the IBS (37 ± 11 years), precisely controlled, intermittent distention stimuli were administered in 2-mmHg increments every 30 seconds using a computerized visceral stimulator. Subjects verbally defined their pain threshold, defined as a score of 3.0 on a 0–5-point visual analog scale, before each trial. A computer-controlled random tracking procedure then increased or decreased pressure to maintain an intensity rating of 3.0 over 30 stimulus trials (total duration of 15 minutes).

Pressure decreased significantly from stimulus 1 to stimulus 15, whereas the volume required to maintain the intensity rating increased from stimulus 1 to stimulus 15 (Figure 11.2). The volume required to maintain a constant intensity level was significantly lower in patients with the IBS (110 ± 83 ml) than in controls (155 ± 78 ml), but there was no significant difference in the pressure or intensity between patients and controls. Thus, when repeated rectal stimulation was administered at the pain threshold, significant decreases in intrabag pressure — the parameter that was systematically varied — were required to maintain a

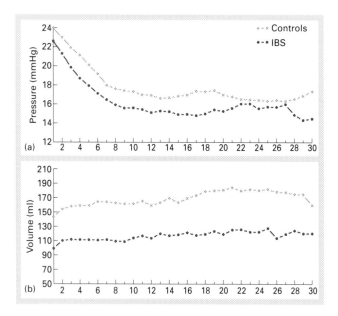

Fig. 11.2 (a) Repeated intermittent balloon distentions resulted in progressive decreases in the pressure required to maintain a constant pain-intensity rating in both patients with the IBS and healthy controls. (b) Simultaneously, intraballoon volumes increased over the 30 distention trials.

constant intensity over time. Interestingly, simultaneous increases in the corresponding volumes were observed. These findings suggest that repeated stimulus presentation may lead to sensitization of perception. The dissociation between pressure and volume with repeated distentions suggests that the rectum adapts over time, i.e., the pressure needed to maintain a constant pain intensity gradually decreased, even though volume increased, thus requiring a greater volume to produce similar or decreased pressures.

Methodologic considerations

Recent technological developments in the field of visceral sensation and perception have brought numerous methodologic issues to the fore. These issues will influence dramatically how quickly and efficiently we are able to advance empiric knowledge in this area. While a complete evaluation of these psychophysical methods cannot be undertaken in this chapter, several critical methodologic issues will be addressed.

Pressure-dependent versus volume-dependent stimuli

Rectal perception of distention stimuli is thought to depend on rectal compliance, which is generally estimated by means of a pressure/volume coefficient. This coefficient can be determined by either pressure- or volume-dependent rectal distention. To date, most laboratories have relied on the more traditional volume-dependent stimuli to determine sensory thresholds. The development of the computerized visceral stimulator/barostat has made it possible to deliver automated, precise stimuli for pressure or volume distention. In theory, the two methods, assuming that they are equally accurate, should provide similar estimations of rectal compliance and similar determinations of perception thresholds. In application, however, the accuracy and applicability of these methods, in the research setting and in clinical diagnostics, may differ.

Our recent data [49] suggest that pressure- and volume-dependent distention stimuli are equally accurate in determining sensory thresholds in healthy subjects and patients with the IBS (Figure 11.3). Although we observed no consistent differences between volume- and pressure-dependent threshold determinations in either group, volume-dependent distentions enhanced the discrimination between groups. This study also emphasized the importance of using the maximal pressure resolution when evaluating between-group differences. Both stepwise and phasic pressure-dependent distentions require a maximal step rate of 1 mmHg to

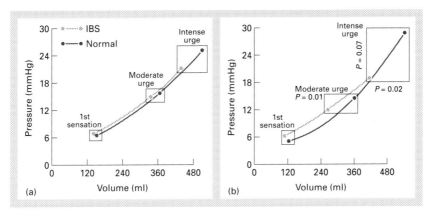

(a)

(b)

Fig. 11.3 (a) Cumulative stepwise pressure-dependent balloon distention and (b) cumulative stepwise volume-dependent balloon distention in patients with the IBS and healthy controls. No threshold differences were found between groups using pressure-dependent stimuli. The pressure–volume curve shifted to the left for patients with the IBS, using volume-dependent stimuli.

yield resolution for detection of group differences. An alternative strategy would be the use of ramp distentions at a fixed flow rate.

These data do not address the physiologic relevance of pressure-dependent versus volume-dependent stimuli for the determination of visceral sensory thresholds. It has been proposed [50] that pressure is the most relevant physiologic stimulus due to the role of mechanoreceptors in visceral sensation. However, data on this issue are lacking. Theoretically, pressure-dependent distentions should yield more consistent results when comparisons are made between groups and between repeated measures over time. For instance, a consistent pressure-dependent distention of 10 mmHg should yield comparable stimulation of stretch receptors across individuals regardless of factors such as the luminal diameter. In contrast, a volume-dependent distention of 50 ml may produce dramatically different stimulation across individuals because of anatomic variations. Additionally, pressure-dependent threshold tracking accounts for dynamic changes in muscle tension within the lumen by adjusting the volume in response to variations in muscle tone, whereas a constant volume distention allows uncompensated pressure changes. Muscle tension has been suggested [51] as a more meaningful dependent measure; it is derived from the law of Laplace, which states that tension is a function of the pressure within the lumen and the luminal diameter. It is important to note, however, that variance may increase with attempts to estimate luminal diameters.

Cumulative stepwise versus intermittent phasic distention

Variations in somatosensory thresholds depend on the characteristics of the stimulus presented, but limited data are available regarding stimulus presentation and its effects on visceral sensory thresholds. Most laboratories routinely perform both cumulative stepwise distentions and discrete phasic distentions to determine anorectal function. Physiologically, cumulative distentions may stimulate the movement and accumulation of solids and liquids in the gut, whereas intermittent distentions may simulate the more rapid dispersion of luminal contents. Additionally, cumulative and phasic distentions may stimulate different neural pathways and result in dramatically different mechanisms being studied. Therefore, both distention methods may yield relevant, independent information on sensory function in the gut, especially in patient groups.

A direct comparison of these two techniques is methodologically difficult and may be influenced by the duration of the stimulus, the interstimulus interval, the rate of inflation, differences in predistention levels, and adaptive relaxation of the lumen. Figure 11.4 illustrates two possible paradigms for comparing pressure- and volume-dependent distentions (other possibilities exist). Paradigm 1 shows a distention method that uses a square-wave stimulus presentation of equal stimulus duration but which fails to control for the infusion rate, interstimulus interval, and predistention effects. Paradigm 2 compares cumulative stepwise pressure distention and intermittent ramp distention. The use of a controlled ramp distention minimizes differences related to rate-dependent mechanisms between the two methods, which becomes extremely important at higher thresholds that require larger inflation volumes. The ramp distention technique does not control for differences in the stimulus duration or for predistention effects, but does control for differences in the interstimulus interval. Although these two methods may not be directly comparable, their relative contributions to perception thresholds can be determined in a straightforward manner. Subjective responses should be obtained at a consistent point within the stimulus interval, and volume and pressure should be compared directly. Data suggest that the influence of volume and pressure on the perception threshold is paradigm dependent. Using paradigm 1, M. Delvaux (per-

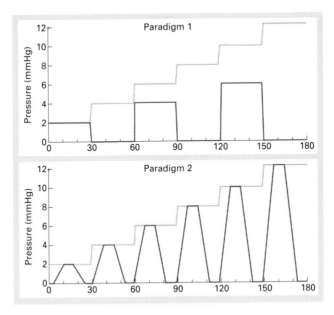

Fig. 11.4 Two paradigms for comparing cumulative stepwise (light lines) and intermittent phasic (dark lines) balloon distentions. Paradigm 1 uses a square-wave stimulus presentation; paradigm 2, an intermittent controlled ramp stimulus.

sonal communication, 1994) found no significant differences in volume or pressure at the thresholds for first sensation, urge, and discomfort between stepwise and phasic distentions.

Using paradigm 2, we [52] recently observed significant differences between stepwise and phasic distentions. In 16 healthy volunteers (35 ± 11 years) a 2 × 2 balanced-squares design with repeated measures was used to analyze the differences between intermittent and stepwise pressure-dependent distentions at two different interstimulus intervals (30 and 60 seconds). Distention stimuli were increased in 2-mmHg increments. Pressure was increased linearly over an 8-second period and maintained at the peak pressure for 8 seconds during phasic distention. A 10 × 15-cm infinitely compliant bag was positioned in the rectum 10 cm from the anal verge. Pressure, volume, and the volume:pressure ratio (compliance index) at each sensory threshold were compared.

Compliance curves shifted to the left with phasic distentions, resulting in increased pressures per unit of volume (Figure 11.5). Consequently, perception thresholds at moderate and intense urge occurred at significantly lower volumes during phasic distention. There was no difference between the two methods in pressure values at each sensory threshold, and the interstimulus interval had no significant effect on any of the variables.

Anorectal motor activity differed dramatically in response to stepwise and phasic distentions. During cumulative stepwise distention, rectal pressure and external anal sphincter (EAS) pressure increased progressively. Internal anal sphincter (IAS) pressure showed a sustained

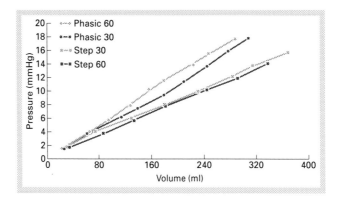

Fig. 11.5 Results in a representative subject, showing the shift to the left in the compliance curve with phasic balloon distentions compared with cumulative stepwise distentions.

relaxation, followed by a slow recovery period. The EAS showed tonic baseline increases, and sphincter contraction was noted with each distention. Phasic contractile activity subsided at the highest distention level. During phasic distentions, rectal pressure increased following each distention. Discrete IAS relaxations were also seen, followed by a pressure-dependent overshoot. These data show that different stimulus characteristics may lead to variations in the dynamic response of the gut wall to distention, influencing both perception and motor activity.

Our results also suggest that stepwise and phasic distention stimuli are not directly comparable, and that under certain circumstances they may result in dramatically different physiologic and perception responses. The method of distention and the paradigm used for each method depend on the system studied and the question to be addressed. For example, signal detection paradigms require the presentation of multiple discrete stimuli and the use of phasic distentions. Additional studies are needed to clarify the physiologic relevance of these differences and to evaluate the responsible mechanisms.

Rates of distention influence perception

Visceral perception thresholds and compliance curves are influenced by distention rates. Sun et al. [40] found that rectal perception thresholds were lower for slow than for fast infusion rates, using ramp infusions of water. Rapid infusion rates resulted in higher pressures at similar volumes compared with slower rates, producing a significant shift to the left in the pressure–volume curve. We have noted a similar result using cumulative stepwise infusions of air with a computer-controlled barostat. Volume-dependent distentions were increased in increments of 20 ml and compared after 5, 30, and 60 seconds. Incremental distentions at 5-second intervals resulted in significantly higher pressure at similar volumes. This observation suggests that sensory thresholds are influenced not only by the infusion rate, but also by the interstimulus interval. Additionally, rapid distentions elicited increased contractile activity for up to 20 seconds after the initial infusion and resulted in transient shifts in perception thresholds. This observation appeared to be limited to shorter distention intervals since no significant differences were observed between 30- and 60-second intervals. Nevertheless, it is critical that perception reports be obtained at consistent points within the stimulus interval (preferably at least 25 seconds postinflation). These data suggest that perception thresholds in the distal bowel may be stretch-rate dependent and further emphasize the importance of standardizing rates of inflation in studies of visceral sensation.

Conclusion

Tremendous progress has been made over the past decade that has enhanced our understanding of the structure, pharmacology, and electrophysiology of the neural mechanisms influencing visceral sensation and perception. Investigators have gained exciting insights into the GI tract as a sensory organ. Until recently, these advances have not been integrated in *in vivo* investigations of visceral perception. Methodologic and technical advances have enabled investigators to begin the arduous task of unraveling these complex brain–gut interactions. However, much remains to be learned about the role of visceral afferents and reflex pathways in visceral perception. As basic scientists make this knowledge available, the applied physiologist is charged with integrating these neurophysiologic data with human behavior. This process will require a thorough understanding of the dynamic properties of smooth muscle within the GI tract and the psychophysics of sensation and perception from the viscera.

References

1 Grundy D. Mechanoreceptors in the gastrointestinal tract. *J Smooth Muscle Res* 1993;**29**:37–46.
2 Sengupta JN, Saha JK, Goyal RK. Stimulus-response function studies of esophageal mechanosensitive nociceptors in sympathetic afferents of opossum. *J Neurophysiol* 1990;**64**:796–812.
3 Cannon B. Method of stimulating autonomic nerves in unanaesthetized cat with observations on the motor and sensory effects. *Am J Physiol* 1933;**105**:366–72.
4 White JC. Sensory innervation of viscera: studies on visceral afferent neurones in man based on neurosurgical procedures for the relief of intractable pain. *Nerv Mental Dis Proc* 1943;**23**:373–90.
5 Stulrajter V, Pavlasek J, Strauss P, Duda P, Gokin AP. Some neuronal, autonomic, and behavioural correlates to visceral pain elicited by gall-bladder stimulation. *Act Nerv Super (Praha)* 1978;**20**:203–9.
6 Ren K, Randich A, Gebhart GF. Effects of electrical stimulation of vagal afferents on spinothalamic tract cells in the rat. *Pain* 1991;**44**:311–19.
7 Randich A, Thurston CL, Ludwig PS, Timmerman MR, Gebhart GF. Antinociception and cardiovascular responses produced by intravenous morphine: the role of vagal afferents. *Brain Res* 1991;**543**:256–70.
8 Mayer EA, Gebhart GF. Basic and clinical aspects of visceral hyperalgesia. *Gastroenterology* 1994;**107**:271–93.
9 Janig W, Koltzenburg M. On the function of spinal primary afferent fibres supplying colon and urinary bladder. *J Autonom Nerv Syst* 1990;**30**(Suppl.):S89–96.

10 Ness TJ, Gebhart GF. Characterization of superficial T13–L2 dorsal horn neurons encoding for colorectal distension in the rat: comparison with neurons in deep laminae. *Brain Res* 1989;**486**:301–9.

11 Cervero F, Sharkey KA. An electrophysiological and anatomical study of intestinal afferent fibres in the rat. *J Physiol* 1988;**401**:381–97.

12 McMahon SB, Koltzenburg M. Novel classes of nociceptors: beyond Sherrington. *TINS* 1990;**13**:199–201.

13 Collins S. Inflammation in the irritable bowel syndrome. In: Mayer EA, Raybould HE, eds. *Basic and Clinical Aspects of Chronic Abdominal Pain*. Amsterdam: Elsevier, 1993:62–70.

14 Gebhart GF, Randich A. Brainstem modulation of nociception. In: Klemm WR, Vertes RP, eds. *Brainstem Mechanisms of Behavior*. New York: Wiley, 1990:315–52.

15 Coffin B, Azpiroz F, Guarner F, Malagelada J-R. Selective gastric hypersensitivity and reflex hyporeactivity in functional dyspepsia. *Gastroenterology* 1994;**107**:1345–51.

16 Cervero F, Tattersall JE. Somatic and visceral sensory integration in the thoracic spinal cord. *Prog Brain Res* 1986;**67**:189–205.

17 Iggo A. Gastrointestinal tension receptors with unmyelinated afferent fibres in the vagus of the cat. *Q J Exp Physiol Cogn Med Sci* 1957;**42**:130–43.

18 Janig W. Spinal cord integration of visceral sensory systems and sympathetic nervous system reflexes. *Prog Brain Res* 1986;**67**:255–77.

19 Chapman WP, Jones CM. Variations in cutaneous and visceral pain sensitivity in normal subjects. *J Clin Invest* 1944;**23**:81–91.

20 Holdstock DJ, Misiewicz JJ, Waller SL. Observations on the mechanism of abdominal pain. *Gut* 1969;**10**:19–31.

21 Ritchie J. Mechanisms of pain in the irritable bowel syndrome. In: Read NW, ed. *Irritable Bowel Syndrome*. London: Grune & Stratton, 1985:163–72.

22 Crowell MD, Bassotti G, Cheskin LJ, Schuster MM, Whitehead WE. Method for prolonged ambulatory monitoring of high-amplitude propagated contractions from colon. *Am J Physiol* 1991;**261**:G263–8.

23 Bassotti G, Crowell MD, Whitehead WE. Contractile activity of the human colon: lessons from 24 hour studies. *Gut* 1993;**34**:129–33.

24 Manning AP, Thompson WG, Heaton KW, Morris AP. Towards positive diagnosis of the irritable bowel. *BMJ* 1978;**2**:653–4.

25 Ritchie J. Pain from distension of the pelvic colon by inflating a balloon in the irritable colon syndrome. *Gut* 1973;**14**:125–32.

26 Kullmann G, Fielding JF. Rectal distensibility in the irritable bowel syndrome. *Ir Med J* 1981;**74**:140–2.

27 Prior A, Maxton DG, Whorwell PJ. Anorectal manometry in irritable bowel syndrome: differences between diarrhoea and constipation predominant patients. *Gut* 1990;**31**:458–62.

28 Richter JE, Barish CF, Castell DO. Abnormal sensory perception in patients with esophageal chest pain. *Gastroenterology* 1986;**91**:845–52.

29 Lemann M, Dederding JP, Flourie B, Franchisseur C, Rambaud JC, Jian R. Abnormal perception of visceral pain in response to gastric distension in chronic idiopathic dyspepsia: the irritable stomach syndrome. *Dig Dis Sci* 1991;**36**:1249–54.

30 Kellow JE, Phillips SF, Miller LJ, Zinsmeister AR. Dysmotility of the small intestine in irritable bowel syndrome. *Gut* 1988;**29**:1236–43.

31 Hoelzl R, Erasmus L-P, Kratzmair M. Peripheral transduction mechanism in visceral pain perception of irritable bowel patients. In: Singer MV, Goebell H, eds.

Nerves and the Gastrointestinal Tract. Lancaster, UK: Kluwer Academic Publishers, 1989:797–8.

32 Whitehead WE, Engel BT, Schuster MM. Irritable bowel syndrome: physiological and psychological differences between diarrhea-predominant and constipation-predominant patients. *Dig Dis Sci* 1980;**25**:404–13.

33 Musial F, Crowell MD, Enck P. Effects of long term rectal distention on rectal tone. *Gastroenterology* 1994;**106**(Suppl.):A546.

34 Crowell MD, Musial F. Rectal adaptation to distention is impaired in the irritable bowel syndrome. *Am J Gastroenterol* 1994;**89**:1689.

35 Crowell MD, Musial F, Lutz K, Schettler-Duncan VA. Adaptive relaxation of rectal smooth muscle influences visceral perception. *Gastroenterology* 1995;**108**(Suppl.):A587.

36 Musial F, Crowell MD, French AW, Guiv N. Effect of prolonged, continuous distention below defecation threshold on mouth-to-cecum and colonic transit time in pigs. *Physiol Behav* 1992;**52**:1021–4.

37 Klauser AG, Voderholzer WA, Heinrich CA, Schindlbeck NE, Muller-Lissner SA. Behavioral modification of colonic function: can constipation be learned? *Dig Dis Sci* 1990;**35**:1271–5.

38 Lipkin M, Almy T, Bell BM. Pressure–volume characteristics of the human colon. *J Clin Invest* 1962;**41**:1831–9.

39 Schuster MM. Motor action of the rectum and anal sphincters in continence and defecation. In: Code C, Prosser CL, eds. *Handbook of Physiology. Section 6: Alimentary Canal*, Vol. IV. Washington, DC: American Physiological Society, 1968:2121–40.

40 Sun WM, Read NW, Prior A, Daly JA, Cheah SK, Grundy D. Sensory and motor responses to rectal distention vary according to rate and pattern of balloon inflation. *Gastroenterology* 1990;**99**:1008–15.

41 Felt-Bersma RJF, Gort G, Meuwissen SGM. Normal values in anorectal manometry and rectal sensation: a problem of range. *Hepatogastroenterology* 1991;**38**:444–9.

42 Whitehead WE, Schuster MM. Anorectal physiology and pathophysiology. *Am J Gastroenterol* 1987;**82**:487–97.

43 Akervall S, Fasth S, Nordgren S, Oresland T, Hulten L. Rectal reservoir and sensory function studied by graded isobaric distension in normal man. *Gut* 1989;**30**:496–502.

44 Crowell MD, Cheskin LJ, Schuster MM, Whitehead WE. A computer-controlled pump for measurement of muscle tone and sensory thresholds. *Gastroenterology* 1992;**102**(Suppl.):A438.

45 Azpiroz F, Malagelada J-R. Gastric tone measured by an electronic barostat in health and postsurgical gastroparesis. *Gastroenterology* 1987;**92**:934–43.

46 Bell AM, Pemberton JH, Hanson RB, Zinsmeister AR. Variations in muscle tone of the human rectum: recordings with an electromechanical barostat. *Am J Physiol* 1991;**260**:G17–25.

47 Steadman CJ, Phillips SP, Camilleri M, Haddad AC, Hanson RB. Variation of muscle tone in the human colon. *Gastroenterology* 1991;**101**:373–81.

48 Crowell MD, Lutz K, Davidoff A, Whitehead WE. Repeated rectal distention leads to perceptual sensitization. *Gastroenterology* 1995;**108**(Suppl.):A587.

49 Musial A, Musial F, Crowell MD. Comparison of stepwise volume and pressure distention for the determination of sensory thresholds and compliance in the rectum. *Gastroenterology* 1994;**106**(Suppl.):A1041.

50 Whitehead WE, Crowell MD, Davidoff A, Cheskin L, Schuster MM. Pain threshold and muscle tone are lower in sigmoid colon than in rectum. *Gastroenterology* 1994;**106**(Suppl.):A588.

51 Munakata J, Lembo N, Niazi N, Kodner A, Mayer EA. Normosensitive IBS patients show reduced compliance of sigmoid colon. *Gastroenterology* 1994;**106**(Suppl.):A544.

52 Mueller J, Musial F, Kollmannsperger P, Crowell MD. Effects of distention duration on visceral sensory thresholds. *Gastroenterology* 1994;**106**(Suppl.):A1041.

« 12 »
The Effect of Sleep on Gastrointestinal Motility

William C. Orr

Introduction

Sleep and the alterations in gastrointestinal (GI) symptoms and physiologic functioning during sleep have not been salient features of the day-to-day practice of gastroenterologists. In contrast, understanding the neurobiology of sleep and alterations in respiratory function during sleep has become an integral part of the practice of pulmonary medicine and the training of pulmonologists. This is due to the discovery and description of profound alterations in respiratory function associated with sleep and to the description of various clinical conditions associated with these alterations [1]. The ubiquity of sleep apnea, the high incidence of sleep complaints in clinical medicine, and the proliferation of research suggesting the relevance of sleep to clinical medicine have thrust sleep into the daily consciousness of the primary care physician. However, the integration of sleep phenomena into the practice of gastroenterology has not kept pace with their integration into other areas of clinical medicine.

In this chapter, alterations in GI functioning during sleep will be reviewed, with a focus on the relevance of these sleep-related changes to the pathogenesis of disease and clinical symptoms. Interest in sleep and GI functioning has increased substantially over the past several years and, more recently, studies [2] have been conducted that describe specific alterations in sleep patterns in patients with GI disorders. The intention of this chapter is to instill an appreciation of the basics of sleep physiology and to describe how alterations in physiologic functioning during sleep can enhance the understanding of GI disease as well as the practice of GI medicine.

Nocturnal symptoms

Nocturnal symptoms are common in the practice of GI medicine. Nocturnal heartburn and esophagitis, epigastric pain during sleep and peptic ulcer disease, and nocturnal diarrhea in diabetic autonomic neuropathy are commonly encountered associations. Despite these associations, the GI system has been largely ignored in the study of sleep physiology, most likely because of the relative inaccessibility of the alimentary tract to conventional measurement techniques. Advances in technology have allowed access to the luminal GI system either by noninvasive techniques or by intubation techniques that are more easily tolerated by patients. The fundamental question that arises relates to the relationship between the nocturnal symptoms and the pathogenesis, diagnosis, and treatment of the underlying disease.

Perhaps the most familiar nocturnal symptom is the epigastric pain of a patient with duodenal ulcer disease. It is a clinical axiom that burning epigastric pain that characteristically causes awakening from sleep and is relieved with food ingestion signals the presence of a duodenal ulcer. Such patients are usually treated empirically with antacids or acid-suppressing medication, and if there is an acceptable reduction in the epigastric pain, it is presumed that the empiric diagnosis of duodenal ulcer was correct. Other peptic symptoms that are manifest during sleep include those of nocturnal gastroesophageal reflux (GER), such as heartburn, angina-like chest pain, coughing, and wheezing. Although clinicians commonly encounter these symptoms in patients with peptic disease, the specific pathophysiology of sleep-related symptoms has not been sufficiently well understood to alter the management of these patients.

Studies [3–5] have been accumulating to document the importance of nocturnal GER in the pathogenesis of the complications of esophageal acid mucosal contact. In fact, a recent clinical study [6] has documented the importance of the report of nocturnal heartburn in distinguishing esophageal disease from angina or duodenal ulcer. Other studies [5, 7, 8] have documented the importance of nocturnal symptoms such as wheezing and coughing in suggesting a pathogenic role for significant nocturnal GER. Nocturnal diarrhea is a symptom commonly noted in patients with diabetic autonomic neuropathy and in individuals who have undergone an ileoanal anastomosis [9,10]. In fact, some patients who have undergone ileoanal anastomosis have complained of diarrhea and incontinence only during sleep. Nocturnal diarrhea has also been noted in some patients with gluten-sensitive enteropathy [11]. Recently, studies [12] have shown sleep abnormalities in patients with irritable bowel syndrome (IBS) as well as correlations between the quality of sleep and the severity of daytime symptoms.

It would seem apparent from these studies that increasing awareness of the relationship between sleep and GI disease has enhanced our understanding of pathophysiology. In addition, many of these studies enhance diagnosis and treatment by providing an awareness not only of nocturnal symptoms but also of how these symptoms are created by alterations in GI functioning during sleep.

Sleep physiology

To monitor the presence of sleep and the various sleep stages and to correlate these stages with intestinal events, it is necessary to simultaneously record GI motility and the standard parameters used to assess the stages of sleep. These parameters include the electroencephalogram (EEG), the electro-oculogram (EOG), and the submental electromyogram (EMG). The pattern of activity noted on the EEG, EOG, and EMG allows the determination of waking and the various stages of sleep [13, 14]. The waking state and the electrophysiologic changes associated with different sleep stages are shown in Figures 12.1–12.5 [15].

The essential change noted from waking (Figure 12.1) to stage 1 sleep is the gradual disappearance of regular alpha-activity (8–10 Hz) in the EEG. Stage 1 sleep (Figure 12.2) is therefore characterized by a relative

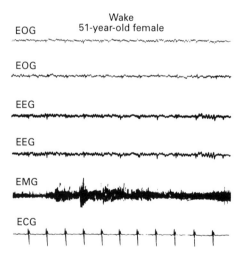

Fig. 12.1 Polysomnographic (EOG, EEG, EMG, electrocardiogram (ECG)) pattern of waking. Note the presence of alpha-activity (8–10 Hz), the absence of eye movements, and tonic activity in the chin EMG (time 20 seconds). (From Orr [15]. In: Schuster MM, ed. *Atlas of Gastrointestinal Motility in Health and Disease*. Media, PA: Williams & Wilkins, 1993.)

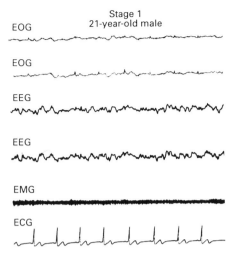

Fig. 12.2 Stage 1 sleep. Note the absence of alpha-activity and the predominance of theta-activity (4–7 Hz) in the EEG and a reduction in the tonic activity of the chin EMG (time 20 seconds). (From Orr [15].)

absence of alpha-activity and a predominance of theta-activity (4–7 Hz) in the EEG and slow-rolling eye movements in the EOG. Stage 2 sleep (Figure 12.3) is characterized by the presence of sleep spindles, which are short bursts of EEG activity in the range of 12–14 Hz. Stages 3 and 4 sleep (Figure 12.4) are characterized by an increasing dominance in the EEG of slow waves in the range of 0.5–3 Hz. These waves are referred to as delta-waves; hence, stages 3 and 4 sleep are usually combined and referred to as slow-wave sleep, or delta-sleep. Rapid eye movement (REM) sleep

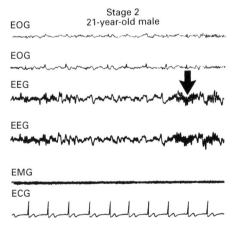

Fig. 12.3 Stage 2 sleep. Note the presence of sleep spindles (bursts of 12–14 Hz activity) (time 20 seconds) in the EEG (arrow). (From Orr [15].)

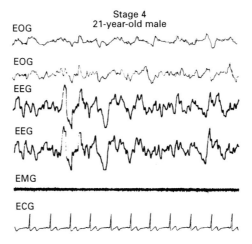

Fig. 12.4 Stages 3 and 4 sleep. Note the predominance of high-voltage, slow-frequency (0.5–3 Hz) activity in the EEG. Stage 3 contains 20–50% of these EEG delta-waves, and stage 4 contains 50% or more in a 30-second or 1-minute epic of sleep (time 20 seconds). (From Orr [15].)

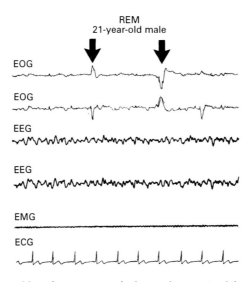

Fig. 12.5 REM sleep. Note the presence of a low-voltage, mixed-frequency EEG, conjugate eye movements (arrows), and diminished tonic activity in the EMG (time 20 seconds). (From Orr [15].)

(Figure 12.5) is characterized by the appearance of low-voltage, mixed-frequency activity in the EEG, suppression of chin EMG activity, and bursts of conjugate eye movements.

Stages 1–4 sleep are commonly referred to collectively as non-REM (NREM) sleep. Periods of REM and NREM sleep alternate throughout the

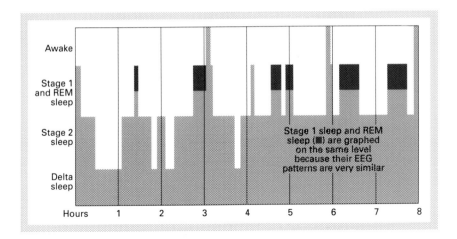

Fig. 12.6 A sleep histogram depicting time and sleep stage in a healthy young adult.

night, with REM periods noted approximately every 90 minutes (Figure 12.6). In the adult population, REM sleep generally accounts for approximately 18–20% of a normal night's sleep; this percentage remains fairly stable throughout life, whereas the percentage of slow-wave sleep diminishes gradually with age [16].

Profound physiologic changes take place during sleep, particularly during REM sleep [17]. Respiratory, metabolic, and thermal regulatory responses are substantially altered during REM sleep [17, 18]. For example, it has been shown that during REM sleep, mammals are poikilothermic, with temperature regulation similar to that of cold-blooded species, and that the regulation of blood gases and pH via the respiratory system is unresponsive to typical stimuli that alter the rate of respiration (e.g. hypoxia and hypercapnea). Studies [18] have shown that during REM sleep, the carbon dioxide response curve is markedly depressed, as is the hypoxic drive. Data [19] are also available to show significant alterations in the autonomic regulation of heart rate during sleep.

Very few studies have examined GI function as it may relate to sleep. The invasive measures necessary to monitor GI motility make it difficult to obtain normal sleep data. It has been the experience in our laboratory that although GI motility can be measured for sustained periods during sleep, evaluation of GI motility during REM sleep remains elusive. Recently, we have been somewhat more successful in obtaining data on GI motility during REM sleep, and these studies will be reviewed subsequently.

Swallowing and esophageal function during sleep

Swallowing is perhaps the single most obvious human function that is clearly related to intestinal motility. The swallow initiates the digestive process. Clearly, swallowing is important in maintaining adequate nutrition, but it also serves a protective function, since it is critical in facilitating the clearance of refluxed gastric contents [20, 21]. Swallowing and the subsequent initiation of the peristaltic wave are integral to producing both volume clearance and acid neutralization subsequent to GER [21, 22]. The clearance of refluxed gastric contents depends on adequate motor functioning of the pharynx and esophagus. Although esophageal function does not appear to be altered during sleep, the swallowing frequency is markedly decreased, and there is virtually no salivary flow [23–26]. Studies from our laboratory [25, 27] have shown that the clearance time of infused acid during sleep is significantly prolonged compared to the clearance time of infusions accomplished in the waking state.

Esophageal motor function has not been shown to exhibit any particularly significant alterations during sleep, and lower esophageal sphincter (LES) pressure and peristaltic amplitudes have not been demonstrated to be significantly altered when individuals were studied at 10 AM and at 10 PM [28]. Propagation data for the morning and the evening were similarly unaffected in this investigation.

LES function during sleep has been shown to be associated with sleep-related GER. Despite a gradual rise in LES pressure during the sleeping interval [29], transient relaxations of the LES are the most common mechanism of reflux during sleep [30, 31]. Although these events occur relatively infrequently during sleep, they have been shown to be most commonly associated with a transient arousal from sleep [30, 32]. The actual stimulus initiating this response has not yet been determined. Although most episodes of reflux are associated with transient arousal responses, reflux events have been identified in our laboratory in the absence of an arousal response. These differences are shown in Figures 12.7 and 12.8 [15]. In the former figure, it can be seen that the drop in esophageal pH coincides with a transient arousal response (as indicated by the movement artifact in the tracing). In Figure 12.8, the drop in pH is noted to be without any alteration in the sleep tracing.

Gastroesophageal reflux and acid clearance during sleep

GER is recognized as a common phenomenon. It frequently occurs

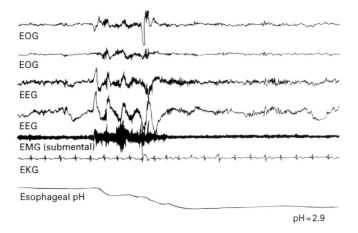

Fig. 12.7 Sleep-related GER. Note arousal response simultaneous with decrease in esophageal pH. (From Orr [15].)

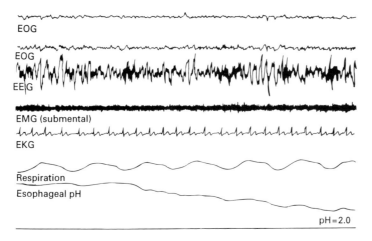

Fig. 12.8 Sleep-related GER without associated arousal response. (From Orr [15].)

postprandially and may or may not be associated with the symptom of heartburn. GER itself may be considered a physiologic phenomenon that occurs in most individuals after ingestion of a meal. Pathologic reflux is recognized when the frequency of GER and reflux symptoms becomes problematic for the patient.

Recently, attention has been focused on the importance of different patterns of GER associated with waking and sleeping. These patterns were documented in studies involving 24-hour monitoring of the distal esophageal pH. In a landmark study [33], Johnson and DeMeester described two patterns of reflux. Reflux in the upright position occurs most often postprandially and usually consists or two or three reflux episodes that are rapidly resolved to a pH of 4 or greater. Reflux in the supine position is usually associated with sleep and with a prolonged acid clearance time [3, 33].

These studies by Johnson, DeMeester, and colleagues have documented significant increases in acid mucosal contact time in patients with esophagitis, and these differences have been most apparent in the supine position or during the sleeping interval, i.e., there was a greater difference between patients and control subjects in the supine than in the upright position. These investigators have speculated that the prolongation of acid clearance during sleep (supine position) results in greater damage to the esophageal mucosa. Several studies have associated sleep-related GER with more severe esophageal mucosal damage, as documented endoscopically. Johnson and DeMeester [33] reported a greater incidence of grades I–III esophagitis in individuals with both upright and supine reflux; Janssens et al. [34] reported similar data. In a recently published study [4], we confirmed that prolonged acid clearance during sleep and the occurrence of longer (>5 minutes) episodes of acid clearance in the supine position best differentiate patients with esophageal mucosal damage from those without such damage.

The importance of swallowing and salivary secretion in the acid clearance and neutralization process has been well described [22, 35]. Of particular relevance to this discussion is that both swallowing frequency and salivation have been shown to be markedly depressed during sleep and, as a result, one would expect a prolongation of acid clearance during sleep to occur with sleep-related episodes of GER [24, 26]. Studies from our laboratory have focused specifically on the parameters of esophageal acid clearance during sleep, and we have developed a model that incorporates the clearance of infused acid during sleep in assessing the effects of sleep on the acid clearance process. This model allows the precise timing of infusions of acid into the distal esophagus during specific periods of documented sleep (i.e. REM versus NREM sleep). The volume of each infusion can be precisely controlled, as well as the exact pH of the infusate. This model also permits a precise comparison of acid clearance during waking and during the different stages of sleep.

This series of investigations has led to a variety of conclusions concerning the effect of sleep on the acid clearance process. Several of our studies have documented that various stimuli in the distal esophagus can produce afferent feedback to the central nervous system (CNS), resulting in an arousal from sleep, which, as suggested above, will produce more prompt acid clearance. Our initial study [27] suggested that an arousal from sleep following the infusion of acid was an important parameter in producing prompt acid clearance. In a subsequent study [25] in healthy volunteers, all subjects were initially shown to be Bernstein negative, i.e., they were unable to distinguish an infusion of acid from water into the distal esophagus. Neither solution produced any noticeable response. However, during sleep the infusion of acid produced a significantly greater percentage of arousal responses than did water. We have also shown that the swallowing rate is markedly enhanced with acid stimulation during sleep.

This study documented that responsiveness to acid, a noxious stimulus to the esophagus, was clearly different during sleep and in the waking state. Responsiveness to esophageal acid mucosal contact was shown to be enhanced under the circumstance of depressed consciousness, which would present a much greater risk of pulmonary aspiration. We then conducted a series of studies to assess other parameters thought to be related to esophageal clearance and mucosal damage. In one study [36], the volume of refluxate in the distal esophagus was assessed to determine whether smaller volumes were more or less rapidly cleared and whether the larger volumes produced a more rapid arousal response. It was hypothesized that larger volumes would create a greater risk of pulmonary aspiration and would therefore produce a more rapid arousal response. Volumes of 5, 15, and 25 ml of 0.1 N hydrochloric acid were infused during waking and sleep on separate occasions. The results indicated that during sleep the largest volume was indeed associated with a shorter arousal latency and a shorter clearance time. These differences were not apparent in the waking state, once again confirming that communication between esophageal receptors and the CNS is enhanced during sleep.

Another important factor in the production of mucosal damage, not only to the esophagus but also to the lungs, is the pH of the refluxant. In a study [37] using the model noted above, infusions into the distal esophagus of equivalent volumes (15 ml) of differing pH (1, 3, 5) were accomplished during waking and sleep. Again, as hypothesized, a lower pH was associated with a more rapid clearance time and a shorter arousal response time, compared with higher pH infusions.

These data indicate that sleep is indeed associated with a more prolonged acid clearance time compared with waking, secondary to the natural consequences of a depressed level of consciousness (i.e. a decreased rate of swallowing). In addition, these studies document a 'fail-safe' system of sensory communication between receptors in the distal esophagus and the CNS. pH levels in the distal esophagus produce differential arousal responses during sleep that can be interpreted as protective of the esophageal mucosa and the tracheobronchial tree.

Very few studies have been conducted to describe the functioning of the upper esophageal sphincter (UES) during sleep. One recent study [38] described some alteration in the UES during sleep, particularly REM sleep. Only a modest decline in the resting pressure was noted during REM sleep; this is somewhat surprising as the cricopharyngeus is a skeletal muscle and REM sleep is generally associated with an inhibition of postural skeletal muscles. From a purely behavioral standpoint, it makes sense that the UES would maintain resting pressure during REM sleep, because it protects the lungs from the aspiration of refluxed gastric contents.

Gastric and small bowel motility during sleep

Few, if any, studies have evaluated spontaneous gastric motility during sleep. Goo *et al.* [39] showed pronounced differences in solid-phase emptying in the morning (8 AM) compared with the evening (8 PM) in normal controls (Figure 12.9). This suggests a marked circadian alteration

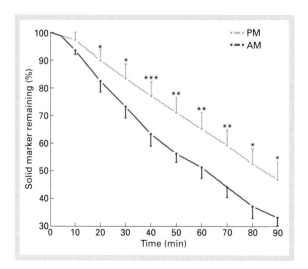

Fig. 12.9 Solid-phase morning (AM) and evening (PM) emptying curves. Significant differences in mean percentage retention values were noted at all timing intervals after 10 minutes. P values (two-tailed paired t test): $*0.02 < P > 0.01$; $**0.01 < P > 0.001$; $***P < 0.001$. (From Goo *et al.* [39].)

in antral motility. We [40] recently published a study in healthy volunteers that described changes during sleep in the gastric basic electrical rhythm as reflected by the electrogastrogram (EGG). This study revealed decreased amplitude in this measure during sleep.

The delay in gastric emptying as a function of time of day suggests that drug absorption may be altered depending on the time of day that medications are taken. Although relatively few drugs are absorbed in the stomach, the rate of gastric emptying into the small bowel would obviously ultimately control the delivery of the drug to the absorptive areas of the small bowel. Thus, rapid absorption of the drug would be best accomplished by administering the medication when gastric emptying is most rapid, for example in the morning. On the other hand, if the peak effect is desired in the early morning hours, the best time to administer the drug would be in the late evening or at bedtime. For example, asthmatics frequently have nocturnal attacks. These attacks usually occur in the very early morning hours, around 4 AM. To time theophylline administration to reach a peak blood level at about that time, it would be best to delay the absorption as long as possible during the sleeping interval. This can be done by taking the medication just before bedtime.

Alterations in small bowel motility during sleep are primarily a reflection of changes in the incidence and propagation of the migrating motor complex (MMC). The MMC is a fasting sequence of motor activity most notable in the distal stomach and the small bowel. Subsequent to food ingestion, there is an interval of quiescence with essentially no detectable motor activity. This period of quiescence, which is referred to as phase I of the MMC, is followed by a period of sporadic motor activity, referred to as phase II. Phase III is characterized by a phasic burst of peristaltic motor activity that usually begins in the antrum and proceeds into the colon (see discussion in Chapter 8). Finch *et al.* [41] have described a relationship between sleep stage and duodenal motility that probably reflects an alteration in the periodicity of phase III of the MMC. In addition, the authors described a periodicity of approximately 90 minutes that was shared by body movement and duodenal motor activity. They interpreted this to reflect the control of these activities by a CNS mechanism [42, 43] that regulates other body functions in a 90-minute cycle.

Prolonged monitoring of the small and large bowel using a variety of sophisticated techniques has allowed a more comprehensive description of intestinal motor activity during waking and sleep. On the basis of these studies, tonic activity in the stomach and small bowel has been described in terms of a basic electrical rhythm and more phasic phenomena, such as the MMC [44]. These studies have highlighted the complexity and variability of the motor activity of the small bowel. Thompson and Wingate [44] found that sleep prolonged the interval between motor complexes in the small intestine. A subsequent study by the same group [45] revealed a decrease in the number of contractions of a specific type in the jejunum associated with sleep. Duodenal ulcer disease and vagotomy did not alter these findings, suggesting that the phenomenon is independent of vagal control and unaffected by duodenal disease. Kumar *et al.* [46] have described the obvious circadian rhythm in the propagation of the MMC, with the slowest velocities occurring during sleep. This finding appears to be the result of a circadian rhythm rather than a true modulation by sleep. Confirmation of these results has come from a study by Kellow *et al.* [47], who also noted that esophageal involvement in the MMC was decreased during sleep, with a corresponding tendency for MMCs to originate in the jejunum.

In another study, Kumar *et al.* [48] examined the relationship between the MMC cycle and REM sleep. They found a significant reduction in both the MMC length and the duration of phase II of the MMC during sleep. The MMCs were distributed equally between REM and NREM sleep, with no obvious alteration in the parameters of the MMC by sleep stage. These data provide evidence of periodic activity in the gut during sleep, but they are also consistent with the notion that the two cycles (the MMC and the REM cycle) are independent. These data would appear to conflict with those described previously, which suggested a relationship between sleep stage and duodenal phase III MMC activity. The same group of investigators [49] has examined how the presence or absence of food in the GI tract alters small bowel motility during sleep. A late evening meal restored phase II activity of the MMC, which is normally absent during sleep.

Kellow *et al.* [50] have examined the occurrence of small bowel motor activity in patients with IBS during waking and sleep. They conducted a prolonged study of continuous recordings from the small bowel that documented a decreased propagation velocity of the MMC during sleep. They did not document any difference in the MMC pattern between the IBS patients and the controls during sleep, but they noted marked differences during waking, including a shorter duration of postprandial motor activity in the IBS patients and shorter MMC intervals in the diarrhea-predominant IBS patients.

Colonic motility during sleep

Relatively few studies have reliably and accurately documented colonic motility during sleep. Numerous technical problems plague the study of colonic activity during sleep, including accurate probe placement and stability of probe placement; problems concerning appropriate data analysis and interpretation are numerous as well. Although several studies have been published that describe colonic function during sleep, they appear to be somewhat contradictory and are difficult to assimilate.

Adler *et al.* [51] have described a decrease in colonic motor function during sleep; these findings have been confirmed by other studies [50, 52, 53], which included measurement of activity in the transverse, descending, and sigmoid colon. Bassotti *et al.* [52] demonstrated an inhibition of the colonic motility index in the transverse, descending, and sigmoid colon, with a marked increase in activity on awakening. This could explain the common urge to defecate on awakening in the morning. A study by Crowell *et al.* [53] showed high-amplitude peristaltic colonic contractions to be virtually absent during sleep. The incidence of these contractions was markedly increased postprandially and just before a bowel movement, suggesting that these contractions are specifically related to colonic transit. Neither of these studies attempted to document sleep with standard polysomnographic measurements.

Furukawa *et al.* [54] measured colonic activity from the cecum to the rectum continuously for 32 hours. They also monitored subjects polysomnographically. Their findings further document the decrease in colonic motor activity during sleep, but the study also described an interesting abolition in propagating waves during slow-wave sleep. During REM sleep, the frequency of these events increased significantly. A recent study [55] of colonic myoelectrical activity in humans suggested a decrease in long spike-burst activity during sleep. It is not clear from this study whether the results indicate a true physiologic alteration during sleep or whether they simply reflect a variation of colonic activity independent of sleep, such as a normal circadian rhythm.

Anorectal activity during sleep

Orkin and colleagues [56, 57] have conducted numerous studies monitoring anal canal motility during sleep. These investigators have demonstrated a rectal motor complex (RMC), which they described as a periodic spontaneous rectal contraction. In studies during sleep and waking they have determined that the RMC occurs more frequently during sleep, but the direction of its propagation has not been determined to be consistently proximal or distal. In addition, these investigators have determined that the rectoanal inhibitory response to rectal distention remains during REM sleep. In a study from our laboratory [58] with 10 normal volunteers, a marked decrease in the external anal sphincter response to rectal distention was demonstrated during sleep. However, the normal internal anal sphincter inhibition associated with rectal distention was not altered. These results confirmed that the external anal sphincter response to rectal distention is most likely a learned response, whereas the internal anal sphincter response appears to be a reflex in that it is not altered by changes in the state of consciousness. In an ambulatory study that included monitoring of anorectal function, Kumar *et al.* [12] demonstrated that external anal sphincter contractions occurred periodically during sleep. The spontaneous contractions were associated with a rise in anal canal pressure, but internal anal sphincter contractions were shown to occur independently of external anal sphincter activity. Of interest is the fact that the spontaneous relaxation of the internal anal sphincter, referred to as the 'sampling reflex', occurred frequently in the waking state but was markedly reduced during sleep.

Sleep and irritable bowel syndrome

The introduction to this chapter mentioned that sleep alterations have been noted in patients with IBS. Kumar *et al.* [59] found patients with IBS to have a rather remarkable increase in the percentage of REM sleep. This is an extraordinary finding considering that the REM sleep literature is replete with alterations resulting from pharmacologic agents as well as endogenous and exogenous stressors, but the changes that have been documented are almost invariably a *decrease* in REM sleep. It is rare to note increases in REM sleep associated with any particular stimulus or medical condition. In addition, a recent study [2] has shown that sleep disturbances are correlated with an exacerbation of abdominal pain in patients with IBS.

These studies are just an example of how integrating the study of GI motility during waking and sleeping can appreciably enhance our understanding of a very common and perplexing GI disease.

Summary

This chapter has documented the effect of sleep on GI motility. It seems clear at this point that the most clinically relevant work relates to the esophagus, particularly to the occurrence of nocturnal GER. Complications such as esophagitis, Barrett's metaplasia, and the respiratory sequelae of laryngopharyngitis and bronchoconstriction appear to be associated with sleep-related GER. Gastric emptying is clearly altered as a function of time of day, and the amplitude of the basic electrical rhythm as measured by the EGG appears to be significantly altered as a function of sleep. Both small bowel and colonic motor activity are altered by sleep, and studies have demonstrated that clusters of small bowel contractions associated with pain in IBS patients disappear during sleep. Colonic and anorectal functioning is less thoroughly investigated and consequently less well understood, and greater elucidation of these sleep-related alterations awaits further research.

References

1 Kryger MH, Roth T, Dement WC, eds. *Principles and Practice of Sleep Medicine*, 2nd edn. Philadelphia: WB Saunders Co, 1994.

2 Goldsmith G, Levin JS. Effect of sleep quality on symptoms of irritable bowel syndrome. *Dig Dis Sci* 1993;**38**:1809–14.

3 DeMeester TR, Johnson LF, Joseph GJ, Toscano MS, Hall AW, Skinner DB. Patterns of gastroesophageal reflux in health and disease. *Ann Surg* 1976;**184**:459–70.

4 Orr WC, Duke JC, Imes NK, Mellow MH. Comparative effects of H_2-receptor antagonists on subjective and objective assessments of sleep. *Aliment Pharmacol Ther* 1994;**8**:203–7.

5 Jacob P, Kahrilas PJ, Herzon G. Proximal esophageal pH-metry in patients with 'reflux laryngitis.' *Gastroenterology* 1991;**100**:305–10.

6 Andersen LI, Madsen PV, Dalgaard P, Jensen G. Validity of clinical symptoms in benign esophageal disease, assessed by questionnaire. *Acta Med Scand* 1987;**221**:171–7.

7 Berquist WE, Rachelefsky GS, Rowshan N, Siegel S, Katz R, Welch M. Quantitative gastroesophageal reflux and pulmonary function in asthmatic children and normal adults receiving placebo, theophylline, and metaproterenol sulfate therapy. *J Allergy Clin Immunol* 1984;**73**:253–8.

8 Harper PC, Bergner A, Kaye MD. Antireflux treatment for asthma: improvement in patients with associated gastroesophageal reflux. *Arch Intern Med* 1987;**147**:56–60.

9 Sleisenger MH, Fordtran JS, eds. *Gastrointestinal Disease: Pathophysiology/Diagnosis/Management*, 3rd edn. Philadelphia: WB Saunders Co, 1983.

10 Metcalf AM, Dozois RR, Kelly KA, Beart RW Jr, Wolf BG. Ileal J pouch–anal anastomosis: clinical outcome. *Ann Surg* 1985;**202**:735–9.

11 Cooper BT, Holmes GKT, Ferguson R, Thompson RA, Allan RN, Cooke WT. Gluten-sensitive diarrhea without evidence of celiac disease. *Gastroenterology* 1980;**79**:801–6.

12 Kumar D, Waldron D, Williams NS, Browning C, Hutton MRE, Wingate DL. Prolonged anorectal manometry and external anal sphincter electromyography in ambulant human subjects. *Dig Dis Sci* 1990;**35**:641–8.

13 Anch AM, Browman CP, Mitler MM, Walsh JK. *Sleep: A Scientific Perspective.* Englewood Cliffs, NJ: Prentice-Hall Inc, 1988.

14 Orr WC. Utilization of polysomnography in the assessment of sleep disorders. *Med Clin North Am* 1985;**69**:1153–67.

15 Orr WC. Effect of sleep and circadian rhythms. In: Schuster MM, ed. *Atlas of Gastrointestinal Motility in Health and Disease.* Media, PA: Williams & Wilkins, 1993:268–76.

16 Carskadon MA, Dement WC. Normal human sleep: an overview. In: Kryger MH, Roth T, Dement WC, eds. *Principles and Practice of Sleep Medicine*, 2nd edn. Philadelphia: WB Saunders Co, 1994:16–25.

17 Parmeggiani PL. The autonomic nervous system in sleep. In: Kryger MH, Roth T, Dement WC, eds. *Principles and Practice of Sleep Medicine*, 2nd edn. Philadelphia: WB Saunders Co, 1994:194–203.

18 Douglas NJ. Control of ventilation during sleep. In: Kryger MH, Roth T, Dement WC, eds. *Principles and Practice of Sleep Medicine*, 2nd edn. Philadelphia: WB Saunders Co, 1994:204–11.

19 Vanoli E, Adamson PB, Lin B, Pinna GD, Lazzara R, Orr WC. Heart rate variability during specific sleep stages: a comparison of healthy subjects with patients after myocardial infarction. *Circulation* 1995;**91**:1918–22.

20 Katzka DA, DiMarino AJ. Pathophysiology of gastroesophageal reflux disease: LES incompetence and esophageal clearance. In: Castell DO, ed. *The Esophagus.* Boston: Little Brown & Co, 1992:449–61.

21 Helm JF, Dodds WJ, Riedel DR, Teeter BC, Hogan WJ, Arndorfer RC. Determinants of esophageal acid clearance in normal subjects. *Gastroenterology* 1983;**85**:607–12.

22 Helm JF, Dodds WJ, Hogan WJ, Soergel KH, Egide MS, Wood CM. Acid neutralizing capacity of human saliva. *Gastroenterology* 1982;**83**:69–74.

23 Lear CSC, Flanagan JB Jr, Moorrees CFA. The frequency of deglutition in man. *Arch Oral Biol* 1965;**10**:83–99.

24 Lichter J, Muir RC. The pattern of swallowing during sleep. *Electroencephalogr Clin Neurophysiol* 1975;**38**:427–32.

25 Orr WC, Johnson LF, Robinson MG. Effect of sleep on swallowing, esophageal peristalsis, and acid clearance. *Gastroenterology* 1984;**86**:814–19.

26 Schneyer LH, Pigman W, Hanahan L, Gilmore RW. Rate of flow of human parotid, sublingual, and submaxillary secretions during sleep. *J Dent Res* 1956;**35**:109–14.

27 Orr WC, Robinson MG, Johnson LF. Acid clearance during sleep in the pathogenesis of reflux esophagitis. *Dig Dis Sci* 1981;**26**:423–7.

28 Avots-Avotins AE, Ashworth WD, Stafford BD, Moore JG. Day and night esophageal motor function. *Am J Gastroenterol* 1990;**85**:683–5.

29 Schoeman MN, Tippett MD, Akkermans LMA, Dent J, Holloway RH. Mechanisms of gastroesophageal reflux in ambulant healthy human subjects. *Gastroenterology* 1995;**108**:83–91.

30 Dent J, Dodds WJ, Friedman RH *et al.* Mechanism of gastroesophageal reflux in recumbent asymptomatic human subjects. *J Clin Invest* 1980;**65**:256–67.

31 Dent J, Holloway RH, Toouli J, Dodds WJ. Mechanisms of lower oesophageal sphincter incompetence in patients with symptomatic gastrooesophageal reflux. *Gut* 1988;**29**:1020–8.

32 Freidin N, Fisher MJ, Taylor W *et al.* Sleep and nocturnal acid reflux in normal subjects and patients with reflux oesophagitis. *Gut* 1991;**32**:1275–9.

33 Johnson LF, DeMeester TR. Twenty-four hour pH monitoring of the distal esophagus: a quantitative measure of gastroesophageal reflux. *Am J Gastroenterol* 1974;**62**:325–32.

34 Janssens J, Vantrappen G, Peeters T, Ghillebert G. How do 24-h measurements distinguish the disease spectrum of reflux patients. *Gastroenterology* 1985;**88**:1431.

35 Allen ML, Orr WC, Woodruff DM, Duke JC, Robinson MG. The effects of swallowing frequency and transdermal scopolamine on esophageal acid clearance. *Am J Gastroenterol* 1985;**80**:669–72.

36 Orr WC, Robinson MG, Johnson LF. The effect of esophageal acid volume on arousals from sleep and acid clearance. *Chest* 1991;**99**:351–4.

37 Orr WC, Lin B. The effect of different levels of pH stimulation on esophageal acid clearance during waking and sleep. *Gastroenterology* 1993;**104**:A561 [Abstract].

38 Kahrilas PJ, Dodds WJ, Dent J, Haeberle B, Hogan WJ, Arndorfer RC. Effect of sleep, spontaneous gastroesophageal (GE) reflux, and a meal on UES pressure. *Gastroenterology* 1986;**90**:1481.

39 Goo RH, Moore JG, Greenberg E, Alazraki NP. Circadian variation in gastric emptying of meals in humans. *Gastroenterology* 1987;**93**:515–18.

40 Orr WC, Chen JZD, Lin B, Shadid GL. Alterations in the gastric basic electrical rhythm during sleep. *Gastroenterology* 1994;**106**:A552.

41 Finch PM, Ingram DM, Henstridge JD, Catchpole BN. Relationship of fasting gastroduodenal motility to the sleep cycle. *Gastroenterology* 1982;**83**:605–12.

42 Orr WC, Hoffman HJ, Hegge FW. Ultradian rhythms in extended performance. *Aerosp Med* 1974;**45**:995–1000.

43 Lavie P. Ultradian rhythms in alertness: a pupillometric study. *Biol Psychol* 1979;**9**:49–62.

44 Thompson DG, Wingate DL. Characterisation of interdigestive and digestive motor activity in the normal human jejunum. *Gut* 1979;**20**:A943.

45 Ritchie HD, Thompson DG, Wingate DL. Diurnal variation in human jejunal fasting motor activity. *Proc Am Physiol Soc* 1980(March);**23**:54–5.

46 Kumar D, Wingate D, Ruckebusch Y. Circadian variation in the propagation velocity of the migrating motor complex. *Gastroenterology* 1986;**91**:926–30.

47 Kellow JE, Borody TJ, Phillips SF, Tucker RL, Haddad AC. Human interdigestive motility: variations in patterns from esophagus to colon. *Gastroenterology* 1986;**91**:386–95.

48 Kumar D, Idzikowski C, Wingate DL, Soffer EE. Relationship between enteric migrating motor complex and the sleep cycle. *Am J Physiol* 1990;**259**:G983–90.

49 Kumar D, Soffer EE, Wingate DL, Britto J, Das-Gupta A, Mridha K. Modulation of the duration of human postprandial motor activity by sleep. *Am J Physiol* 1989;**256**:G851–5.

50 Kellow JE, Gill RC, Wingate DL. Prolonged ambulant recordings of small bowel motility demonstrate abnormalities in the irritable bowel syndrome. *Gastroenterology* 1990;**98**:1208–18.

51 Adler HF, Atkinson AJ, Ivy AC. A study of the motility of the human colon: an explanation of dyssynergia of the colon, or of the unstable colon. *Am J Dig Dis* 1941;**8**:197–202.

52 Bassotti G, Bucaneve G, Betti C, Morelli A. Sudden awakening from sleep: effects on proximal and distal colonic contractile activity in humans. *Eur J Gastroenterol Hepatol* 1990;**2**:475–8.

53 Crowell MD, Bassotti G, Cheskin LJ, Schuster MM, Whitehead WE. Method for

prolonged ambulatory monitoring of high-amplitude propagated contractions from colon. *Am J Physiol* 1991;**261**:G263–8.

54 Furukawa Y, Cook IJ, Panagopoulos V, McEvoy D, Sharp D, Simula M. Relationship between sleep patterns and human colonic motor patterns. *Gastroenterology* 1991;**100**:A444.

55 Frexinos J, Bueno L, Fioramonti J. Diurnal changes in myoelectric spiking activity of the human colon. *Gastroenterology* 1985;**88**:1104–10.

56 Orkin MD, Smith LE, Emsellem H, Dent J, Tissaw M. The rectal motor complex: propagation at night. *Dis Colon Rectum* (in press).

57 Orkin BA, Tissaw M. The rectoanal inhibitory reflex: the contractile component and sleep stages. *Gastroenterology* 1994;**107**:1247.

58 Whitehead WE, Orr WC, Engel BT, Schuster MM. External anal sphincter response to rectal distention: learned response or reflex. *Psychophysiology* 1982;**19**:57–62.

59 Kumar D, Thompson PD, Wingate DL, Vesselinova-Jenkins G, Libby CK. Abnormal REM sleep in the irritable bowel syndrome. *Gastroenterology* 1992;**103**:12–17.

« 13 »

Surgical Approach to Gastrointestinal Motility Disorders

James M. Becker

Introduction

In 1899 W.M. Bayless and E.H. Starling wrote, 'In no subject in physiology do we meet with so many discrepancies of fact and opinion as in that of the physiology of the intestinal movements' [1]. Although physiologists and medical professionals today know more about intestinal motility, a great deal remains poorly understood. Motility of the gastrointestinal (GI) tract depends on a highly integrated, coordinated response of the smooth muscle contained within the bowel wall. Our understanding of the mechanisms that control motility — neural and humoral as well as myogenic — in both physiologic and pathologic states is incomplete, although newer electrophysiologic, manometric, and histologic techniques are rapidly expanding our knowledge.

GI motor disorders can be intrinsic to alimentary function or result from surgical manipulation of the bowel or nervous system. These disorders are difficult to diagnose and treat. Surgery is seldom indicated for GI motility disorders. Nevertheless, many motor dysfunctions have been found to be amenable to surgical therapy. For example, the use of modern manometric techniques to evaluate sphincter of Oddi dysfunction has identified specific primary dysmotilities that can be treated by surgical or endoscopic sphincterotomy. A better understanding of the pathophysiologic roles of the esophageal body, lower esophageal sphincter (LES), and stomach in gastroesophageal reflux has provided a firm rationale for the clinical effectiveness of antireflux procedures. Our knowledge of GI physiology also has led to the development of more directed, physiologic procedures. The classic example of such a development is in peptic ulcer surgery: the use of proximal gastric vagotomy instead of truncal vagotomy preserves antral innervation and reduces the incidence of postvagotomy complications. Similarly, newer modalities for evaluating colorectal motility have led to a better grasp of the etiology of severe and debilitating forms of constipation and better outcomes of targeted surgical intervention. This chapter discusses each of these developments in surgical therapy for motor disorders of the GI tract.

The role of surgery in esophageal motor disorders

Myotomy of the pharyngocervical esophageal segment

Cricopharyngeal myotomy has demonstrated efficacy in the treatment of pharyngeal dysphagia, but appropriate indications have not been well defined. Low rates of morbidity and mortality have encouraged the use of this procedure in patients who exhibit problems during the pharyngeal phase of swallowing [2]. However, an overall success rate of only 64% in these cases suggests the need for better patient selection [3, 4].

Carefully performed motility testing combined with videoradiography may demonstrate poor coordination and incomplete relaxation of the upper esophageal sphincter (UES) during swallowing. This abnormality may result in failure of the pharynx to empty, leading to cervical dysphagia, nasal regurgitation, and aspiration. Neoplasia should be ruled out by endoscopy. The presence of a cricopharyngeal bar, a narrowed pharyngoesophageal segment, or Zenker's diverticulum on a barium swallow test is a predictor of successful outcome of myotomy of the pharyngocervical esophageal segment [5–7].

Loss of compliance of the pharyngocervical esophageal segment may be the most common abnormality in patients with pharyngeal dysphagia. Surgical myotomy can increase the diameter of this noncompliant segment and reduce the resistance to bolus transport into the esophagus. In most situations, myotomy can be performed under local anesthesia. Dysphagia and other esophageal motility problems are discussed in detail in Chapter 2.

Myotomy of the lower esophageal sphincter

Although the complete absence of peristalsis in the esophageal body is commonly associated with achalasia, the primary disorder is failure of the LES to relax completely, which can lead to dysmotility of the esophageal body. Esophageal peristalsis sometimes returns in patients with classic achalasia following dilatation or myotomy, providing support for a primary disorder of the sphincter. The inference is that minimal outflow obstruction can have profound effects on the esophageal body and that complete myotomy performed early in the course of the disease may preserve esophageal body function.

Whether to treat esophageal achalasia by endoscopic balloon dilatation or by surgical myotomy remains controversial [8, 9]. There has been one controlled randomized trial, involving 81 patients, comparing the two modalities: as primary therapy for esophageal achalasia, surgical myotomy produced better long-term results. Retrospective series also support the use of surgical myotomy as the initial treatment of choice. These studies were performed before the availability of the more easily placed endoscopic Rigiflex (microvasive) achalasia balloons, which appear to be associated with a lower morbidity rate.

The effectiveness of surgical myotomy depends on the distal extent of the incision. Persistent dysphagia may result when the incision is too short. Conversely, an incision that is too far below the gastroesophageal junction produces severe postoperative gastroesophageal reflux. Newer technology allows myotomy to be performed via a laparoscopic or thoracoscopic approach, avoiding the need for an incision as well as the morbidity associated with open surgery.

Long esophageal myotomy for motor disorders of the esophageal body

Many motility disorders characterized by segmental or generalized simultaneous contractions can cause dysphagia. They include diffuse esophageal spasm, vigorous achalasia, and nonspecific motility disturbances associated with a midesophageal or epiphrenic diverticulum. In patients whose symptoms are not relieved by medical therapy, a long esophageal myotomy is rarely indicated [2]. Use of prolonged ambulatory manometry has greatly improved identification of patients who may benefit from surgical myotomy of the esophageal body.

Before undergoing esophageal myotomy, patients should receive manometric studies to determine the proximal extent of the procedure. To reduce outflow resistance, the myotomy must be extended distally across the LES. As a result, the addition of some form of anatomic antireflux mechanism is warranted to prevent postoperative gastroesophageal reflux. Most experts recommend use of a partial fundoplication to avoid adding resistance that can impair emptying in a myotomized esophagus. Improvements in the results of myotomy have paralleled the improvement in preoperative diagnosis afforded by manometry.

The role of surgery in gastroesophageal reflux disease

About 60% of patients with documented gastroesophageal reflux disease (GERD) have mechanical failure of the LES [2]. In the remaining 40%, reflux may be due to esophageal or gastric pathology. Mechanical failure of the LES is diagnosed on esophageal manometry by a sphincter pressure of less than 6 mmHg, a sphincter length of less than 1 cm exposed to the abdominal positive-pressure environment, and an overall resting sphincter length of less than 2 cm. If any one or a combination of these findings is present, the patient has a mechanically defective sphincter. The esophageal body may compensate for the failure of one or two components, but the presence of all three defects inevitably prolongs esophageal exposure to gastric refluxate [10]. More recently, transient relaxations of the LES (TLESR) have been shown to be a more important cause of reflux than a lax LES. The motility abnormalities contributing to GERD are discussed further in Chapter 3.

The incidence of a mechanically defective sphincter increases progressively with increasing severity of reflux complications, including esophagitis, stricture, and Barrett's esophagus. It is tempting to attribute the loss of sphincter function to the presence of inflammation or tissue destruction. However, defective sphincters have been observed in GERD patients without mucosal injury [11], suggesting that the mechanical defect of the sphincter is a primary disorder along with TLESR.

In the past, the reflux of gastric acid along with pepsin was generally regarded as the major, if not the sole, source of mucosal damage in GERD. Recent studies by Stein *et al.* [11] correlated the presence and severity of reflux complications with increased esophageal exposure to both acid and alkalinity. Furthermore, results of combined esophageal and gastric pH monitoring suggest that the alkaline component is due to excessive reflux of duodenal contents through the stomach into the distal esophagus. These findings indicate that the mechanical characteristics of the LES and the reflux of gastric acid contaminated with duodenal contents are the most important determinants of esophageal mucosal injury in GERD patients. They also may explain why some cases of esophagitis not only do not heal on acid-suppressive therapy, but also progress to a stricture or Barrett's esophagus [11].

It is important to identify GERD patients who have a mechanically defective LES before complications develop [12]. In such patients, surgery is recommended before there is loss of esophageal body function, which may occur with progression of mucosal injury. In patients with increased esophageal exposure to refluxate due to a mechanically defective LES, reconstruction of a functional sphincter by an antireflux procedure is a rational therapy because it effectively abolishes reflux of either acid or alkaline gastric juice in more than 90% of cases.

Prospective studies have shown that the Nissen fundoplication is an effective and durable antireflux repair procedure. It provides symptom relief in more than 90% of patients and is associated with minimal side effects (Tables 13.1 & 13.2 [13]). In recent years, laparoscopic antireflux operations have been performed with increasing frequency and success, making surgery an increasingly appropriate therapeutic alternative. A recently completed, although unpublished, prospective randomized trial comparing laparoscopic versus open Nissen fundoplication demonstrated a shortened length of hospital stay and more rapid return to work with the former procedure, while functional results were equivalent.

Motility disorders following gastric operations

Three general types of motility disturbance follow gastric operations (Table 13.3).
1   Rapid gastric emptying, which manifests as the dumping syndrome or diarrhea, occurs mostly after gastric resection.
2   Gastric emptying slows after truncal vagotomy with or without gastric drainage.
3   Enterogastric reflux occurs after operations that destroy or bypass the pylorus, such as pyloroplasty and gastric resection with gastro-duodenostomy or gastrojejunostomy.

Disorders associated with rapid gastric emptying

The dumping syndrome occurs to a greater or lesser extent in up to 50% of patients after partial gastric resection, in up to 30% after vagotomy and pyloroplasty, and in as many as 5% after proximal gastric vagotomy. It is refractory to dietary manipulation and requires reoperation in only a small proportion of these patients.

In patients with the dumping syndrome, rapid gastric emptying of liquids and solids is usually induced by surgery [14]. The small intestine is suddenly distended by the large volume 'dumped' into it from the stomach. If the prematurely emptied meal is hypertonic, extracellular fluid pours into the intestinal lumen in an attempt to achieve luminal isotonicity. The plasma volume shrinks, as reflected by an increasing

Table 13.1 Comparison of current antireflux procedures. (From DeMeester & Stein [13].)

Operation	Concept of function	Ease of construction	Effectiveness of valve	Outflow resistance	Toleration of tension	Best use
Hill posterior gastropexy	Complex	Difficult	Dependent on intraoperative manometrics	Dependent on degree of imbrication of cardia	Good	Previous gastric resection
Belsey partial fundoplication	Simple	Most difficult	Effective; patients usually able to belch	Lowest	Poor	Poor esophageal pump
Nissen fundoplication	Simple	Average	Most effective; patient unable to belch	Highest; long and tight wrap can cause permanent dysphagia	Fair	Standard antireflux procedure
Collis–Belsey (Pearson procedure)	Simple	Difficult	Effective; patient unable to belch	Low	Best	Poor esophageal pump and short esophagus

Table 13.2 Results of primary surgical antireflux repairs for GERD. (From DeMeester & Stein [13].)

Repair	Source	Number of patients	Follow-up period	Good results (%)	Reflux recurrence (%)	Dysphagia (%)	Gas bloat (%)	Mortality
Belsey	Skinner	632	1–5 years	85	7.0	—	—	1.2
Mark IV	Orringer	892	3–15 years	84	11.0	—	—	1.0
Hill posterior gastropexy	Hill 1967, 1983	149			4.8	2		
	No intraoperative motility	541			4.8		—	0
	Intraoperative motility	191			1.5			
	No intraoperative motility	72	92.6 months	65	4.1	0		0
	Intraoperative motility	83	47 months	89	0	0		0
	Maher 1978	65		82	9.0			4.6
Nissen	Five reports	1141	1–12 years	87	7.0	8 (4/48)	8 (97/1115)	1.0

Table 13.3 Motor disorders following gastric surgery.

Type of motor disorder	Type of procedure
Enterogastric reflux	Pyloric destruction or bypass
Rapid gastric emptying	Gastric resection or vagotomy and drainage
Slow gastric emptying	Truncal vagotomy

hematocrit, rapid pulse, and drop in blood pressure. Vasoactive amines, including substance P, kinins, and glucagon, are released, resulting in cardiovascular effects that occur 10–20 minutes after the meal. In some patients, rapid gastric emptying and carbohydrate absorption may result in rebound hypoglycemia 1.5–3.0 hours after meals, a phenomenon considered to be responsible for the 'late' dumping syndrome.

The early dumping syndrome is characterized by postprandial weakness, tremulousness, and giddiness that may progress to syncope. It is accompanied by digestive symptoms (epigastric fullness, nausea, borborygmi, urgency to pass stool, and diarrhea) and vasomotor phenomena (tachycardia, palpitations, and profuse diaphoresis with flushing and pallor). Because the meal itself brings on these symptoms, patients fear eating and therefore lose weight. Patients with the late dumping syndrome experience symptoms associated with hypoglycemia, including weakness and faintness, which occasionally progress to syncope, profuse perspiration, and hunger. These symptoms are frequently relieved by carbohydrate ingestion.

In general, diarrhea occurs in 20–30% of patients after vagotomy or gastrectomy. The incidence depends on the type of operation: 2–13% of patients become diarrheic after proximal gastric vagotomy and drainage, 20–67% after truncal vagotomy and drainage. The pathophysiology of postvagotomy diarrhea has not been elucidated clearly, but there is little to support a causative role for parasympathetic denervation of the small intestine or colon. Proposed mechanisms [15, 16] include bacterial colonization of the small bowel, resulting in: direct mucosal irritation or deconjugation of bile salts; nontropical sprue or lactose malabsorption; pancreatic insufficiency; early gastric emptying of fluid; increased bile acid levels in the intestine due to changes in biliary kinetics; and rapid small bowel transit of bile acids with incomplete absorption and subsequent colonic irritation.

Treatment

Many treatment approaches have been proposed to control the dumping syndrome. Medical regimens have included multiple, small, dry, isotonic meals in combination with anticonstipant drugs. Dietary management is fundamental, frequently warranting consultation with a dietitian, and is often successful in the treatment of dumping. When diet fails, pharmacotherapy, including anticholinergics, adrenergic agents, 5-HT antagonists, and either insulin or oral hypoglycemics, have been tried without convincing results.

Surgical treatment is reserved for the very few patients with severe dumping syndrome refractory to dietary and medical management. Surgery, which is designed to slow gastric emptying, includes interposition of an antiperistaltic or isoperistaltic segment of the jejunum between the gastric remnant and small bowel, Roux-en-Y gastrojejunostomy, conversion of Billroth II gastrojejunostomy to Billroth I gastroduodenostomy, and pyloric reconstruction (Figure 13.1 [17]). The results of surgery are variable. Few patients are restored to perfect health, and up to 50% of patients have persistent symptoms after reconstructive operations [17].

Recent experimental evidence suggests a role for retrograde electrical pacing of the small bowel in the treatment of postgastrectomy dumping syndrome (Figure 13.2 [18]). In healthy dogs, backward duodenal pacing slows gastric emptying of isotonic solutions [19]; in dogs with Billroth I gastrectomy, backward duodenal pacing slows gastric emptying of

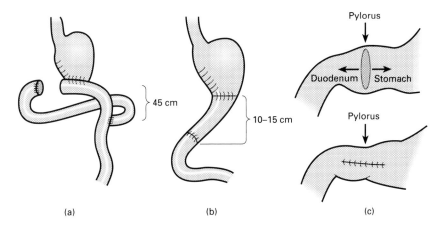

Fig. 13.1 Reconstructive gastric operations: (a) Roux-en-Y gastrojejunostomy; (b) jejunal interposition; and (c) pyloric reconstruction. (From Kelly *et al.* [17].)

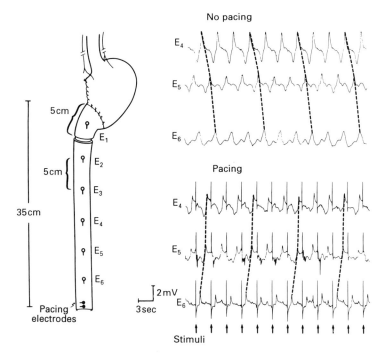

Fig. 13.2 Canine preparation (left) and effect of pacing on recordings of duodenal myoelectric activity (right). Dotted lines depict direction of pacemaker potential propagation. E, recording electrodes. (From Becker *et al.* [18].)

hypertonic instillates and ameliorates dumping [18]. The antidumping effect of such pacing is enhanced when it is applied to the Roux limb of a Roux-en-Y gastrojejunostomy [20]. A major advantage of the technique in humans would be the ability of patients to activate an implanted pacing unit to slow gastric emptying in the immediate postprandial period, after which the unit could be turned off to enable residue and debris to empty from the stomach during the interdigestive period.

The treatment of postvagotomy diarrhea depends on the individual patient. In most patients, fluid-restricted meals and frequent, small feedings will control diarrhea. A trial of pancreatic enzyme supplements should be considered to rule out maldigestion secondary to poor mixing of gastric and pancreatic contents. A lactose-free diet is appropriate for patients with lactose intolerance, a gluten-free diet for celiac disease. Bacterial overgrowth can be treated with antibiotics. If bile salt malabsorption is a factor, cholestyramine may be useful. Cholestyramine is an ion-exchange resin that binds bile salts within the intestinal lumen. Since rapid gastric emptying is likely to be the major pathophysiologic factor, the procedures described above to combat the dumping syndrome are also applicable in diarrheal patients. Surgeons have placed reversed jejunal segments distal to the ligament of Treitz, with variable results.

Disorders associated with slow gastric emptying

If truncal vagotomy is combined with a drainage procedure, the slowed gastric emptying rarely becomes apparent clinically. Gastric stasis persists and becomes difficult to treat in less than 10% of patients after truncal vagotomy. In most patients, a barium contrast study reveals gastric dilatation associated with retained food and delayed emptying of the barium. Gastroscopy may show a dilated stomach and retained food and should rule out a mechanical gastric outlet obstruction. The delay in gastric emptying can be quantified by assessing emptying of radiolabeled solid and liquid meals with a gamma-camera, although normal ranges have not been determined for patients following different types of gastric surgery.

If gastric atony persist for more than 2–3 weeks after gastric surgery, medical therapy should be initiated. Cholinergic and anticholinergic agents have been tried with limited success. Randomized, double-blind trials have reported the efficacy of the dopamine antagonist metoclopramide in acute and chronic postsurgical stasis. More recently, other prokinetic agents — cisapride and erythromycin — have been shown to be effective for postvagotomy gastroparesis, with the former associated with fewer side effects than metoclopramide or erythromycin. A review of medical therapy is found in Chapter 6.

Patients with persistent gastric stasis refractory to an adequate therapeutic trial of metoclopramide for at least 4–8 weeks should receive alternative regimens with other gastrokinetic agents, such as cisapride or erythromycin. Further gastric surgery should be considered only in patients who are refractory to a combination of prokinetic agents (often in large dosages), dietary treatment, and possible acid suppression. Gastric resection is usually necessary, with reconstruction performed as a Billroth II or Roux-en-Y gastrojejunostomy, or a Billroth I gastroduodenostomy. Results of gastric reconstruction for delayed emptying have not been uniformly satisfactory. Nausea and vomiting are usually relieved, but often are replaced by other symptoms, especially the dumping syndrome and diarrhea [4].

Roux stasis syndrome

The combination of vagotomy, distal gastric resection, and Roux-en-Y gastrojejunostomy produces delayed gastric emptying of both solids and liquids. Epigastric fullness, abdominal pain, nausea and vomiting occur postoperatively in 10–50% of patients [21, 22]. Gastric bezoars may form, and severe symptoms can lead to malnutrition and weight loss.

Investigations of this Roux stasis syndrome have revealed that both the postvagotomy proximal gastric remnant and the Roux limb contribute to the emptying delay. Vagotomy diminishes the tone of the remaining stomach; removal of the atonic gastric remnant usually improves symptoms [14, 23]. Scintigraphic studies of the Roux limb have demonstrated delayed transit [24], which may be attributable to altered myoelectric patterns.

In healthy individuals, action potentials, or contractions, in the small intestine, as in the stomach, are controlled by pacesetter potentials that propagate from the duodenum distally down the jejunum [25]. Construction of the Roux limb requires transection of the jejunum, which interrupts the propagation of pacesetter potentials and reduces their frequency in the Roux limb [26]. Ectopic pacemakers then develop in the limb, generating pacesetter potentials that propagate toward the stomach [27]. The orad propagating pacesetter potentials, associated with orad propagating contractions, result in slower transit through the Roux limb. Myoelectric studies in fasting patients have demonstrated a higher frequency of irregular phase III potentials in the Roux limb, which do not propagate as well as potentials in healthy individuals [28, 29].

A new surgical procedure has been designed to prevent the Roux stasis syndrome. Similar to the standard Roux-en-Y construction, the 'uncut Roux' gastroenterostomy theoretically lacks the inherent motor pathophysiology. It is fashioned from a loop gastrojejunostomy with the afferent limb occluded by staples [30] (Figure 13.3 [31]). The staples prevent the flow of biliopancreatic secretions across the gastrojejunostomy (thus preventing alkaline reflux gastritis), but allow normal aboral propagation of pacesetter potentials. The afferent and efferent loops of the gastrojejunostomy are anastomosed proximal to the staple line. In a canine study [32], the uncut Roux operation abolished ectopic pacemakers in the Roux limb and speeded the delayed gastric emptying found with the conventional Roux gastrojejunostomy. The procedure warrants further clinical evaluation of postoperative symptoms, myoelectric activity of the Roux limb, and possible staple-line dehiscence. Early results have been promising.

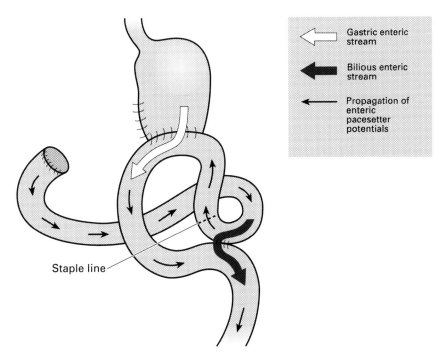

Fig. 13.3 'Uncut Roux' gastroenterostomy. Arrows depict the flow of gastric content and biliopancreatic secretions as well as the direction of propagation of enteric pacemaker potentials. (From Cullen & Kelly [31].)

Enterogastric reflux

In some patients, enterogastric reflux produces no symptoms; in others, refluxed bile may result in bilious vomiting, epigastric pain that is unrelieved by antacids, and endoscopically demonstrable gastritis or esophagitis. Because the syndrome is poorly defined and variable, the incidence of clinically significant enterogastric reflux is difficult to determine. Bilious vomiting occurs in 10–20% of patients after gastric resection or pyloroplasty.

The pathophysiology of reflux gastritis remains enigmatic. Of all the refluxed materials — bile, pancreatic juice, and intestinal chyme — bile acids appear to be the most damaging to the gastric mucosa. Bile acids are capable of breaking the gastric barrier, allowing back-diffusion of acid into the cell, release of intracellular ions into the lumen, histamine release, capillary dilatation, and gastric mucosal hemorrhage. Bile acids also may inhibit gastric motor activity, prolonging contact between bile and the gastric mucosa.

In general, patients with enterogastric reflux develop symptoms within 3 months of the original gastric operation. However, reconstructive procedures have not been performed until a mean of 8 years later. Endoscopy is performed when enterogastric reflux is suspected, but the findings may be difficult to interpret. Reflux of bile into the stomach is seen in more than 60% of patients, and either peristomal or generalized gastritis occurs in 80%. The severity of both symptoms and gastritis, whether assessed endoscopically or histologically, correlates closely with the intragastric concentration of bile acids [33]. No consistent relationship has been found between the extent of gastritis and the severity of the clinical syndrome.

Attempts have been made to quantify more objectively the degree of bile reflux, in the hope that this would improve the identification of patients who will benefit from bile diversionary operations. Technetium-labeled hepatobiliary iminodiacetic acid (HIDA), which is excreted by hepatocytes into bile, has been used as a bile marker. HIDA can be tracked noninvasively through the biliary system and the upper GI tract with a gamma-camera, and the amount of enterogastric reflux quantified. However, this technique has not reliably predicted a successful outcome for diversionary operations. Quantification of excessive bile acids in the gastric remnant has been used to identify postgastrectomy patients with above-normal degrees of reflux and gastritis. Ritchie [33] found that these patients responded favorably to diversionary surgery.

Medical therapy for suspected alkaline reflux gastritis aims at binding the bile salts, improving gastric emptying, or healing and protecting the gastric mucosa. Limited endoscopic or histologic improvement has been seen with cholestyramine, although up to 50% of patients have reported symptomatic improvement. Metoclopramide improves gastric emptying, but limited success in these patients has been reported. Cisapride may promote healing of gastritis. Ursodeoxycholic acid may improve symptoms associated with gastroparesis due to biliary gastritis. Topical prostaglandins, sucralfate, and total parenteral nutrition have been used to promote gastritis healing, but are of no proven benefit.

Reconstructive operations are designed to divert duodenal juices from the gastric remnant. Pyloric reconstruction, jejunal interposition, conversion of Billroth II to I, and Roux-en-Y gastrojejunostomy have been performed. These procedures, particularly the Roux-en-Y diversion, employing at least a 40–45-cm jejunal limb, have produced excellent results, with 65–75% [4, 34] and 85% [35] of patients experiencing long-term symptomatic relief. Many patients appear to improve in the early postoperative period, only to have some or all of their symptoms recur over several years. Nevertheless, the Roux-en-Y diversion results in improvement of abdominal pain, bilious vomiting, and gastritis frequently enough for its use to be recommended in patients with severe complaints suggestive of enterogastric reflux.

Afferent loop syndrome

Afferent loop syndrome is not a disorder of gastric motor function but results from mechanical obstruction of the afferent limb of the gastrojejunostomy after a Billroth II gastrectomy. Because patients can present with bilious vomiting, this syndrome is included in the differential diagnosis of alkaline reflux. Patients describe postprandial upper abdominal pain caused by distention of the partially obstructed afferent limb associated with secretion. Within 30 minutes of a meal, and often with a change in position, the loop suddenly decompresses into the stomach, resulting in the vomiting of bile-stained fluid.

Acute obstruction of the afferent limb occurs in about 1% of cases and may be caused by an afferent loop that is too long, too short, kinked by adhesions, stenosed, herniated, or intussuscepted through the stoma. This condition commonly develops during the first few postoperative weeks and usually requires early reoperation. Chronic afferent loop obstruction can result in bacterial overgrowth, leading to deconjugation of bile salts, diarrhea, steatorrhea, vitamin B_{12} deficiency, and inactivation of lipase, trypsin, and amylase. Both acute and chronic afferent limb syndromes can be treated by revision of the gastrojejunal anastomosis or by conversion of the anastomosis to a gastroduodenostomy or Roux-en-Y gastrojejunostomy.

Disorders of small intestinal motility

Chronic idiopathic intestinal pseudo-obstruction

Chronic idiopathic intestinal pseudo-obstruction is a motor disorder of the small intestine that affects both the fasted and the fed patterns of motility [36]. The usual aboral progression of luminal contents does not occur after a meal because of discoordinated or absent postprandial motility. Because of the absence or relative paucity of migrating motor complexes (MMCs) during the fasted state, stasis develops in the small intestine, resulting in bacterial overgrowth and distention. Delayed gastric emptying is frequently present. Patients frequently receive total parenteral nutrition because of their inability to tolerate oral intake of food.

Limited success has been demonstrated using a combination of total parenteral nutrition and a venting enterostomy. Most patients undergo gastrostomy; jejunostomies and cecostomies also have been used. Because of the global nature of the disorder, surgical resections of portions of the GI tract are associated with frequent postoperative morbidity and high failure rates. A fuller discussion of chronic idiopathic intestinal pseudo-obstruction may be found in Chapter 8.

Small intestinal obstruction

Incomplete or complete mechanical obstruction of the small intestine results most frequently from adhesions, an incarcerated internal or external hernia, or abdominal cancer [37]. Patients with clinically significant small bowel obstruction have an increased incidence of migrating clustered contractions proximal to the obstruction [38], which may be the cause of abdominal cramps. When obstruction is incomplete, these contractions propel intraluminal contents and allow them to pass distal to the point of obstruction. In the presence of unrelieved complete obstruction, the inability of intraluminal contents to pass distally leads to progressive accumulation of intraluminal fluids and distention of the proximal segment of the intestine, resulting eventually in the initiation of retrograde giant contractions (RGCs) in the small intestine as the first phase of vomiting.

Ileus

Postoperative ileus mainly alters motility of the colon and stomach, with more transient disruption of small intestinal motor function [39–41]. It should be remembered that any intestinal anastomosis creates an obstruction and prolongs the return of bowel function beyond the usual effects of ileus. In uncomplicated ileus, in which no small intestinal anastomosis is present, contractile activity returns to the small intestine within 5–10 hours, to the stomach by day 3, and to the colon by day 5. The stomach and colon may become atonic, whereas the small intestine does not. Ingested food and swallowed air are not emptied from the stomach, and excessive gastric dilatation can induce an RGC of the small intestine and vomiting of gastric contents. Although contractile activity returns to the small intestine fairly rapidly after abdominal surgery, MMCs are inhibited for 1–2 days [23, 42].

Postoperative ileus is caused by wide exposure of the abdominal cavity and handling of the intestines. The duration of the ileus appears to be influenced not by the length of the operation or the amount of handling, but rather by the prolonged use of opioid analgesics and by complications, such as infection. The precise mechanism of initiation and continuation of postoperative ileus is not well understood. The rapid recovery of bowel function after laparoscopic operations suggests that postoperative ileus may be induced by the peritoneal incision. Pharmacologic agents that increase contractile activity have been administered in the postoperative period with limited success in reducing the duration of ileus.

Adynamic ileus usually involves the stomach, small intestine, and colon. It is distinguished clinically from a mechanical obstruction of the small bowel by the presence of a large amount of gas in the colon. Initially, the small intestine loses its tone and has minimal or no contractile activity. If the problem is not corrected, progressive dilatation and complete stasis of intestinal contents occur. Frequent causes of adynamic ileus are serious intra-abdominal infection, generalized peritonitis, pancreatitis, and electrolyte abnormalities. Its precise mechanism has not been delineated; it is likely that more than one mechanism is involved. Although these phenomena are not as well documented as in postoperative ileus, MMCs and fed contractions are inhibited during adynamic ileus.

Intestinal transection with anastomosis

The frequency of electrical control activity (ECA), also called slow waves, in the intact small intestine is controlled by a pacemaker in the proximal duodenum. A plateau rate in the duodenum and proximal jejunum decreases progressively along the small intestine. In the intact intestine, ECA and, therefore, contractions propagate distally. After transection and anastomosis, the intestine distal to the anastomosis is no longer entrained by the duodenal pacemaker, and the frequency of ECA decreases to the basal frequency in the remaining small intestine. Because the ECA frequency determines the maximum frequency of contractions [43, 44], the frequency of contractions distal to the anastomosis decreases. If the intestinal transection is in the jejunum, reverse propagation of ECA slows postprandial transit. Resection of the segment involved in reverse propagation of ECA restores transit to normal [45]. Transection also interrupts the distal propagation of MMCs for 30–40 days. During this time, MMCs are initiated distal to the anastomosis and are separate from the usual MMCs initiated in the duodenum. Initiation of the fed pattern of activity is unchanged by transection, as would be suspected from the usual pattern of recovery after intestinal resection. These changes have little impact on intestinal transit and absorption of food.

Small intestinal transplantation

Transplantation of the small intestine is slowly gaining acceptance as a treatment for short gut syndrome, especially when complications associated with total parenteral nutrition occur. Although the transplanted segment of small intestine is extrinsically denervated, the enteric nervous system remains largely intact if the warm ischemic time is kept to a minimum. Animal studies demonstrated the presence of MMCs in isografts and autotransplants of the jejunoileum. MMCs also occurred in the native duodenum, but were not temporally coordinated with MMCs in the transplanted segment. In experiments in dogs, feeding did not interrupt MMCs in the transplanted intestine or induce a fed pattern of contractile activity, except in one study in which dogs were fed a 500-g meal. In rats, *ad libitum* feeding interrupted MMCs and induced a fed pattern of contractile activity. These results suggest that a transplanted small intestine can develop relatively normal patterns of contractile activity.

Disorders of colon and rectal motility

Idiopathic chronic constipation

It is exceedingly difficult to define unequivocally normal bowel function. A normal frequency is generally accepted as ranging from three bowel movements daily to one every third day. Frequency may be altered by dietary factors, particularly the fiber content of the diet. Because of the difficulty of defining a normal pattern, abnormal patterns also are poorly defined. While a stool frequency of fewer than three bowel movements weekly constitutes significant constipation, 7 days between bowel movements is several standard deviations away from normal and satisfies the author's criterion for severe constipation.

A review of the manifold causes of constipation, as well as clinical evaluation and management, may be found in Chapter 10. Since different approaches have been developed for the management of different subgroups of patients with idiopathic chronic constipation, it is increasingly important to establish a correct and specific diagnosis.

Colonic inertia

Constipation may result from an inability of colonic motor activity to propel fecal contents into the rectosigmoid in a timely fashion, a condition called colonic inertia or idiopathic colonic dysmotility. The exact defect in idiopathic colonic dysmotility is poorly understood, but may involve an abnormality of myogenic, neural, or biochemical control.

No consistent defect involving hypermotility or hypomotility of the colon, either in the fasting state or postprandially, has been identified [46, 47]. Abnormalities of the myenteric plexus have been reported: in a histologic study using silver stain, Krishnamurthy *et al.* [48] observed a reduced number of argyrophilic neurons, the presence of abnormal argyrophilic neurons, a decrease in the number of axons, and an increase in the number of variably sized nuclei within the enteric ganglia of severely constipated patients. Our laboratory [49] has since confirmed these observations. While abnormalities of the myenteric plexus would be expected to affect colonic contractility, their precise relationship to idiopathic constipation is not known.

Rectal outlet obstruction

Sarna [50, 51] recently summarized the disorders of the rectal sphincter area that may contribute to constipation. The rectum may be unable to sense the presence of stool and transmit a signal to the higher centers. The internal anal sphincter may not relax in response to rectal distention when stool is propelled into it, or the external anal sphincter fails to relax in response to voluntary neurologic input. Finally, the puborectalis muscle may fail to relax during defecation.

Rectal sensation, as measured by balloon distention, is impaired in many patients with severe constipation. The inability of the rectum to sense the presence of a large volume of feces may be due to rectal adaptation to the continued presence of stools, a neural disorder, or the absence of giant migrating contractions in the distal colon which normally propel stool rapidly into the rectum and distend it. In any individual, it is difficult to know whether the apparent decrease in sensory threshold is a primary or secondary event.

Hirschsprung's disease classically consists of aganglionosis of the rectum and colon and presents in childhood with symptoms of constipation, colonic obstruction, or sepsis due to enterocolitis. In rare cases, Hirschsprung's disease remains undiagnosed until adolescence or adulthood. In such patients, the prolonged partial colonic obstruction is overcome by hypertrophy of the active, normally innervated proximal bowel. In addition, patients can compensate for the obstructed aganglionic bowel by the use of cathartics and enemas. Ultimately, however, the dilated colon may decompensate secondary to the distal physiologic obstruction, and the patient may experience rapidly worsening constipation or even acute obstruction. It is at this advanced stage of Hirschsprung's disease that the adult will present for definitive diagnosis and surgical management. Anorectal manometry, an important diagnostic tool, can demonstrate whether the internal anal sphincter relaxes insufficiently, does not relax at all, or even contracts in response to rectal distention in patients with this deficit.

Pelvic floor outlet obstruction is a rare cause of severe constipation [52]. This diagnosis should not be confused with other problems of the pelvic floor, such as anal pain caused by a hypertrophic internal anal sphincter, anal ulcer, anal stenosis, irritation of the pelvic floor caused by injury or inflammation, and internal intussusception of the rectum causing outlet obstruction. While the mean anorectal angle during the resting state is the same in patients with constipation and healthy subjects, it becomes more acute during defecation in constipated patients, suggesting a greater anatomic resistance to evacuation. In some patients, contraction of the pelvic floor during defecation also may contribute to constipation. Because failure of the puborectalis muscle to relax is commonly associated with other pelvic floor abnormalities, it is unclear whether this finding is of primary or secondary importance. The puborectalis muscle and the external sphincter muscle function as a unit, even though they are separately innervated. When one muscle contracts, the other follows. They also malfunction as a unit and may cause secondary problems. Combined with laxity of the rectosigmoid mesentery and abnormal straining, nonrelaxation of the pelvic floor during defecation may eventually lead to internal intussusception, anterior rectocele, and even rectal prolapse [53, 54].

Surgical treatment

Hirschsprung's disease

If a clear diagnosis of adult Hirschsprung's disease can be made by anorectal manometry, or perhaps by a full-thickness biopsy, surgery is generally indicated. The surgical management of adult Hirschsprung's disease is controversial (Table 13.4) [55]. The Soave endorectal pull-through has produced good results in pediatric patients and, because the dissection is performed within the endorectal plane, there is no risk of pelvic nerve injury. In adults, long-term results with this procedure have been satisfactory, but the incidence of postoperative complications is much higher than that reported in children. The increased risk of complications may argue against use of the Soave procedure in adults, particularly if it is performed by a surgeon with limited experience in this technique. Increasing experience with endorectal pull-through procedures for chronic ulcerative colitis and familial polyposis coli should reduce the morbidity rate associated with essentially the same operation in adults with Hirschsprung's disease.

The Duhamel retrorectal pull-through procedure has a long-term efficacy rate of 91% and the advantage of avoiding an extensive pelvic dissection. The frequency of major postoperative complications is less than with the endorectal pull-through (10% versus 25% in adults,

Table 13.4 Results of surgical treatment in 199 adults with Hirschsprung's disease. (From Wheatley *et al.* [55].)

Procedure	Number	Complications	Results
Endorectal pull-through	32	Major: 8 (25%) Minor: 4 (13%)	Good: 27 (85%) Fair: 2 (6%) Poor: 3 (9%)
Duhamel procedure	58	Major: 6 (10%) Minor: 1 (2%)	Good: 53 (91%) Fair: 4 (7%) Poor: 1 (2%)
Swenson procedure	30	Major: 10 (33%) Minor: 2 (7%)	Good: 24 (80%) Fair: 6 (20%)
Low anterior resection	18	Major: 8 (6%) Minor: 0 (0%) Death: 1 (6%)	Good: 13 (67%) Fair: 2 (11%) Poor: 3 (17%)
Colectomy	15	Major: 4 (27%) Minor: 0 (0%) Death: 1 (7%)	Good: 10 (67%) Fair: 1 (7%) Poor: 4 (26%)
Posterior anorectal myectomy	38	Major: 0 (0%) Minor: 1 (3%)	Good: 21 (55%) Fair: 2 (5%) Poor: 15 (40%)
Posterior anorectal myectomy and low anterior resection	8	Major: 0 (0%)	Good: 8 (100%)

respectively). As with the latter, the most prevalent complication of the Duhamel procedure is anastomotic disruption, leading to abscess or fistula formation.

The Swenson pull-through procedure is associated with major complications in 33% of patients, including impotence in 7%, according to several series in adult patients. Satisfactory long-term results were reported in only 80% of patients.

Recent reports have advocated posterior anorectal myectomy as the initial approach to adult Hirschsprung's disease. This procedure is easy to perform, does not require pelvic dissection, and is associated with a low morbidity rate. Although 40% of recipients are treatment failures, many are managed relatively easily with a subsequent anterior resection or pull-through procedure.

Low anterior resection and left hemicolectomy or subtotal colectomy have been advocated for the treatment of adult Hirschsprung's disease, but they do not address the fundamental problem of rectal aganglionosis with spasm. Their use has been largely abandoned.

In summary, although controversial, anorectal myectomy appears to be a reasonable first-line surgical therapy for short-segment adult Hirschsprung's disease. The best long-term results are obtained with a Soave endorectal or a Duhamel retrorectal pull-through operation.

Pelvic floor outlet obstruction

Surgery has not been a successful treatment option. Puborectalis muscle incision and myectomy have produced variable results and may result in a patient who is incontinent of solid stool. Excellent long-term results have been reported recently [56] with biofeedback techniques, including outpatient methods [52, 57], with restoration of normal bowel function.

Idiopathic colonic dysmotility

Definitive surgery is reserved for individuals with severe chronic idiopathic constipation who are truly refractory to medical management, including dietary manipulation and the use of stool softeners, anticonstipant medications, and enemas. In patients with an unequivocal diagnosis of colonic inertia with normal anorectal function, several procedures have been advocated. Segmental colectomy appeared promising in patients with apparent segmental dilatation of part of the colon, but results have been disappointing. Total abdominal colectomy with ileorectal anastomosis has been successful in 66–100% (average: 88%) of patients with severe idiopathic constipation.

In our laboratory [49], a series of 12 patients received a diagnosis of primary colonic dysmotility without anorectal dysfunction based on physiologic, radiographic, and histologic testing (Table 13.5). These patients received standard treatment with total abdominal colectomy and ileorectal anastomosis and were followed carefully for 2 years or more. In all patients, histologic analysis with silver staining revealed defects in the myenteric plexus. These patients did not require cathartic or antidiarrheal medications and had normal stool frequency at 24 months post-operatively. Ninety-two per cent of patients were extremely satisfied and 8% were satisfied with their outcome. There were no treatment failures.

Until better methods for localization and documentation of segmental colonic motility are available, total abdominal colectomy with ileorectal anastomosis appears to be the most effective operation when anorectal manometric findings are normal. A high percentage of patients have good or excellent long-term results with this approach.

Table 13.5 Surgical treatment of colonic dysmotility: 24-month functional results. (Data from Zenilman et al. [49]; © 1989, American Medical Association.)

Nocturnal stools		1/12 (8%)
Minor leakage		2/12 (17%)
Dietary modification		3/12 (25%)
Anticonstipant medication		0/12 (0%)
Stool consistency	Formed	9/12 (75%)
	Soft	3/12 (25%)
	Liquid	0/12 (0%)
Patient satisfaction	Excellent	11/12 (92%)
	Good	1/12 (8%)
	Poor	0/12 (0%)

Motor disorders of the biliary tract

Over the past decade, the development of biliary manometry, biliary scintigraphy, and ultrasonography to assess dynamic changes in the sphincter of Oddi, gallbladder volume, and bile flow have led to an increased understanding of biliary tract motility [58–60].

Sphincter of Oddi dysfunction is usually seen in women following cholecystectomy. It affects approximately 6000 new patients in the USA annually [61], constituting 15% of all patients with postcholecystectomy pain and less than 1% of patients who undergo cholecystectomy. The pain is frequently biliary-like and is associated with recurring bouts of epigastric or right upper quadrant pain, which often radiates to the back and is exacerbated by meals. The pain may be followed by nausea and vomiting and is accompanied rarely by fever, jaundice, or frank pancreatitis. Some patients may have intermittent or constant abnormalities of liver enzymes, particularly serum alkaline phosphatase. Others may have intermittent elevations of serum amylase levels. Before sphincter of Oddi dysfunction is considered, the possibility of retained common bile duct stones should be excluded by cholangiography. Other upper GI tract disorders with a similar clinical presentation also should be excluded, including peptic ulcer, gastritis, pancreatitis, and irritable bowel syndrome.

Clinical evaluation

The clinical evaluation of patients with sphincter of Oddi dysfunction should include a history and physical examination, liver function tests, and measurement of serum amylase levels. At present there is no definitive diagnostic standard, but many diagnostic tests have been proposed. Most current methods used to diagnose and treat sphincter dysfunction are largely unproven, and most reports are based on uncontrolled studies. Only in the past several years have new approaches to the problem been developed.

Previously, the diagnosis of sphincter of Oddi dysfunction or papillary stenosis could be made only in the operating room, and then with very imprecise techniques. In general, the decision to perform a surgical sphincteroplasty was based on the finding of resistance to flow of a column of contrast material introduced through a T-tube into the distal common bile duct. In some cases the contrast study was combined with intraoperative manometry. A presumptive diagnosis of sphincter stenosis was suggested if resistance exceeded $30\,cmH_2O$ in the distal bile duct in the absence of impacted stones. The diagnosis was confirmed by an inability to pass a 3-mm Bakes dilator through the sphincter of Oddi into the duodenum or an inability to pass a 2-mm lacrimal probe into the pancreatic duct transduodenally. Neither technique ensured either a diagnosis of papillary stenosis or a good result following surgical sphincteroplasty.

A radiographic diagnosis is based on the demonstration of a dilated common bile duct and delayed biliary drainage after endoscopic retrograde cholangiopancreatography (ERCP) or intravenous cholangio-graphy (Figure 13.4). A number of factors suggest that the diameter of the common bile duct may not be useful in making a diagnosis of sphincter of Oddi stenosis: variations in normal duct size, controversy over the existence of postcholecystectomy dilatation, and a normal-sized common bile duct in the presence of severe stenosis.

Delayed emptying of the common bile duct in excess of 45 minutes following ERCP may be suggestive of sphincter of Oddi dysfunction. This test is poorly standardized, however, with limited data to support its use.

A new approach to documenting delayed common duct emptying is nuclear scintigraphy [62]. Hepatobiliary scintigraphy (Figure 13.5) essentially entails no morbidity or mortality. Unlike intravenous chol-angiography, it can be performed in the presence of an elevated serum bilirubin level; unlike ERCP, it is easily performed in most hospitals. The technique can be standardized and provides quantitative as well as qualitative information. Using this technique, delayed biliary-to-bowel transit can be demonstrated in patients whose ducts are not opacified on

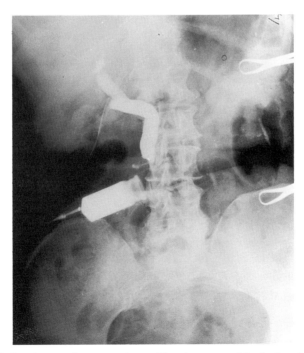

Fig. 13.4 Cholangiogram demonstrating a dilated common bile duct and delayed biliary drainage.

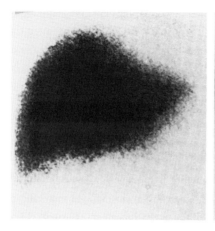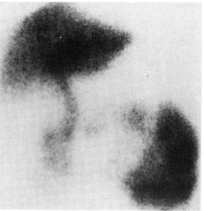

Fig. 13.5 Nuclear scintigram demonstrating delayed emptying of the common bile duct.

ERCP and in those who cannot tolerate endoscopic manometry because of severe stenosis of the sphincter of Oddi.

Scintigraphy appears to be less sensitive than biliary manometry: it has a reported sensitivity of about 83% in identifying patients with partial obstruction of the distal common duct and a false-positive rate of 10–15%. Another disadvantage is that it frequently does not differentiate parenchymal liver disease from common duct pathology. Thus, hepatobiliary scintigraphy may be useful as a screening modality or in institutions where endoscopic manometry and ERCP cannot be performed. It also may provide an objective measure of therapeutic response.

Provocative testing, such as the morphine–prostigmine test, has been used for decades to establish the diagnosis of papillary stenosis or sphincter of Oddi dysfunction. Patients are administered the medications and then observed to determine whether their typical pain is reproduced along with a rise in pancreatic- or liver-associated enzymes, or both. Early reports supported the clinical usefulness of these tests, but more recent prospective studies [63, 64] have shown them to be neither specific nor sensitive for sphincter dysfunction. Nitroglycerin also has been used to evaluate the pain associated with sphincter of Oddi dysfunction. It has been postulated that nitroglycerin-sensitive pain is attributed to dyskinesia of the sphincter, whereas nitroglycerin-insensitive pain is attributed to stenosis of the papilla.

Another noninvasive diagnostic approach is the combined use of ultrasound evaluation of the bile duct and pancreatic stimulation, either with a fatty meal or with intravenous cholecystokinin octapeptide (CCK_8). Some studies suggest that both fatty meals and CCK_8 can cause dilatation of the common bile duct in an unobstructed duct, but not in a nonobstructed one. Obstruction may be secondary to a structural problem, such as a stone, or to a functional problem, such as sphincter of Oddi dysfunction. Cholangiography should be performed initially, to rule out a structural lesion. A recent study [62] suggests that fatty-meal scintigraphy has a sensitivity of 67% and a specificity of 100% for diagnosing a mechanical or functional obstruction of the duct.

A similar approach uses ultrasonography to assess changes in the diameters of the pancreatic and bile ducts after stimulation of pancreatic secretion by secretin. Warshaw *et al.* [64] reported pancreatic duct dilatation in 10 of 12 (83%) symptomatic patients who were found at surgery to have sphincter of Oddi stenosis. On repeat testing after surgical sphincteroplasty, no ductal dilatation was demonstrated after secretin stimulation. Surgical sphincteroplasty successfully prevented recurrent pancreatitis and ameliorated pain in 90% of patients with a positive test result. The success rate was only 29% in patients who tested negative. While this test may be useful, it requires further evaluation.

The development of ERCP has provided a nonsurgical method for diagnosing sphincter of Oddi dysfunction. ERCP can be used to assess the ease of cannulation of the papilla as well as the appearance of the papilla, to provide anatomic definition after instillation of a contrast agent into the pancreaticobiliary ducts, and to evaluate the ductal emptying rate. In addition, pressure and motility patterns of the sphincter of Oddi zone can be measured directly by ERCP manometric techniques. Only biliary manometry has demonstrated value in assessing the possibility of sphincter dysfunction. However, the procedure is invasive and difficult to perform; the patient is sedated and generally not experiencing acute pain during the study. Because of insufficient data on sphincter of Oddi pressures in normal individuals, asymptomatic patients after cholecystectomy, and patients with other causes of abdominal pain, the data generated in patients with sphincter dysfunction may be difficult to interpret.

To avoid the problems of sedation, limited sampling, and procedure-related morbidity, techniques have been developed for placing an indwelling microtransducer catheter into the common duct during ERCP. The endoscope is removed, and the transducer remains in place. The patient can then be studied under various conditions without sedation.

Motility disorders in sphincter of Oddi dysfunction

Four motility abnormalities are characteristic in patients with suspected sphincter of Oddi dysfunction:

1 an elevated basal pressure;
2 a paradoxical response to CCK_8;
3 retrograde propagation of phasic waves;
4 an increased frequency of phasic wave contractions (tachyoddia).

An increase in basal pressure may result from spasm or fibrosis involving the terminal bile duct or pancreatic duct. The elevation appears to correlate most closely with papillary or sphincter dysfunction and to predict most accurately a good outcome following endoscopic or surgical sphincterotomy. Differences in the basal pressures of the sphincter of Oddi and common bile duct have been noted among control subjects, probably owing to the use of different types of catheters and infusion techniques in various studies. However, cumulative data suggest that a sphincter of Oddi basal pressure greater than 40–45 mmHg is abnormally elevated.

Normally, the phasic activity of the sphincter of Oddi in humans is abolished by intravenous pulse doses of CCK_8. However, paradoxical increases in phasic wave contractions have been observed following such administration in a number of patients with papillary stenosis. According to one proposed explanation, the effect of CCK on the sphincter of Oddi is mediated by the stimulation of inhibitory nerves that override the direct excitatory effect of CCK on the smooth muscle of the sphincter. In the presence of impaired inhibitory sphincter innervation, CCK would act directly on smooth muscle and cause sphincter contraction. Impaired inhibitory innervation may also account for the elevated basal sphincter pressures in many of these patients.

Antegrade propagation of phasic waves predominates in the normal sphincter of Oddi in humans, a process apparently controlled by a myogenic pacemaker. Predominantly retrograde propagation was identified initially in patients with common bile duct stones, but also has been reported in patients with sphincter of Oddi dysfunction.

Phasic wave contractions occurring at a rate of more than 10/min have been observed in patients with papillary dysfunction. This increased frequency may result in shortening of the diastole, or the filling phase of the sphincter, and thus in decreased biliary emptying.

Treatment

Treatment options for sphincter of Oddi dysfunction include pharmacotherapy and surgical or endoscopic sphincterotomy. Small uncontrolled series have suggested that calcium channel blockers, by causing
the sphincter of Oddi to relax, induce dose-dependent decreases in
sphincter pressure and motor activity in healthy controls as well as
patients with sphincter dysfunction. It also has been suggested that
nitroglycerin alleviates abdominal pain and relaxes the sphincter, as
determined by endoscopy. Controlled trials of medical therapy are
obviously needed. Other agents that may be useful include anticholinergics, cerulein, and pancreatic enzyme supplements.

Studies [63, 65] have reported symptomatic relief with endoscopic
sphincterotomy in patients with sphincter of Oddi dysfunction. A good
outcome after this procedure has been reported primarily in older
patients with a dilated common bile duct and decreased emptying after
ERCP. In a prospective randomized study by Geenen *et al.* [63], endoscopic sphincterotomy reduced pain sensations over a 4-year follow-up
period in most patients with elevated sphincter of Oddi pressures, while
sham procedures improved symptoms in only a few patients (Figure
13.6). Sphincterotomy did not improve symptoms, however, in patients
with normal sphincter pressures. These findings were not reproduced in
several retrospective studies.

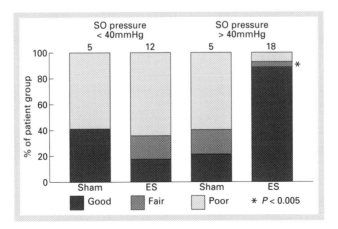

Fig. 13.6 Endoscopic sphincterotomy (ES) resulted in reduction of pain sensation over
a 4-year follow-up period in most patients with high sphincter of Oddi pressure, while
sham procedures improved symptoms in few. (Reprinted with permission from the
New England Journal of Medicine. Geenen *et al.* [63]; © 1996, Massachusetts Medical
Society.)

At present, there is no consensus as to the parameters that best predict a successful outcome with endoscopic sphincterotomy (Table 13.6 [66]; Figure 13.7). In patients with suspected sphincter dysfunction, endoscopic sphincterotomy is associated with a 0.4% mortality rate. However, the complication rate may be as high as 10–15% when the procedure is performed to correct sphincter dysfunction, compared with a 6% rate in operations to treat retained gallstones.

Other endoscopic procedures have been advocated for the treatment of papillary dysfunction. Balloon dilatation for sphincter of Oddi dysfunction has been attempted, but is associated with an unacceptably high complication rate. A trial of temporary pancreatic stent placement may identify patients who would benefit from pancreatic duct sphincterotomy. However, indwelling stents are potentially dangerous and have not been tested systematically.

Until endoscopic techniques that disrupt the sphincter of Oddi were developed, surgical sphincteroplasty was performed in patients with suspected papillary stenosis. The technique was modified by some surgeons to include division of the septum lying between the distal common bile duct and the pancreatic duct. In the largest such series, reported by Moody *et al.* [67], 36 of 83 (43%) patients experienced no pain 10 years after surgery, 27 (33%) experienced occasional pain, and 20 (24%) had no relief of pain. The most difficult aspect of this type of surgical treatment is patient selection.

Whether this operation provides better overall results than endoscopic sphincterotomy is questionable. With both surgical and endoscopic

Table 13.6 Milwaukee biliary classification to differentiate stenosis and dyskinesia of the sphincter of Oddi. (From Hogan & Geenen [66].)

Biliary group I	Biliary group II	Biliary group III
Biliary-type pain *plus* all of the findings listed below	Biliary-type pain *plus* one or two of the findings listed below	Biliary-type pain alone

FINDINGS
- Abnormal LFTs: AP and AST > twice normal on two occasions
- Dilated common bile duct (>12 mm) by ultrasound
- Delayed drainage of radiocontrast after ERCP (>45 minutes)

AP, alkaline phosphatase; AST, aspartate aminotransferase; ERCP, endoscopic retrograde cholangiopancreatography; LFTs, liver function tests.

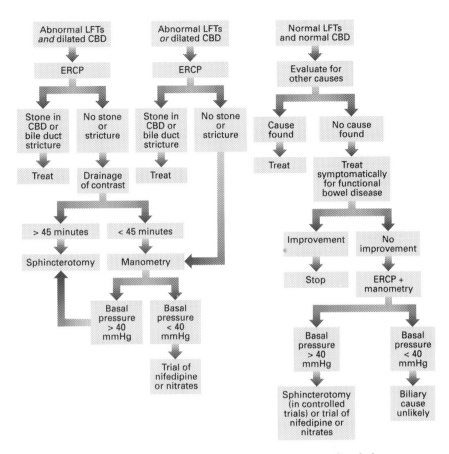

Fig. 13.7 Flow diagram for the management of biliary-type pain after cholecystectomy. CBD, common bile duct; ERCP, endoscopic retrograde cholangiopancreatography; LFTs, liver function tests.

sphincterotomy, the restenosis rate appears to be relatively high, possibly because of incomplete sectioning of the sphincter. It may be that surgical sphincteroplasty permits more extensive sectioning of the sphincter. Nevertheless, it would seem reasonable to perform the less morbid endoscopic procedure first. If symptoms are unrelieved or recur, and subsequent evaluation shows restenosis of the endoscopic sphincterotomy, then a surgical sphincteroplasty may be considered.

Summary

Developments in diagnostic technique have enabled better identification of the underlying pathophysiology in patients with GI symptoms. These newer technologies also have resulted in better identification of patients who may benefit from surgical treatment, resulting in enhanced clinical outcomes. In addition, treatment results have improved as a result of newer operative techniques, such as laparoscopic or thoracoscopic myotomy of the LES in patients with achalasia and endoscopic sphincterotomy for dysfunction of the sphincter of Oddi.

References

1 Becker JM. Motility disorders of the gastrointestinal tract. *Surg Clin North Am* 1993;**73**:1081–346.

2 DeMeester TR. The role of surgery in motor disorders of the upper gastrointestinal tract. In: Fisher RS, Krevsky B, eds. *Motor Disorders of the Gastrointestinal Tract: What's New and What to Do.* New York: Academy Professional Information Services Inc, 1993:85–91.

3 Ellis FH Jr, Olsen AM, Schlegel JF, Code CF. Surgical treatment of esophageal hypermotility disturbances. *JAMA* 1964;**188**:862–6.

4 Hurwitz AL, Duranceau A. Upper-esophageal sphincter dysfunction: pathogenesis and treatment. *Am J Dig Dis* 1978;**23**:275–81.

5 Bonavina L, Khan NA, DeMeester TR. Pharyngoesophageal dysfunction: the role of cricopharyngeal myotomy. *Arch Surg* 1985;**120**:541–9.

6 Ellis FH Jr, Crozier RE. Cervical esophageal dysphagia: indications for and results of cricopharyngeal myotomy. *Ann Surg* 1981;**194**:279–89.

7 Cook IJ, Blumbergs P, Cash K *et al.* Zenker's diverticulum: evidence for a restrictive cricopharyngeal myopathy. *Gastroenterology* 1989;**96**:A98.

8 Csendes A, Velasco N, Braghetto I, Henriquez A. A prospective randomized study comparing forceful dilatation and esophagomyotomy in patients with achalasia of the esophagus. *Gastroenterology* 1981;**80**:789–95.

9 Csendes A, Braghetto I, Henriquez A, Cortes C. Late results of a prospective randomised study comparing forceful dilatation and oesophagomyotomy in patients with achalasia. *Gut* 1989;**30**:299–304.

10 Zaninotto G, DeMeester TR, Schwizer W, Johansson KE, Cheng S-C. The lower esophageal sphincter in health and disease. *Am J Surg* 1988;**155**:104–11.

11 Stein HJ, DeMeester TR, Naspetti R, Jamieson J, Perry RE. Three-dimensional imaging of the lower esophageal sphincter in gastroesophageal reflux disease. *Ann Surg* 1991;**214**:374–84.

12 Stein HJ, Eypasch EP, DeMeester TR, Smyrck TC, Attwood SEA. Circadian esophageal motor function in patients with gastroesophageal reflux disease. *Surgery* 1990;**108**:769–78.

13 DeMeester TR, Stein JH. Surgical treatment of gastroesophageal reflux disease. In: Castell DO, ed. *The Esophagus.* Boston: Little, Brown and Co, 1992:579–625.

14 McKelvey ST. Gastric incontinence and post-vagotomy diarrhoea. *Br J Surg* 1970;**57**:741–7.

15 Strauss R, Wise L. New concepts in the prevention, causes and treatment of post-vagotomy diarrhea. *Curr Surg* 1978;**35**:77–84.

16 Bond JH, Levitt MD. Use of breath hydrogen (H_2) to quantitate small bowel transit time following partial gastrectomy. *J Lab Clin Med* 1977;**90**:30–6.

17 Kelly KA, Becker JM, Van Heerden JA. Reconstructive gastric surgery. *Br J Surg* 1981;**68**:687–91.

18 Becker JM, Sava P, Kelly KA, Shturman L. Intestinal pacing for canine post-gastrectomy dumping. *Gastroenterology* 1983;**84**:383–7.

19 Kelly KA, Code CF. Duodenal-gastric reflux and slowed gastric emptying by electrical pacing of the canine duodenal pacesetter potential. *Gastroenterology* 1977;**72**:429–33.

20 Cranley B, Kelly KA, Go VLW, McNichols LA. Enhancing the anti-dumping effect of Roux gastrojejunostomy with intestinal pacing. *Ann Surg* 1983;**198**:516–24.

21 Britton JP, Johnston D, Wand DC, Axon AT, Barker MC. Gastric emptying and clinical outcome after Roux-en-Y diversion. *Br J Surg* 1987;**74**:900–4.

22 Gustavsson S, Ilstrup DM, Morrison P, Kelly KA. Roux-Y stasis syndrome after gastrectomy. *Am J Surg* 1988;**155**:490–4.

23 Eckhauser FE, Knol JA, Raper SA, Guice KS. Completion gastrectomy for post-surgical gastroparesis syndrome: preliminary results with 15 patients. *Ann Surg* 1988;**208**:345–53.

24 Perino LE, Adcock KA, Goff JS. Gastrointestinal symptoms, motility, and transit after Roux-en-Y operation. *Am J Gastroenterol* 1988;**83**:380–5.

25 Hermon-Taylor J, Code CF. Localization of the duodenal pacemaker and its role in the organization of duodenal myoelectric activity. *Gut* 1971;**12**:40–7.

26 Richter HM III, Kelly KA. Effect of transection and pacing on human jejunal pacesetter potentials. *Gastroenterology* 1986;**91**:1380–5.

27 Karlstrom LH, Soper NJ, Kelly KA, Phillips SF. Ectopic jejunal pacemakers and enterogastric reflux after Roux gastrectomy: effect of intestinal pacing. *Surgery* 1989;**106**:486–95.

28 Fich A, Neri M, Camilleri M, Kelly KA, Phillips SA. Stasis syndromes following gastric surgery: clinical and motility features of 60 symptomatic patients. *J Clin Gastroenterol* 1990;**12**:505–12.

29 Mathias JR, Fernandez A, Sninsky CA, Clench MH, Davis RH. Nausea, vomiting and abdominal pain after Roux-en-Y anastomosis: motility of the jejunal limb. *Gastroenterology* 1985;**88**:101–7.

30 Van Stiegmann G, Goff JS. An alternative to Roux-en-Y for treatment of bile reflux gastritis. *Surg Gynecol Obstet* 1988;**166**:69–70.

31 Cullen JJ, Kelly KA. Gastric motor physiology and pathophysiology. In: Becker JM, ed. Motility disorders of the gastrointestinal tract. *Surg Clin North Am* 1993;**73**:1145–60.

32 Miedema BW, Kelly KA. The Roux stasis syndrome: treatment by pacing and prevention by use of an 'uncut' Roux limb. *Arch Surg* 1992;**127**:295–300.

33 Ritchie WP Jr. Alkaline reflux gastritis: an objective assessment of its diagnosis and treatment. *Ann Surg* 1980;**192**:288–98.

34 Boren CH, Way LW. Alkaline reflux gastritis: a reevaluation. *Am J Surg* 1980;**140**:40–5.

35 Sawyers JL, Herrington JL, Buckspan GS. Remedial operation for alkaline reflux gastritis and associated postgastrectomy syndromes. *Arch Surg* 1980;**115**:519–24.

36 Telford GL, Walgenbach-Telford S, Sarna SK. Pathophysiology of small intestinal motility. In: Becker JM, ed. Motility disorders of the gastrointestinal tract. *Surg Clin North Am* 1993;**73**:1193–9.

37 Sarr MG, Tito WA. Intestinal obstruction. In: Zuidema GD, ed. *Shackerford's Surgery of the Alimentary Tract*, Vol. 5, 372–413. 3rd edn. Philadelphia: WB Saunders Co, 1991.

38 Summers RW, Yanda R, Prihoda M, Flatt A. Acute intestinal obstruction: an electromyographic study in dogs. *Gastroenterology* 1983;**85**:1301–6.

39 Condon RE, Sarna SK. Motility after abdominal surgery. *Clin Gastroenterol* 1982;**11**:609–20.

40 Livingston EH, Passaro EP Jr. Postoperative ileus. *Dig Dis Sci* 1990;**35**:121–32.

41 Waldhausen JHT, Shaffrey ME, Skenderis BS II, Jones RS, Schirmer BD. Gastrointestinal myoelectric and clinical patterns of recovery after laparotomy. *Ann Surg* 1990;**211**:777–85.

42 Bueno L, Fioramonti J, Ruckebusch Y. Postoperative intestinal motility in dogs and sheep. *Am J Dig Dis* 1978;**23**:682–9.

43 Sarna SK. *In vivo* myoelectric methods, analysis and interpretation. In: Wood JD, ed. *Handbook of Physiology: Motility and Circulation*, Vol. 1. Bethesda, MD: American Physiological Society, 1989;817–63.

44 Sarna SK, Otterson MF. Small intestinal physiology and pathophysiology. *Gastroenterol Clin North Am* 1989;**18**:375–404.

45 Eagon JC, Cullen JT, Kelly KA. Ectopic jejunal pacemakers after bowel transection and their relationship to transit. *Gastroenterology* 1993;**104**:A501.

46 Shouler P, Keighley MRB. Changes in colorectal function in severe idiopathic chronic constipation. *Gastroenterology* 1986;**90**:414–20.

47 Krevsky B, Malmud LS, Maurer AH *et al*. The effect of oral cisapride on colonic transit. *Aliment Pharmacol Ther* 1987;**1**:293–304.

48 Krishnamurthy P, Schuffler MD, Rohrmann CA, Pope CE II. Severe idiopathic constipation is associated with a distinctive abnormality of the colonic myenteric plexus. *Gastroenterology* 1985;**88**:26–34.

49 Zenilman ME, Dunnegan DL, Soper NJ, Becker JM. Successful surgical treatment of idiopathic colonic dysmotility. *Arch Surg* 1989;**124**:947–51.

50 Sarna SK. Physiology and pathophysiology of colonic motor activity, part 1 of 2. *Dig Dis Sci* 1991;**36**:827–62.

51 Sarna SK. Physiology and pathophysiology of colonic motor activity, part 2 of 2. *Dig Dis Sci* 1991;**36**:998–1018.

52 Fleshman JW, Dreznik Z, Meyer K, Fry R, Carney R, Kodner IJ. Outpatient protocol for biofeedback therapy of pelvic floor obstruction. *Dis Colon Rectum* 1992;**35**:1–7.

53 Martelli H, Devroede G, Arhan P, Duguay C. Mechanisms of idiopathic constipation: outlet obstruction. *Gastroenterology* 1978;**75**:623–31.

54 Read NW, Timms JM, Barfield LJ, Donnelly TC, Bannister JJ. Impairment of defecation in young women with severe constipation. *Gastroenterology* 1986;**90**:53–60.

55 Wheatley MJ, Wesley JR, Coran AG, Polley TZ Jr. Hirschsprung's disease in adolescents and adults. *Dis Colon Rectum* 1990;**33**:622–9.

56 Bleijenberg G, Kuijpers HC. Treatment of the spastic pelvic floor syndrome with biofeedback. *Dis Colon Rectum* 1987;**30**:108–11.

57 Wexner SD, Cheape JD, Jorge JMN, Heymen S, Jagelman DG. Prospective assessment of biofeedback for the treatment of paradoxical puborectalis contraction. *Dis Colon Rectum* 1992;**35**:145–50.

58 Becker JM, Moody FG. Sphincter of Oddi and biliary motility. In: Condon RE, DeCosse J, eds. *Surgical Care II*. Philadelphia: Lea & Febiger, 1985:40–55.

59 Parodi JE, Becker JM. Biliary motility. *Curr Opin Gastroenterol* 1989;**5**:606–16.

60 Parodi JE, Becker JM. Gallbladder and sphincter of Oddi motility. *Curr Opin Gastroenterol* 1990;**6**:668–76.

61 Steinberg WM. Sphincter of Oddi dysfunction: a clinical controversy. *Gastroenterology* 1988;**95**:1409–15.

62 Lee RGL, Gregg JA, Koroshetz AM, Hill TC, Clouse ME. Sphincter of Oddi stenosis: diagnosis using hepatobiliary scintigraphy and endoscopic manometry. *Radiology* 1985;**156**:793–6.

63 Geenen JE, Hogan WJ, Dodds WJ, Toouli J, Venu RP. The efficacy of endoscopic

sphincterotomy after cholecystectomy in patients with sphincter-of-Oddi dysfunction. *N Engl J Med* 1989;**320**:82–7.

64 Warshaw AL, Simeone J, Schapiro RH, Hedberg SE, Mueller PE, Ferrucci JT. Objective evaluation of ampullary stenosis with ultrasonography and pancreatic stimulation. *Am J Surg* 1985;**149**:65–72.

65 Neoptolemos JP, Bailey IS, Carr-Locke DL. Sphincter of Oddi dysfunction: results of treatment by endoscopic sphincterotomy. *Br J Surg* 1988;**75**:454–9.

66 Hogan WJ, Geenen JE. Biliary dyskinesia. *Endoscopy* 1988;**20**:179–83.

67 Moody FG, Becker JM, Potts JR. Transduodenal sphincteroplasty and transampullary septectomy for postcholecystectomy pain. *Ann Surg* 1983;**197**:627–36.

« 14 »
The Future of Gastrointestinal Motility

Malcolm C. Champion and William C. Orr

It is anticipated that rapid advances will occur in our understanding of the pathophysiology, diagnosis, and treatment of gastrointestinal (GI) motility disorders. This chapter reviews the future of GI motility and is based on discussion and contribution from all of the textbook authors.

At least three themes appear to be common to all areas of GI motility.
1 There is a need for better definition and consistency in the classification of motility disorders. This will lead to greater uniformity in patient classification and consequently more reliable results in therapeutic trials.
2 There is general concern over the lack of correlation between symptoms and objective parameters of motility abnormality. This is particularly the case in diffuse esophageal spasm, noncardiac chest pain, functional dyspepsia, gastroparesis, and the irritable bowel syndrome (IBS). An understanding of the relationship between symptoms and specific motility abnormalities will be enhanced by the burgeoning of research into the mechanisms of visceral sensation.
3 Expanded options for the treatment of GI motility disorders can be anticipated. New drugs are particularly needed for esophageal motility disorders, functional dyspepsia, IBS, and constipation.

Esophageal motility disorders

Esophageal manometry will continue to expand our knowledge base in esophageal motility disorders. It is anticipated that both 24-hour ambulatory pH monitoring and manometry will be increasingly utilized to establish more reliably the relationship between symptoms and motility disorders. In the future, the use of esophageal balloon distention and the role of bolus transit time in the esophagus or, alternately, the assessment of contractile amplitudes and esophageal clearance will become better defined as to their proper utilization in delineating esophageal motility abnormalities. Furthermore, more sophisticated techniques will be utilized to determine the actual statistical relationship between symptoms and physiologic events, such as reflux or an esophageal motor abnormality. Defining an actual cause-and-effect relationship has proven to be elusive, and much more work needs to be done utilizing appropriate methodologies to define the true relationship between physiologic events and symptoms [1].

The upper esophageal sphincter (UES) remains a poorly understood structure, and patients with UES dysfunction are often referred to either a gastroenterologist, neurologist, speech pathologist, or ear, nose, and throat surgeon. More sophisticated methodologies are being applied to measuring the UES, including both manometric and radiologic technologies; these efforts should be encouraged. By using newer sensors and automated computerized evaluation of the oropharynx, simultaneous manometry, and video swallowing methodologies, advances will almost certainly be forthcoming [2]. These technologies, however, need to be developed into more user-friendly applications. The importance of lower esophageal acidification and spasm of the UES, and their respective roles in producing symptoms such as globus, should be better defined. We need to understand much more about the role of the UES in producing dysphagia, and work needs to be done in terms of defining these phenomena as well as developing new methodologies and technologies to treat dysphagia. The need for a team approach in diagnosing and treating dysphagia is essential.

The present long list of pharmacotherapeutic options for diffuse esophageal spasm (DES) suggests that we have no really effective treatment for this disorder. More successful pharmacologic approaches to DES and other esophageal dysmotilities need to be developed. Thus, advances in both technology and pharmacotherapy are needed to advance beyond the relatively unsatisfactory level of treatment that currently exists.

Gastroesophageal reflux disease (GERD)

There are several potential areas for expansion in our understanding of the pathophysiology of GERD. The role of nitric oxide (NO) in the relaxation of the lower esophageal sphincter (LES) will become better defined. Clinical investigation will evaluate whether pharmacotherapy to block the NO receptors or modulate the synthesis of NO will be of therapeutic benefit. Delineation of the mechanisms of transient relaxations of the LES (TLESRs) will continue. Its role in the development of GERD may be clarified by use of prolonged monitoring in the ambulatory setting. Trigger mechanisms for TLESR need to be better understood, and the exact roles of gastric emptying and gastric fundic tone, as well as the association between TLESRs and reflux, need to be better defined. Clearly, however, the discovery and elucidation of the role of TLESRs in the pathogenesis of GERD represents a major advance [3].

Prolonged (24-hour) ambulatory pH monitoring will become better accepted as the standard test for defining GERD. There needs to be a better understanding of the relationship between results of 24-hour ambulatory pH recording, endoscopic evaluation, and symptom occurrence. Combined 24-hour ambulatory pH and motility studies will remain a focus only for specialized centers, and it is anticipated that these ambulatory studies will enhance our understanding of how reflux relates to both mucosal damage and symptom occurrence.

Other putative mechanisms in the pathogenesis of GERD that require further clarification include the role of esophageal bicarbonate production, the importance of bile, and the circumstances under which bile becomes toxic to the esophageal mucosa. These insights will be important in patients with principally bile reflux. Should patients with documented bile and acid reflux receive acid-suppressive therapy? Wider clinical application of the bile monitor probe will also help to clarify the importance of bile in the pathogenesis of esophagitis [4].

The exact impact of over-the-counter (OTC) H_2 receptor antagonists on the referral pattern and treatment of GERD will be an interesting development over the next 5 years. It remains to be seen whether this will result in more self-medication for milder symptoms. Although the natural history of GERD is not well understood, it is not unreasonable to assume that some patients will subsequently present to physicians with more advanced disease. Will there be fewer visits to primary care physicians and fewer referrals to specialists?

Even though cisapride has been shown to be effective, continued development of drugs specifically designed to correct the motility abnormalities associated with GERD should be encouraged. The role of cisapride in combination with acid-suppressing agents for both acute and maintenance therapy should be investigated further, in light of recent promising results [5, 6]. What is the optimal role of surgery in the treatment of GERD? With evidence mounting that a combination of acid suppression and prokinetic treatment can markedly reduce relapse rates, can this approach be justified economically in light of the increasing influence of managed care?

The use of proton pump inhibitors (PPIs) as primary therapy is becoming a common practice which needs to be further refined. Would a low-dose regimen of a PPI be beneficial? Further investigation is warranted into whether relapse rates in GERD are proportional to the degree of acid suppression in acute treatment. Some preliminary data suggest that maximal acid suppression is associated with higher relapse rates [7, 8]. This may be due to a selection bias with more severe patients receiving PPI therapy. Some have suggested that a rebound hyperacidity phenomenon following discontinuation of treatment may explain relapse, but a recently published study does not confirm this speculation [9].

Respiratory symptoms, noncardiac chest pain, and other atypical manifestations of GERD need to be identified and properly treated. This will require increasing utilization of 24-hour pHmetry to identify patients in whom the relationship between gastroesophageal reflux and a particular symptom can reasonably be established. There remains a poor relationship between esophageal motility disorders and noncardiac chest pain, and this issue needs further elucidation.

The role of chronic acid suppression, laser therapy, and antireflux surgery in the management of Barrett's esophagus should become defined over the next 5 years. Dating back to the early 1970s, there has been an increase in the incidence of adenocarcinoma of the distal esophagus and proximal stomach. This has paralleled the advent of more potent acid suppression, with either H_2 antagonists or the PPIs. The increased incidence in distal esophageal adenocarcinoma is remarkable in that this has been accompanied by a concomitant decrease in incidence of squamous carcinoma of the esophagus and adenocarcinoma of the distal stomach. Is this due to the occurrence of unrecognized Barrett's esophagus, and does this suggest a more aggressive approach to the recognition of Barrett's esophagus? What are the implications for surveillance protocols for Barrett's esophagus? These questions and issues are under investigation, and more definitive answers should be forthcoming in the next few years [10].

Functional dyspepsia

There is a general consensus that functional dyspepsia or nonulcer dyspepsia (NUD) needs a more useful definition. This is particularly important in multicenter studies on functional dyspepsia. It was also felt that functional dyspepsia describes a heterogeneous group of patients. The classification of dyspeptic patients into ulcer-like, GERD-like, and motility-like subgroups has been suggested as useful in defining treatment strategies, for example using a prokinetic agent in patients with motility-like dyspepsia. Although results utilizing a similar diagnostic scheme have not been particularly encouraging [11], much more work needs to be done.

The pathophysiology of functional dyspepsia remains poorly understood, and progress has been slow due to the lack of consensus as to a precise definition of this condition. There is also a lack of correlation between symptoms and motility abnormalities in functional dyspepsia patients. It is possible that not all the motility abnormalities in functional dyspepsia may be identified by current diagnostic techniques. Whether the application of multiple techniques (e.g. gastric emptying study, antroduodenal motility, and electrogastrography (EGG)) in the same patient will define these motility abnormalities better remains to be demonstrated.

It is important to emphasize that at this time there are no rational or scientific data to support the eradication of *Helicobacter pylori* in patients with dyspeptic symptoms. However, there are some potentially interesting new therapeutic agents for functional dyspepsia. Fedotozine and the motiloids have been studied recently. Their exact role in management needs to be elaborated, as well as the role of antidepressants.

Symptom evaluation and the establishment of therapeutic endpoints in clinical studies of dyspeptic patients are critical factors in understanding pathogenesis and determining efficacious treatments. Future therapeutic trials should also include evaluation of the quality of life of the patient as well as the psychological status.

Gastroparesis

Gastric emptying studies have become well established for the assessment of gastroparesis, but there remain many limitations. If a gastric emptying study is abnormal, it confirms delayed emptying but gives no information about the underlying disorder or any abnormality in wall motion or electrical activity. There is a general concern about the lack of uniformity of gastric emptying studies. The need for each center to develop its own normal controls is important but often not accomplished [12]. It is anticipated that differences in age and gender will become more important in the evaluation of gastric emptying, since it has been shown that the rate of gastric emptying in females may be decreased as much as 40% compared with males [13]. The sensitivity of gastric emptying studies and the poor correlation of symptoms with gastric emptying need to be explored further. These problems highlight the difficulty of conducting multicenter studies without a standard protocol and a set of normal values established at each center.

The potential clinical application of dynamic antral scintigraphy, which is used to define the contraction amplitude while a gastric emptying test is being performed, needs to be determined [14]. In the future, the role of intraluminal gastric emptying measurement using a nasogastrically placed gamma probe should be elucidated. Whether this can be applied not only to stationary monitoring of gastric emptying but also to ambulatory monitoring needs to be explored. In addition to ambulatory gastric emptying [15], the importance and feasibility of ambulatory monitoring of pyloric function is being explored [16].

EGG will become more established as a means of assessing gastric functioning in the next few years. There is a definite need for standardized normal values and a more standardized methodology and equipment in correlating gastric motility with EGG and in correlating these measures with scintigraphic measures of gastric emptying. Is it possible that a noninvasive measure such as the EGG could be used clinically to assess gastric emptying?

The use of conventional ultrasonography is limited as a means of gastric emptying assessment. This is because the accuracy is very much operator dependent and the technique is limited to the emptying of liquids. The role of intraluminal ultrasound in evaluating gastric emptying, via either an endoscope or a nasogastric tube, needs to be further explored, as does the use of magnetic resonance imaging [17].

Manometric measurement of gastric motility, either by using pressure transducers to assess circumferential forces or axial force transducers to measure push forces, is available and needs to be better understood. Further development of the combination of these two manometric measurements will further help us in understanding both normal and abnormal gastric physiology [18]. There will be increasing use of combined studies. Early results of the combined use of manometry, radionuclide gastric emptying, and EGG have been particularly promising. Further work will likely occur since techniques for ambulatory monitoring are now available.

There is a need for further expansion in the understanding of presently available prokinetic agents. Metoclopramide remains the sole available parenterally administered prokinetic agent. Erythromycin has shown some promise as a parenteral prokinetic agent, but there are only a few open studies demonstrating its efficacy. Domperidone has yet to be approved in the USA but is widely used in other countries. Similarly cisapride has received approval for the treatment of gastroparesis in most countries except for the USA, where it has only received approval for

GERD. Clinical observations suggest that the effective therapeutic doses of presently available prokinetic agents for the treatment of gastroparesis often appear to be higher than those recommended in the prescribing information. There is a need for more comparative trials of prokinetic agents, as well as studies on the efficacy of combining prokinetic agents, particularly in severe refractory gastroparesis. In diabetic patients, the dosage of prokinetic agents often has to be increased with time, probably due not to tachyphylaxis but to disease progression. However, further investigation of tachyphylaxis is needed, with recent data demonstrating that chronic dosing of erythromycin results in some downregulation of the motilin receptor [19].

The efficacy of erythromycin as a gastric prokinetic agent has led to the development of several motilin agonists, the motiloids. Several uncontrolled studies, but few placebo-controlled or long-term studies, have demonstrated the efficacy of erythromycin. Whether there will be any better controlled studies with erythromycin is doubtful as interest will focus on the newer motiloids. Manipulation of the 5-hydroxytryptamine (5-HT) receptors to improve gastric emptying appears to involve both 5-HT_3 antagonism and 5-HT_4 agonism. There is a definite need for the rapid development of newer prokinetic drugs with more specific action, for example, on fundal hypomotility or pyloric spasm, or by stimulating or inhibiting the gastric pacemaker.

There is a limited role for surgery in the treatment of gastroparesis. Presently, surgery is limited to the placement of jejunal tubes for nutritional support, often via the laparoscope. Attempts at gastric pacing by using externally placed electrodes have been disappointing both in clinical and in animal studies. However, preliminary data from the University of Virginia appear to offer some promise [20].

Intestinal pseudo-obstruction

The diagnosis of chronic intestinal pseudo-obstruction (CIPO) remains one of exclusion. Patients present with symptoms of obstruction but on investigation there is no evidence of mechanical obstruction. Many patients with intestinal dysmotility do not fit into this rather narrow definition of CIPO. For this reason, it may be conceptually more useful to create a broader definition of intestinal dysmotility. A subgroup of patients with the IBS, particularly those with pain and bloating, may fit into a broader definition, since these patients have no evidence of mechanical or structural abnormalities of the luminal GI tract. A consensus conference to better define the criteria for diagnosing patients with

CIPO and related dysmotility conditions could be quite beneficial.

In patients with possible CIPO, an initial transit study that is subsequently confirmed by manometry is currently the 'gold standard' for evaluation. Manometric evaluation of the antrum and small bowel should become more uniform and standardized over the next few years. Certainly, obtaining gastric antral data as part of this assessment appears to be important. Manometry should be able to differentiate normal from abnormal motility, but is unlikely to be helpful in differentiating myopathic from neuropathic CIPO. The final diagnostic test is the laparoscopic full-thickness biopsy, which at present is usually performed only at the time of placement of a feeding jejunostomy. Unfortunately, in the 1990s, there is a major problem with having these biopsies prepared and interpreted by a trained neuropathologist. There also needs to be refinement in the techniques for preparing these specimens and a consensus on the diagnostic criteria for CIPO. There is a definite need for a data bank and also a group of trained and dedicated pathologists across North America to be able to interpret these specimens, possibly supported by a national reference laboratory.

Over the past few years there has been a trend away from using total parenteral nutrition in CIPO. More patients are receiving enteral nutrition, often through a feeding jejunostomy. The role of venting ostomies for decompression should become better defined. Cisapride has been shown to be effective in the management of CIPO, although the optimal dosage is not clear. There are data to suggest that leuprolide and octreotide may be useful in CIPO, and additional research should clarify the utility of these agents. Narcotic analgesics should be avoided; often, by the time some patients are assessed at specialized centers, there is addiction to narcotics. The exact role of small intestinal transplantation should become better defined and whether a small bowel transplant on its own or the combination of liver and small bowel has a better success rate also needs to be elucidated.

Role of sleep in GI motility disorders

Our understanding of the pathophysiology of GI motility disorders will continue to be enhanced by investigations into the effects of sleep on GI functioning. For example, 24-hour esophageal pH monitoring has shown that the pattern of gastroesophageal reflux during sleep (i.e. in the supine position) is associated with a prolonged esophageal acid clearance time. This prolongation, as noted in Chapter 12, increases the risk for more severe complications of GERD. Sleep research is being conducted in the lower as well as upper GI tract, with similar potential for contributing to our better understanding of GI diseases.

Irritable bowel syndrome

Although we have learned much about the epidemiology of the IBS, its diagnosis, and the circumstances under which it presents to specialists, much work needs to be done to determine its pathogenesis and optimal treatment.

Manometry of the colon and small intestine has led to a variety of hypotheses, but results have not been reproducible or definitive concerning pathophysiology. The development of the barostat as a technique to evaluate visceral sensation shows considerable promise in defining more specific abnormalities in IBS. In the future, distention of the intestine by pressure, not by volume, may result in more reproducible results.

There is at present much interest in the role of afferent nervous system and higher cortical centers in IBS. The processing of afferent sensory input by these higher cortical centers has led to the notion of the hypersensitive gut. The concept is not a new one, but has undergone revival, spearheaded by the observation that balloon distention within the gut produces symptoms at lower volumes in IBS patients than in controls. A number of observations have suggested that the small bowel and colon appear to be hypersensitive to various stimuli, including physical and emotional stress, drugs, food, and distention.

There have been interesting developments in the role of sleep disorders in patients with the IBS. The association of increased REM sleep with IBS raises the question: is this a priming effect that occurs during sleep which manifests as symptoms during the day?

The pharmaceutical industry is already intensely investigating 5-HT agonists and antagonists and their role in reducing gut hypersensitivity. This area is complex, and many receptors have been discovered in the enteric and central nervous systems; it is doubtful that a specific receptor will be identified whose stimulation or suppression will correct the often paradoxical phenomena of the IBS. One has only to consider that the same individual can have constipation and diarrhea, hard and loose stools, straining and urgency, and many other seemingly unrelated symptoms.

There will be continuing work on the relationship between psychosocial factors and the somatic symptoms of the IBS. The evidence thus far would suggest that there are independent variables that come together in patients seen in tertiary care centers. The debate will continue, however, since many cling to the notion that psychosocial disturbances may cause or at least unmask somatic symptoms. The conundrum has been neatly put by Almy [21], who asked whether the manifestations of the IBS are a qualitative or quantitative departure from the psychophysiologic reactions of normal individuals.

Considerable work will be required to develop cost-effective means by which IBS patients presenting to physicians can be managed. In tertiary research centers, much effort has been expended on drug trials and various psychological treatments. These will necessarily continue, but will lead to solutions only for a rather small proportion of the mass of IBS sufferers. We know that many individuals who experience symptoms of IBS do not see physicians and most of those who do are not satisfied by an encounter with a primary care physician. Nonetheless, drugs are widely used without sufficient validation, and there is great variability as to what constitutes a cost-effective workup. In keeping with trends in medicine, over the next 5 years there will be a great deal of research on the manifestations and management of the IBS in primary care practice.

Constipation

Normal bowel habits can vary from twice a day to three times a week. This observation, along with the recognition that up to one-third of patients with self-reported constipation fail to meet the generally accepted criteria for constipation, emphasizes the need for greater standardization. The most useful definition of constipation (stool frequency? straining?) remains unclear. Likewise, the most appropriate means of evaluating bowel habits remains equally vague. The definition of constipation can be made historically or from daily bowel logs and frequency of evacuation. The most critical parameters appear to be difficulty in achieving evacuation and stool consistency. However, better techniques are needed for quantifying the difficulty or straining associated with evacuation. Better quantitative measures are also needed to evaluate stool consistency.

Chronic constipation has a complex pathophysiology that is known to be associated with other disease entities such as diabetes. Additional investigations of these interactions are needed to increase our understanding of the mechanisms involved and potential interventions. Colonic inertia has been associated with both idiopathic constipation and functional outlet obstruction. Complex reflex pathways within the enteric nervous system in the rectum and colon may account for these abnormalities. However, the precise relationship between these disorders will require further investigation. Alterations in sensory thresholds found in patients with functional outlet obstruction may be primary or secondary. New methods for evaluating sensory dysfunction in these patients should help clarify these issues in the future.

Advances in the evaluation of constipation will require simpler quantitative tests that ideally would require less radiation exposure. Colonic transit studies using radio-opaque markers should be standardized as to the number and type of markers, the pattern of ingestion, and the number and timing of X-rays. As with gastric emptying studies, cinegraphic evaluations will require much greater standardization on such issues as whether the isotope should be loose or bound to some form of particulate matter.

The question remains of the diagnostic utility of colonic motility studies. A primary benefit of motility studies will be to develop subgroups of patients with constipation who may require different types of intervention. The exact usefulness of anorectal manometry and whether it is helpful in patient management will require carefully designed outcome studies based on physiologic subgroups. Defecography and expulsion testing is another promising area, but has been poorly standardized. The role of electromyographic studies of the pelvic floor muscles during rectal balloon expulsion needs to be elaborated, as well as their role in the complete evaluation of patients with chronic constipation. Again, outcome studies evaluating the influence of these diagnostic tests on clinical decision making and therapeutic intervention will be required.

There is a definite need for improved laxatives that are less toxic and have fewer side effects. Presently available laxatives also need to be re-evaluated. Adequate data are currently lacking on the specific problems associated with laxatives such as the anthraquinolones. Future studies also should focus on the most appropriate fiber supplements. Hydration of the stool appears to be particularly important in the treatment of constipation, but data on the differing ability of fibers to retain fluids are currently inadequate. An exciting area for future developments should be new drugs that have a direct action on the colonic enteric nervous system. Biofeedback techniques should also provide improved therapy for patients with skeletal muscle dysfunction. However, these methods must become more standardized and available. Finally, the role of surgical intervention must be better delineated with well-designed outcome studies.

Visceral sensation and functional bowel disorders

Integrating information from basic research into clinical investigations should be the main thrust in the area of visceral sensation and perception. Advances in basic research should continue to enhance our understanding of visceral afferents and their role in pain transmission and control. Advances should include further elucidation of the role of mechanical sensory afferents, multimodal mucosal afferents, and the interaction between sympathetic and parasympathetic afferent pathways.

A number of theories on pain transmission and control warrant further exploration. These different theories can be broadly subgrouped into intensity, specificity, convergence, and plasticity theories. Incorporation and evaluation of the tenets of these theories in the evaluation of pain transmission may yield valuable information on potential interventions in the future. Additional data are needed to increase our understanding of smooth-muscle tone and reflex pathways and their role in the transmission of sensory information from the gut. This includes the effect of viscoelastic properties on sensation and perception and the influence of the autonomic nervous system on dynamic properties of smooth muscle.

The understanding of so-called functional bowel disorders such as IBS and functional dyspepsia appears to be linked to our enhanced understanding of visceral sensation and perception. Numerous studies have established that many patients with IBS have a diminished pain threshold and an enhanced sensation of luminal distention [22]. Understanding this aspect of bowel function, as well as how it is altered by efferent activity from the central nervous system, will advance our knowledge of the pathogenesis of functional bowel disorders [23]. New methodologic advances should incorporate psychophysical techniques into the study of visceral sensation and perception [24, 25]. This incorporation should result in the utilization of more sensitive qualitative and quantitative measurement scales and a better understanding of afferent responses to different stimuli. Perception of stimuli from the gut is not static. As recent studies have shown, future investigations must focus on the dynamic properties of sensation and perception (e.g. sensitization and habituation). Finally, increased emphasis on standardization of procedures should result in more reproducible measures and increased clinical application.

Rapid technological advances in hardware and software designed specifically to present visceral stimulation and record responses should continue. Computerized pumps are now available that allow multiple stimuli to be delivered and recorded simultaneously. Computerized devices are also allowing continuous monitoring and recording of sensation from subjects over prolonged periods, thus enabling a better understanding of the dynamics of sensation and perception from the gut. There should be an increased emphasis on solving the technical problems and limitations associated with these new devices. It is also critical to focus on standardizing the procedures and equipment used in these investigations.

Conclusions

The future appears to hold many exciting challenges for physicians and scientists working in the area of GI motility. The development of technology to assess various aspects of intestinal electrical activity and motility will continue to provide opportunities to expand our understanding of the mechanisms of motor activity in the GI tract. Advances in the understanding of motility from a cellular to a whole organ basis will undoubtedly result in additional pharmacologic treatments for motility disorders.

The relatively poor correlation between objective parameters of dysmotility and symptoms clearly needs and will obtain greater focus in the coming years. This conundrum continues to confound our understanding of the relationship between intestinal motility and the clinical symptoms ostensibly associated with motor abnormalities. The development of techniques to assess visceral sensation, and a burgeoning of research in this area, will certainly continue and very likely result in major advances in this area in the coming years.

Advances in the understanding of the pathophysiology of so-called functional bowel disorders will be aided by more precise definitions of these conditions and by a better understanding of the mechanisms of visceral sensation. It is anticipated that a better understanding of the mechanisms of visceral sensation will lead to pharmacologic alterations in the threshold of sensation for luminal distention. Such developments could result in effective pharmacologic treatments for some of the most common complaints encountered in clinical medicine. Perhaps the most imposing challenges relate to better understanding of the relationship between motility abnormalities and symptom production, and the most effective means of treating these conditions, be it by altering the motility itself or the visceral afferent sensory thresholds.

References

1 Orr WC. The physiology and philosophy of cause and effect. *Gastroenterology* 1994;**107**:1898–901.

2 Castell JA, Dalton CB, Castell DO. Pharyngeal and upper esophageal sphincter manometry in humans. *Am J Physiol* 1990;**258**:G173–8.

3 Mittal RK, Holloway RH, Penagini R, Blackshaw LA, Dent J. Transient lower esophageal sphincter relaxation. *Gastroenterology* 1995;**109**:601–10.

4 Vaezi MF, Singh S, Richter JE. Role of acid and duodenogastric reflux in esophageal mucosal injury: a review of animal and human studies. *Gastroenterology* 1995;**108**:1897–907.

5 Kimmig JM. Treatment and prevention of relapse of mild oesophagitis with omeprazole and cisapride: comparison of two strategies. *Aliment Pharmacol Ther* 1995;**9**:281–6.

6 Vigneri S, Termini R, Leandro G *et al.* A comparison of five maintenance therapies for reflux esophagitis. *N Engl J Med* 1995;**333**:1106–10.

7 Hetzel DJ, Dent J, Reed WJ *et al.* Healing and relapse of severe peptic esophagitis after treatment with omeprazole. *Gastroenterology* 1988;**95**:903–12.

8 Tytgat GNJ, Anker Hansen OJ, Carling L *et al.* Effect of cisapride on relapse of reflux oesophagitis, healed with an antisecretory drug. *Scand J Gastroenterol* 1992;**27**:175–83.

9 Orr WC, Mellow MH, Grossman MR. Patterns of 24-hour esophageal acid exposure after acute withdrawal of acid suppression. *Aliment Pharmacol Ther* 1995;**9**:571–4.

10 Spechler SJ. Complications of gastroesophageal reflux disease. In: Castell DO, ed. *The Esophagus.* Boston: Little, Brown & Co, 1992:543–56.

11 Talley NJ, Weaver AL, Tesmer DL, Zinsmeister AR. Lack of discriminant value of dyspepsia subgroups in patients referred for upper endoscopy. *Gastroenterology* 1993;**105**:1378–86.

12 House AA, Champion MC, Chamberlain M. A national survey of radionuclide gastric emptying in Canada. *Am J Gastroenterol* 1994;**89**:1639.

13 Hutson WR, Roehrkasse RL, Wald A. Influence of gender and menopause on gastric emptying and motility. *Gastroenterology* 1989;**96**:11–17.

14 Vekemans MC, Parkman H, Van Cauteren *et al.* Dynamic antral scintigraphy to characterize gastric antral motility in functional dyspepsia. *J Nucl Med* 1995;**36**:1579–86.

15 Ritter M, Heimbucher J, Hoeft SF *et al.* Ambulatory measurement of gastric emptying: introduction of an intragastric gamma detecting probe. *Gastroenterology* 1995;**108**:A1242.

16 Sun WM, Smout A, Malbert C, *et al.* Relationship between surface electro-gastrography and antroduodenal pressures. *Am J Physiol* 1995;**268**:G424–30.

17 Schwizer W, Maecke H, Fried M. Measurement of gastric emptying by magnetic resonance imaging in humans. *Gastroenterology* 1992;**103**:369–76.

18 Camilleri M. Appraisal of medium-and long-term treatment of gastroparesis and chronic intestinal dysmotility. *Am J Gastroenterol* 1994;**89**:1769–74.

19 Bologna SD, Hasler WL, Owyang C. Down-regulation of motilin receptors on rabbit colon myocytes by chronic oral erythromycin. *J Pharmacol Exp Ther* 1993;**266**:852–6.

20 Lin ZY, Pan J, McCallum RW, Chen J. Do gastric myoelectrical abnormalities predict delayed gastric emptying? *Gastroenterology* 1995;**108**:A639.

21 Almy TP. The irritable bowel syndrome: back to square one? *Dig Dis Sci* 1980;**25**:401–3.

22 Accarino A, Azpiroz F, Malagelada JR. Selective dysfunction of mechanosensitive intestinal afferents in irritable bowel syndrome. *Gastroenterology* 1995;**108**:636–43.
23 Trimble KC, Farou R, Pryde A, Douglas S, Heading RC. Heightened visceral sensation in functional gastrointestinal disease is not site-specific evidence for a generalized disorder of gut sensitivity. *Dig Dis Sci* 1995;**40**:1607–13.
24 Mayer EA, Gebhart GF. Basic and clinical aspects of visceral hyperalgesia. *Gastroenterology* 1994;**107**:271–93.
25 Mayer EA. Gut feelings: what turns them on? *Gastroenterology* 1995;**108**:927–40.

Index